T020929

KT-548-153

4/07

Critical Care in Childbearing for Midwives

Edited by

Mary Billington and Mandy Stevenson

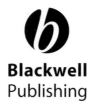

Blackwell
Publishing

© 2007 by Blackwell Publishing Ltd

Blackwell Publishing editorial offices:
Blackwell Publishing Ltd, 9600 Garsington Road, Oxford OX4 2DQ, UK
Tel: +44 (0)1865 776868
Blackwell Publishing Inc., 350 Main Street, Malden, MA 02148-5020, USA
Tel: +1 781 388 8250
Blackwell Publishing Asia Pty Ltd, 550 Swanston Street, Carlton, Victoria 3053, Australia
Tel: +61 (0)3 8359 1011

The right of the Author to be identified as the Author of this Work has been asserted in
accordance with the Copyright, Designs and Patents Act 1988.

All rights reserved. No part of this publication may be reproduced, stored in a retrieval system,
or transmitted, in any form or by any means, electronic, mechanical, photocopying, recording or
otherwise, except as permitted by the UK Copyright, Designs and Patents Act 1988, without
the prior permission of the publisher.

First published 2007 by Blackwell Publishing Ltd

ISBN-13: 978-1-4051-1638-1

Library of Congress Cataloging-in-Publication Data
Critical care in childbearing for midwives / edited by Mary Billington and Mandy Stevenson.
p. ; cm.
Includes bibliographical references and index.
ISBN-13: 978-1-4051-1638-1 (pbk. : alk. paper)
ISBN-10: 1-4051-1638-2 (pbk. : alk. paper)
1. Midwives.   2. Pregnancy—Complications   3. Critical care medicine.
I. Billington, Mary.   II. Stevenson, Mandy. [DNLM: 1. Pregnancy Complications.
2. Pregnancy, High-Risk.   3. Critical Care.   4. Midwifery.   WQ 240 C9335 2007]
RG950.C75 2007
618.2'028—dc22
2006019914

A catalogue record for this title is available from the British Library

Set in 10/12 pt Palatino
by Graphicraft Limited, Hong Kong, China
Printed and bound in Singapore
by COS Printers Pte Ltd

The publisher's policy is to use permanent paper from mills that operate a sustainable
forestry policy, and which has been manufactured from pulp processed using acid-free and
elementary chlorine-free practices. Furthermore, the publisher ensures that the text paper
and cover board used have met acceptable environmental accreditation standards.

For further information, visit our subject website: www.blackwellnursing.com

Contents

Preface

It may seem anomalous to publish a book titled *Critical Care in Childbearing for Midwives* at a time when the Royal College of Midwives (2005) has launched the Campaign for Normal Birth. Some would argue that the time spent preparing this text would have been better spent promoting 'normality'. However, it is important to distinguish between the majority of women with uncomplicated pregnancies, who have the potential to give birth normally to healthy babies, and the small but growing minority who, for a variety of reasons, have the potential to become critically ill during childbearing.

The aim of this book is to provide a source of reference for midwives involved in the care of the latter group of women. It may also have relevance for nurses working in intensive and high dependency care settings who are involved in the care of childbearing women who are transferred to these areas. The need for such a book was identified by one of the editors, Mandy Stevenson, when developing a course for qualified midwives following a request from a local maternity service for a course to support the development of a 'high risk' midwifery team. Key texts for the course were (and still are) obstetric texts that focus on medical disorders and high risk pregnancy (for example, de Swiet 2002; James et al. 1999; Nelson-Piercy 2002; Gilbert & Harmon 2003), and nursing texts on critical care (for example, Woodrow 2000; Urden et al. 2002). What was lacking was literature that combined the two and considered issues from a midwifery perspective. We hope that this publication will go some way towards meeting this identified shortfall.

References

Gilbert, E. and Harmon, J. (2003) *Manual of High Risk Pregnancy and Delivery*. Mosby, St Louis.

James, D., Steer, P., Weiner, C. and Gonik, B. (1999) *High Risk Pregnancy: Management options*. W.B. Saunders, London.

Nelson-Piercy, C. (2002) *Handbook of Obstetric Medicine*. Martin Dunitz, London.

Royal College of Midwives (2005) Campaign for normal birth. http://www.rcmnormalbirth.org.uk

de Swiet, M. (2002) *Medical Disorders in Obstetric Practice*. Blackwell Science, Oxford.

Urden, L., Stacy, K. and Lough, M. (2002) *Thelans Critical Care Nursing Diagnosis and Management*. Mosby, St Louis.

Woodrow, P. (2000) *Intensive Care Nursing: A framework for practice*. Routledge, London.

Contributors

Mary Billington MSc, BA, PGCEA, ADM, RM, RN
Principal Lecturer – Midwifery. School of Health and Social Care, University of Greenwich, London, UK.

Angela Bromley BSc, RM, RN
Practice Development Midwife. Queen Elizabeth Hospital, Woolwich, London, UK.

Priscilla Dike MSc, BSc, PG Dip (HE), Diploma in Tropical Nursing, RM, RN
Senior Lecturer – Midwifery. School of Health and Social Care, University of Greenwich, London, UK.

Terry Ferns MA, PG Dip (HE), Diploma in Professional Practice, RN
Senior Lecturer – ITU. School of Health and Social Care, University of Greenwich, London, UK.

Sarah Gregson MSc, RM, RN
Consultant Midwife. Maidstone and Tunbridge Wells NHS Trust, Kent, UK.

Tina Heptinstall MSc, BSc, PGCEA, ADM, RM, RN
Senior Lecturer – Midwifery. School of Health and Social Care, University of Greenwich, London, UK.

Pat Jackson MA, BA, MTD, RM, RN
Senior Lecturer – Midwifery. School of Health and Social Care, University of Greenwich, London, UK.

Nick Rowe ODP (Anaesthetics and Recovery)
Senior Theatre Practitioner/Operating Department Assistant. Chelsfield Park Hospital, Orpington, Kent, UK.

Lynne Spencer MSc Humanistic Integrative Psychotherapy, Advanced Diploma in Psychotherapy, Postgraduate Certificate in Couples Counselling, Diploma in Individual and Group Supervision, MA Education, PGCEA, ADM, RM, RN
Campus Head of Student Affairs. Medway Campus, University of Greenwich, Chatham Maritime, Kent, UK.

Dianne Steele MSc, BSc, PGCEA, RM, RN
Senior Lecturer – Midwifery. University of East Anglia, Norwich, Norfolk, UK.

Mandy Stevenson MSc, BSc, PG Dip (Education), Dip HE, RM, RN
Senior Lecturer – Midwifery. School of Health and Social Care, University of Greenwich, London, UK.

1 Introduction

Mandy Stevenson and Mary Billington

Although the majority of women have uncomplicated pregnancies and give birth normally to healthy babies, a small but growing minority have the potential to become critically ill during childbearing. This chapter seeks to put forward a definition of midwifery critical care and to provide the context for midwives' involvement in caring for critically ill women in childbearing.

Defining critical care

In the United Kingdom, there is no clear definition of what 'critical care' is within midwifery or what situations constitute critical care. In light of this deficit, wider exploration of the term critical care may identify the relevant components pertinent to formulating a midwifery-relevant definition. A concept analysis of the terms 'critical' and 'care' (Walker & Avant 1988) find that the commonalities drawn from paper and Internet definitions indicate that 'life threatening' and 'constant observation and monitoring' are the defining attributes that reflect the complexities of critical care provision within any situation. Mosby (1986) provides a definition that corresponds to these components by indicating that critical care provision is "constant, complex, detailed health care as provided in various acute life threatening conditions." Obstetric disorders such as pre-eclampsia, HELLP syndrome (*h*aemolysis, *e*levated *l*iver *e*nzymes, *l*ow *p*latelets) or massive postpartum haemorrhage correspond with the life-threatening component of the above definition (Fraser & Cooper 2003), whilst the aspect of 'complex health care' could represent the provision of invasive and non-invasive procedures and care provision within the delivery suite. Central venous pressure monitoring to evaluate fluid management may be viewed as one such invasive procedure. A specific definition for midwifery critical care could reflect the attributes drawn earlier and could bear a resemblance to "the provision of concentrated care (physical, psychological and social) on a one to one basis in an acute situation where a woman's condition has or is at risk of deteriorating and where advanced management such as drug therapy, more intensive forms of monitoring and inter-pretation of results are required on a frequent basis."

Terminology can, however, provide a confusing view on what care is actu-ally being provided. The term intensive care is often interchanged with the term critical care or high dependency care. Hence the consistent use of appropriate terminology needs to be addressed within clinical practice and documented evidence. For the purpose of this book, the authors have adopted the term crit-ical care.

Midwives caring for critically ill women

Midwives are increasingly in contact with women who have the potential to become critically ill due to a variety of reasons. Better neonatal and paediatric care means that women with, for example, cardiac or respiratory disorders, who in the past would not have survived to the age of childbearing, now do so, and with their fertility intact. Advances in fertility treatments also mean that women who may have unrecognised problems can achieve pregnancies. Furthermore, there has been a gradual increase in the age of childbearing, with more women than ever before having children in their late thirties and forties (Office of National Statistics 2005). It is important to recognise that childbearing will be uncomplicated for many of these women but it is equally important to be aware that for some women their age and/or health status makes them more likely to become critically ill.

The report of the Standing Nursing and Midwifery Advisory Committee (1998), *Midwifery: Delivering our future*, recognised that midwives are working in many different ways, which includes caring for critically ill mothers. Becoming a member of a 'high risk midwifery team' or a midwife with critical care skills and knowledge may be viewed as responding to the call of providing woman-centred care (Department of Health 1993) in addition to developing higher level clinical expertise to provide high quality specialist services.

Lee (2000) reporting Yiannouzis at a meeting of the Forum on Maternity and the Newborn of the Royal Society of Medicine, considered the growing trend for critically ill childbearing women being cared for by midwives in obstetric high dependency units. This, it was argued, should enable ill women to "receive the best of both types of care: the 'high tech', reflecting advances in science and technology, combined with the 'high touch' approach evident in a true woman-centred philosophy."

It could be assumed that all midwives are equipped for and capable of pro-viding critical care. However, this assumption is inaccurate as, at the point of qualification, such skills are not a requirement to register (Nursing and Midwifery Council 2004). Due to the evolution of pre-qualifying midwifery programmes, which do not require students to possess a first level nursing qualification, more midwives in clinical practice will not have experienced critical care unless it was specifically placed within their programme and even then the experience may have only been a short, mainly observational placement.

The Confidential Enquiries into Maternal Deaths for the triennium 2000–2002 (Lewis 2004) recognised that many women who died had higher risk pregnancies, complications or underlying medical conditions that required specialist obstetric or multidisciplinary care. In most cases midwives provided the important continuity, supportive link and point of contact between a woman and a number of different health care professionals. However, one recommendation from the report indicates that all health professionals should receive regular and updated training on the signs and symptoms of critical illness, from both obstetric and non-obstetric causes. It is imperative, therefore, that midwives have confidence in this role, both to provide high standards of care and, when necessary, to challenge other practitioners so that they can truly act as an advocate for women.

Midwives possess an individual responsibility to identify any shortfalls in their knowledge base and should update their skills as part of their continuing professional development (Nursing and Midwifery Council 2004), while employers should aid the continuing professional development of midwives to improve care delivery and clinical risk management (Lewis 2004).

Suboptimal care has been blamed in many instances for the deterioration and/or demise of women related to childbirth. Of the 261 women who died from *direct* and *indirect* causes, 67% were considered to have some form of suboptimal clinical care (Lewis 2004). Examples indicate that staff had failed to recognise and act on common signs of critical illness that were not specifically related to obstetric practice, such as pyrexia or tachycardia. This lack of attention to basic assessment findings could cause the women to require more intensive care in a dedicated unit away from their baby and midwifery support. The report does not differentiate clearly between the professionals involved in providing suboptimal care. However, it is important that midwives possess the competencies to recognise that a woman's condition is deteriorating and that prompt referral needs to take place. With education and training, midwives can develop both the competencies and opportunities to provide care to women who can then remain in a familiar environment in close contact with their babies on the delivery ward, whilst still receiving both critical- and midwifery-specific care and management.

The Royal College of Medicine and Royal College of Obstetricians and Gynaecologists (1999) report appears to be the first UK-based policy document to support the ethos of midwives being educated to provide high dependency care to critically ill women. Prior to the publication of the report, it had been suggested all midwives were able to work interchangeably in any part of the midwifery services (Bryar 1995). This assumption could be viewed as problematic as not all midwives have acquired the relevant skills and knowledge in their education to provide optimal care within the critical care arena. This potential lack of education to gain appropriate knowledge and understanding could impact upon clinical practice by causing a delay in summoning other appropriate specialists, initiating treatment or in failing to recognise the severity of a condition.

Critical care in childbearing for midwives

A significant development in line with the increasing rate of critically ill women has been the development of high risk/critical care teams. The rationale behind the evolution of such teams is primarily to enable the provision of greater continuity of care. Midwives can care for the ill woman in a majority of situations in the delivery ward as opposed to being cared for by nurses in the intensive treatment unit (ITU). Chapter 2 provides evidence of the development of one such team in a NHS trust, while Chapter 3 investigates the concept of autonomous practice in relation to the midwife providing care for critically ill women.

   An overview of some of the more common causes of critical illness in childbearing is provided in Chapters 4–8, which variously consider a range of medical and haematological disorders (Chapters 4 and 5), hypertensive disorders (Chapter 6) and obstetric haemorrhage (Chapter 7), as well as an overview of the various causes of shock (Chapter 8). The next chapters provide information on aspects of management and care, namely fluid replacement and therapy (Chapter 9), specialist technology and skills (Chapter 10), anaesthesia and resuscitation (Chapter 11), pain management (Chapter 12), and transfer to the intensive treatment unit (Chapter 13). Last, but by no means least, Chapter 14 considers the psychological needs and care of women (and their families) who experience critical illness during childbearing.

References

Bryar, R. (1995) *Theory for Midwifery Practice*. MacMillan Press, London.
Department of Health (1993) *Changing Childbirth*. Her Majesty's Stationery Office (HMSO), London.
Fraser, D. and Cooper, M. (2003) *Myles Textbook for Midwives* (14th edn). Churchill Livingstone, Edinburgh.
Lee, B. (2000) Life threatened by birth: mothers in high dependency obstetric care *RCM Midwives Journal*, **3** (9): 282–3.
Lewis, G. (2001) *Why Mothers Die 1997–1999: The Confidential Enquiries into Maternal Deaths in the United Kingdom*. Royal College of Obstetricians and Gynaecologists (RCOG) Press, London.
Lewis, G. (2004) *Why Mothers Die 2000–2002: Report on Confidential Enquiries into Maternal Deaths in the United Kingdom*. Royal College of Obstetricians and Gynaecologists (RCOG) Press, London.
Mosby (1986) *Mosby's Medical and Nursing Dictionary* (2nd edn). C.V. Mosby, St Louis.
Nursing and Midwifery Council (2004) *Standards of Proficiency for Pre Registration Midwifery*. Nursing and Midwifery Council (NMC), London.
Office of National Statistics (2005) *Age specific fertility rates, 1994–2004*. www.statistics.gov.uk
Royal College of Midwives and Royal College of Obstetricians and Gynaecologists (1999) *Towards safer childbirth. Minimum standards for the organisation of labour wards. Report of a joint working party*. Royal College of Midwives and Royal College of Obstetricians and Gynaecologists (RCOG) Press, London.
Standing Nursing and Midwifery Advisory Committee (1998) *Midwifery: Delivering our future*. Department of Health, London.
Walker, L. and Avant, K. (1988) *Strategies for Theory Construction in Nursing* (2nd edn). Appleton & Lange, Connecticut.

2 A Team Approach to Providing Care for the Critically Ill Woman

Sarah Gregson

Successive Confidential Enquiries into Maternal Deaths (CEMD) in the United Kingdom (Department of Health 1996, 1998; Lewis 2001, 2004) have found that substandard care is a factor in up to 67% of all maternal deaths in the UK. For the years 1997–1999, this rose to 80% (Lewis 2001) due to conditions such as hypertensive disorders of pregnancy – including severe pre-eclampsia, eclampsia and HELLP syndrome (*h*aemolysis, *e*levated *l*iver *e*nzymes, *l*ow *p*latelets) – but fell to 46% during 2000–2002 (Lewis 2004). Recurring problems in relation to management of these conditions include failure to recognise the severity of the condition, delay in calling for senior help, delay in initiating treatment, failure to involve other appropriate specialists, lack of team work and poor management of blood pressure and fluid balance.

Cordingley and Rubin (1997) found that approximately one intensive treatment unit (ITU) admission will arise per 1000 deliveries and it has been suggested that maternity services should make provision for up to ten high dependency cases per thousand deliveries per year (Royal College of Midwives (RCM) & Royal College of Obstetricians and Gynaecologists 1999). According to an audit carried out in the southeast of England (Sauter 1999), individual hospital trusts have had a variable response to making provision for the care of women who become critically ill as recommended in successive CEMD. Most maternity units do provide a designated room or area where women who are seriously ill can be cared for, but the question of who actually provides the care for these women and what sort of experience and training they have had is an issue that requires careful consideration (Gregson 2003). This chapter discusses how a team approach provides optimum care for women who become critically ill during childbearing, and gives practical advice how this can be achieved.

This chapter will consider the rationale for a midwifery high dependency team, the practical process of setting up such a team and an evaluation of how one such team has improved care.

Rationale behind a midwifery high dependency team

The obstetrician is recognised as the lead professional for women with complicated pregnancies (Department of Health 1993), but there are occasions when an individual doctor might not have the necessary clinical experience in caring for a woman who becomes critically ill. This situation may occur because less than 1% of women become critically ill during pregnancy (Cordingly & Rubin 1997) and, of course, may be compounded by the recent reduction in doctors' working hours.

In a survey of junior obstetric doctors, Ennis (1991) found that a small proportion claimed to have received little or no supervision, and that over half felt inadequately prepared to carry out their duties in the obstetric unit, which highlights a serious deficiency in practice. 'Out of hours' (i.e. after 17:00 hours and at weekends) most labour wards will not have a consultant on site, unless they are specifically called in, and successive Confidential Enquiries (Department of Health 1996, 1998; Lewis 2001, 2004) have highlighted the fact that on occasions junior obstetric staff have failed to recognised the severity of a woman's condition until it is too late.

The ethos of midwifery care in many maternity services during the 1980s and early 1990s was that midwives should be able to work interchangeably in any part of the maternity services, but this meant that on occasions women who were critically ill were being cared for by midwives without the necessary skills and training to ensure that optimum care was being delivered. An average size maternity unit that has 3500 deliveries per year may employ around 100 midwives, which means that an individual midwife may not experience caring for a critically ill woman more than once every few years. Successive CEMD have demonstrated that the combination of inexperienced doctors and *inexperienced* midwives, particularly 'out of hours', could potentially be disastrous for a woman who becomes critically ill.

The CEMD have also recommended that a multidisciplinary team approach from obstetricians, midwives and anaesthetists should be adopted to ensure that optimum care is given to women who become critically ill during childbirth. However, until the late 1990s, there was very little debate in the midwifery literature as to what contribution midwives could make, probably because efforts were being concentrated on the age-old struggle of being recognised as 'experts' of normal childbirth with little time or energy left to devote to other causes. The first policy document to discuss midwives and high dependency care for critically ill mothers in any depth – *Towards safer childbirth* (RCM & Royal College of Obstetricians and Gynaecologists 1999) – was not published until 1999. This report was written jointly by the Royal College of Obstetricians and Gynecologists, the Royal College of Midwives and the Royal College of General Practitioners. It states that:

> ". . . as far as midwifery cover for such [high dependency care] units is concerned, it will be necessary to develop a cadre of midwives who have particular experience and expertise in the management of the critically ill woman."

This report marked a turning point for midwives with the recognition that a midwifery qualification does not automatically mean that an individual midwife will have all the knowledge and skills to work in any part of maternity services without any additional training.

It was with these aims that an intrapartum critical care initiative was developed at North Staffordshire NHS Trust (McLachlan et al. 1996) and a midwifery team for high risk pregnancies was developed at Chelsea and Westminster NHS Trust (Bradshaw et al. 1995). Some maternity services have followed this lead and set up initiatives of their own, but there are still many maternity units in the UK that have no special arrangements for caring for women who become critically ill during childbirth (Sauter 1999).

Setting up a midwifery high dependency team

In 1996–1997 Queen Mary's Sidcup NHS Trust developed a midwifery high dependency team in response to the poor management of a woman with severe pre-eclampsia. This chapter continues with an analysis of some of the issues that need to be considered when setting up such a team and how these were addressed.

Literature search

At the onset of any proposal for changing practice or service development, it is important to ascertain whether similar ideas have been previously explored. A literature search can often reveal previously unknown initiatives, which can in turn lead to a refinement of the original plan and develop an awareness of some of the problems that can be avoided.

In 1996 the idea of a midwifery high dependency team was relatively unusual, apart from the well-known Silver Star team at the John Radcliffe Hospital in Oxfordshire (a multidisciplinary initiative caring for women with medical conditions throughout the antenatal period). However, a literature search revealed that Chelsea and Westminster maternity services had recently developed a midwifery group practice approach to caring for women throughout pregnancy, labour and the pueperium (Bradshaw et al. 1995). Following a visit to the John Radcliffe Hospital and a discussion with a senior midwife at the Chelsea and Westminster Hospital regarding the workings of their team, it was decided that the midwifery high dependency team at Queen Mary's Sidcup NHS Trust would be delivery suite based. It was felt that this was where the greatest difference could be made to the care of women who are critically ill within the available resources.

A proposal for developing a midwifery high dependency team was written and presented to the Director of Midwifery at Queen Mary's. This proved an effective way of ensuring that the rationale for setting up the team was clearly thought out and that attention was given to any financial implications involved. From the beginning it was recognised that the team should be a multidisciplinary initiative, so circulation of the completed business plan/proposal for change was circulated to key senior staff including midwifery managers, consultant obstetricians and consultant anaesthetists.

Management of change

The issue of change management has been well documented and discussed and it is commonly known that certain factors will influence how well a new project or service development is accepted or rejected. In the initial stages of change, an important factor is to ensure that 'key players' are identified and their support for the project is obtained. It is also vital that all staff in the unit, not just those directly involved in the formation of the team, are made aware of the aims and objectives of the new development and how it will improve the existing services. Groups can be powerful promoters and supporters of the change process if they lend their weight to its promotion (Wilson 1990).

With this in mind, the proposal was discussed and approved at the monthly care group meeting attended by the senior midwifery managers and the consultant obstetricians. Once support from these key people had been obtained, the initiative was presented to all staff at a large unit meeting and the importance of the project and need for change was emphasised by including a case analysis of a recently mismanaged case of severe pre-eclampsia.

Working arrangements

As the new service needed to be provided within the existing budget, it was decided that staff would be recruited from the core midwifery staff. A group of approximately six whole-time equivalent midwives would form the team, ensuring that at least one member of the team would be working on the delivery suite for each shift, thus providing a 24-hour service. This would mean that team members would still be a part of the core delivery suite staff, but would be available to give high dependency midwifery care to any woman if the need arose. The high dependency midwife would be able to refer directly to a consultant obstetrician where appropriate and could also suggest involvement of other specialists such as an anaesthetist or haematologist where necessary. A number of midwives would be rotated into and out of the team approximately every year so that skills and knowledge would be disseminated and the perception of the team as an elitist group would be avoided.

Selection of the team leader and team members

The criteria for joining the midwifery high dependency team were:

- At least 18 months' post-qualification experience
- Willingness to undertake extra study
- Enthusiasm for the scheme
- 'Direct entrant' midwives were also included, but it was acknowledged that they might need extra support due to a lack of previous nursing experience

Midwives who wished to join the high dependency team were asked to apply in writing, giving reasons why they felt they should be considered. The selection process was then carried out by two midwifery managers, one of whom was the labour ward manager, on the basis of the written applications. Ten midwives (approximately six whole-time equivalents) were finally selected from the 16 original applicants.

A knowledgeable and enthusiastic leader is vital to the success of a project. Hugman and Hadley (1993) found that where active facilitation of the group occurred it made an observable positive difference as to how the group behaved and worked.

With the benefit of hindsight, the selection process for appointing team members would have been improved by involving the team leader in the process. Her lack of involvement at this stage led to feelings of marginalisation, which might have resulted in reduced commitment to the project. Furthermore, the midwives expressed disappointment that an interview was not included in the selection process as they felt that this would have given a more robust impression of the selection process, particularly for those who were not initially selected to be members of the team.

Education and training

It should be acknowledged that the midwifery high dependency team at Queen Mary's Sidcup NHS Trust was initially implemented with minimal 'in house' training from a consultant obstetrician, consultant anaesthetist and an ITU sister. However, forming the team with such minimal training at the onset could be justified by the fact that previously women who became critically ill were cared for by midwives who had not even had this basic training.

Whilst much of the learning would come from experience at the bedside it was felt that improving knowledge was a fundamental requisite to making a midwifery high dependency team effective, especially as team members might on occasion be in a position requiring them to challenge inappropriate medical care. This issue was highlighted in the 1998 CEMD (Department of Health 1998), which states that midwives caring for critically ill women must be able to assert their views on behalf of the woman if inappropriate decisions are being made. Whilst the challenging of medical care can sometimes be difficult (Strong & Robinson 1990; Mackay 1993; Oakley 1994), a sound knowledge of physiological aspects and contemporary management of conditions that may lead to critical illness enables midwives to feel more confident and able to take an equal responsibility in ensuring high standards of care are maintained.

The training of team members therefore needed to be approached from two angles. Practical training was required to learn how to use specialist equipment such as central venous pressure monitors and sophisticated monitoring equipment. Academic study was also essential to underpin this practical experience and develop knowledge of physiology, psychology and management of conditions that may lead to critical illness.

There was collaboration with the University of Greenwich to set up a course that would underpin clinical experience for team members. The result was the 'Care of the critically ill woman in childbearing' course, which gives 30 credits at level 3 and can be undertaken as a stand alone course or part of a post-registration degree programme for qualified midwives. Financial constraints and service needs meant that only four midwives at a time could undertake the course, but after the first year it was possible to ensure that all new team members could undertake this course fairly soon after joining the team.

Useful practical experience was also gained by establishing links with the intensive care unit at Queen Mary's and arrangements were made for team members to work two shifts on the intensive care unit when they initially joined the team and then every year thereafter. This gave team members valuable experience in caring for critically ill patients, especially in relation to managing multiple intravenous lines, central venous pressure lines and accurate charting of observations.

In any hospital there is a wealth of experience and knowledge that can be utilised for education and training, without undergoing extra expenditure apart from replacement costs. Senior staff from different departments, including obstetricians, anaesthetists, a haematologist, biochemist, the resuscitation officer and a senior sister from intensive care, gave generously of their time to encourage and teach the group, and these sessions were extremely valuable in enabling the midwives to feel more confident in their new role.

Guidelines for referral

At the onset of planning a midwifery high dependency team it is crucial that written guidelines for referral to the team should be decided in order to prevent inappropriate use of the team, and also for appropriate referral to the intensive care unit. It is important that these are written with input from all members of the multidisciplinary team, including midwives, obstetricians and anaesthetists and that they are displayed where they are immediately accessible to all staff.

Box 2.1 shows the guidelines devised at Queen Mary's for referral to the midwifery high dependency team. Box 2.2 shows the definitions of conditions included in the referral guidelines and Box 2.3 shows criteria for transfer to the ITU.

Financial implications

Financial constraints are a reality in the modern National Health Service. However it is possible to set up a maternity high dependency team with minimal extra costs involved. At Queen Mary's, costs were kept to a minimum by recruiting the team members from the existing staff complement and it is only in exceptional circumstances such as sickness that 'on call' arrangements are made. When there are no 'high risk' women to look after, the team midwife works as a core member of the delivery suite staff. Extra funding is required for training, such as external study days, but it has been estimated that this works out at less than £200 per month, which should be offset against the fact that the team provides care for several women each year who would have previously required transfer to intensive care.

Box 2.1   Guidelines for referral to the midwifery high dependency team (see Box 2.2 for definitions).

Severe pre-eclampsia
Eclampsia
Severe haemorrhage
HELLP syndrome
Disseminated intravascular coagulation
All women requiring a central venous pressure line
A critically ill woman whose diagnosis may be unclear but does not yet require transfer to ITU
Request from consultant obstetrician or consultant anaesthetist

The high risk team midwife will help stabilise and treat the following conditions whilst transfer to ITU is being arranged:

Major trauma
Post-anaesthetic complications (e.g. Mendelson's syndrome)
Pulmonary embolism
Diabetic coma/diabetic ketoacidosis
Anaphylactic shock
Septic shock
Amniotic fluid embolism
Myocardial infarction
Cerebrovascular accident
Cardiac arrest

Box 2.2   Definitions of some of the conditions listed in the referral guidelines.

Severe pre-eclampsia

Blood pressure (BP) > 170/110 on two occasions 4 hours apart, or a diastolic BP > 120 mmHg once only
plus
Proteinuria > 3 g/24 h (or protein > + + on dipstick testing)
or
Diastolic BP > 90 mmHg
plus
Proteinurea (as above)
plus one of the following:
Oliguria < 500 ml/24 h
Severe intractable headache
Epigastric pain

Thrombocytopaenia ($< 100 \times 10^9$/L)
Pulmonary oedema

Eclampsia
Convulsions in the presence of pre-eclampsia

Severe primary haemorrhage
Acute blood loss of > 1500 ml or an unmeasured loss requiring supportive measures to maintain a stable BP

Disseminated intravascular coagulation
Any two of the following:

Thrombocytopaenia ($< 100 \times 10^9$/L)
Low fibrinogen (< 300 mg/dl)
Prolonged prothrombin time (> 14 seconds)
Prolonged partial thromboplastin time (> 40 seconds)

Sepsis
Two or more of the following presenting on the same day:

Temperature > 38°C or < 36°C
Heart rate > 90 beats/min
Respiratory rate > 20/min
White cell count > 18 or $< 4 \times 10^9$/L or 10% immature forms

Severe sepsis
Sepsis in association with one of the following:

Organ dysfunction (e.g. cardiac failure leading to pulmonary oedema, renal failure leading to oliguria, liver failure leading to alterations in liver function tests)
Hypoperfusion (e.g. lactic acidosis, oliguria or an acute alteration in mental status)
Hypotension (systolic BP < 80 mmHg or a drop of 40 mmHg or more in the absence of another cause)

HELLP syndrome
One from each of the categories below:

Haemolysis:
    Abnormal peripheral smear
    Raised total bilirubin (> 12 mg/L)
Elevated liver enzymes:
    Raised ALT (alanine aminotransferase) (> 70 u/L)
    Raised gamma GT (glutamyl transferase) (> 70 u/L)
Low platelets:
    ($< 100 \times 10^9$/L)

Box 2.3   Criteria for the transfer of high risk patients from the high dependency midwifery team to intensive care or other specialist units.

1   Patients requiring ventilation
2   Patients requiring inotropic support
3   Any patient who develops severe organ failure
4   Patients requiring intra-arterial monitoring

Transfer policy

1   The consultant obstetrician, consultant anaesthetist, senior midwife and any other appropriate specialist (e.g. haematologist) should be involved in the decision to make a transfer
2   A senior anaesthetist, operating department assistant, senior midwife and a porter are the minimum staff required for performing the transfer. On occasions it may be appropriate to involve the PAR (patient at risk) team with the transfer
3   The patient will usually be transferred on the theatre trolley. Ensure the accompanying oxygen cylinder on the bottom of the trolley is full
4   Ensure that relatives are informed
5   The high dependency trolley and any other appropriate equipment, such as emergency drugs (kept in the drug cupboard) will need to accompany the patient
6   Monitoring of the patients condition will need to be continued using the datascope monitor (NB this is the only time the monitor may be unplugged from mains electricity)
7   Communication: intensive care staff should be alerted when the patient is leaving the delivery suite. Detailed handover to intensive care staff will be the responsibility of the senior midwife, senior obstetrician and senior anaesthetist involved
8   Temperature control of the patient may be facilitated using a space blanket
9   If staffing levels permit, the high risk team midwife should stay with their patient whilst on intensive care

---

Does a midwifery high dependency team make a difference?

Having discussed the case for developing a high dependency team and describing how this was done at Queen Mary's Sidcup NHS Trust, it is now important to ask what differences such a team can make to the quality of care given to women who become critically ill during childbirth. The concluding part of this chapter will examine how the midwifery high dependency team has changed the way in which the women who become critically ill are cared for at Queen Mary's Hospital.

During 2002, 84 women were cared for by the midwifery high dependency team. Not surprisingly the most common conditions that occurred were severe pre-eclampsia and severe postpartum haemorrhage, but there was also a range of other conditions including HELLP syndrome, unstable supraventricular tachycardia, metabolic acidosis following a 'flu-like' illness, severe asthma and eclampsia. Some of these women were extremely ill but team members, working in partnership with obstetricians and anaesthetists, were experienced enough to know when to seek advice from senior medical staff, which meant that the women could be safely managed on the delivery suite. Two women were transferred to the intensive care unit, one who required ventilation for severe pneumonia, and the other with recurring seizures of unknown origin. Without the midwifery high dependency team it is likely that another four women would have required transfer to intensive care (three with severe pre-eclampsia and one with a major haemorrhage), but were instead cared for on the delivery suite, where they experienced less anxiety and did not have to undergo the trauma of being separated from their babies. Not only did this mean considerable cost savings within the trust, but more importantly released intensive care beds for other patients that needed them.

Multidisciplinary working

Successive Confidential Enquiries have recommended that there should be a greater emphasis on teamwork between the different professions involved in caring for women who become critically ill and this has been echoed by policy documents such as *First Class Delivery* (Audit Commission 1997), *Towards safer childbirth* (RCM & Royal College of Obstetricians and Gynaecologists 1999) and *Changing childbirth* (Department of Health 1993). The latter document states that a woman:

> "... should feel confident that the professionals are working in harmony, as a team, supporting her and her family with clear patterns of referral and a smooth transfer of information and responsibility."

This is particularly pertinent when complications occur.

At Queen Mary's, the high dependency team consisted of midwives only for the first two years, although there was also considerable collaboration with and support from the obstetricians and obstetric anaesthetists, especially with regard to providing training and education for team members. More recently, the group has evolved to become a multidisciplinary high risk team, consisting of a consultant obstetrician and two consultant obstetric anaesthetists, as well as the midwives. This expansion of the group has contributed to wide ranging improvements in care, some of which will be discussed below.

Clinical governance and risk management

A risk management approach to maternity care has prevailed in the UK since the 1980s and the Clinical Negligence Scheme for Trusts (CNST) has been adopted as a generic framework for all risk management activities. However, there have not always been systems in place to ensure that health professionals involved in an adverse event take part in a critical event analysis.

At Queen Mary's, the maternity high risk team meetings have now become an essential part of the clinical governance and risk management framework of the maternity services. Every 6–8 weeks the group meets primarily to review the case notes of every woman cared for by the team during the previous two months. Prior to the meeting, the notes of each woman are summarised by the consultant obstetrician, using a chart for easy reference (Table 2.1). Each case is then presented and discussed, with input from the obstetricians, midwives and obstetric anaesthetists. Minutes of the meetings are circulated throughout the maternity unit and the risk manager also receives a copy, enabling her to follow through problems and recommendations where necessary. The multidisciplinary framework of the meetings has made a great difference, not just from an educational point of view, but also in ensuring that protocols are continuously evolving with input from all disciplines, as recommended in several policy documents including *Changing childbirth* (Department of Health 1993), *First Class Delivery* (Audit Commission 1997) and *Towards safer childbirth* (RCM & Royal College of Obstetricians and Gynaecologists 1999).

At the meetings new initiatives are also put forward and discussed. For example, in 2003 the anaesthetists instigated an early warning system that allowed women with potential serious anaesthetic and medical problems to be identified early on in pregnancy, thus allowing proper planning between the obstetricians, anaesthetists and midwives to take place. A documented plan of care for each individual is kept in a folder on the delivery suite and also in the woman's notes.

Emergency equipment and drugs

Busy labour wards often have problems with getting equipment repaired and checked regularly. There is usually a large number of staff working in this area and individuals often assume someone else has done a task unless they are given specific responsibility. The midwifery high dependency team has made important improvements with regard to the equipment used in the high dependency room because there is now a dedicated group who are responsible for ensuring that it is checked regularly and laid out in a logical order. There are also simple, clear instructions for setting up certain pieces of equipment such as central venous pressure lines and blood-warming devices. A drug cupboard in the high dependency room now contains emergency drugs, with laminated cards giving doses and instructions on how to prepare them; obstetric intensive care charts have been created, allowing observations and fluid management to be charted clearly. These are all fairly simple changes, which have minimal resource implications, but collectively have made a real difference in minimising delay in giving emergency treatment where necessary.

Improved environment

Having a dedicated group of midwives who are responsible for caring for women who become ill during childbearing has also meant that attention has been focused

Table 2.1 Framework for case analysis at high risk team meetings (initials and dates have been removed to preserve patient confidentiality). Reproduced with kind permission from Mark Waterstone, consultant obstetrician, Queen Mary's S dcup NHS Trust.

Patient initials	Delivery date	Primary condition	Secondary condition	Other condition	Predictable	When	Preventable?	Delivery type	Relevant factors
		Fluid overload			No	N/a	Yes	Em c/s	Twins with one trisomy 13
		Moderate PET			No	N/a	No	Em c/s	Excessive use of Mg ? unnecessary c/s
		PPH 12 000	Total abdominal hysterectomy		Yes	AN	No	El c/s	Major communication error but outcome would have been the same
		PPH 1300	Tx 4 units		No	N/a	Possibly	El c/s	No ivi synto
		PPH 1740			Possibly	AN	No	El c/s	Low anterior fibroid cons underestimated loss by 500 ml
		Fluid overload			No	N/a	Yes	Em c/s	Over-reaction to 1500 ml loss at c/s; given 4 litres of crystalloid and 2 units of blood unnecessarily
		PPH 1650 ml			No	N/a	No	Em c/s	Nil to note
		PPH 3000 ml			No	N/a	No	Em c/s	Unexpected adherent placenta. Well managed

on improving the environment of care for these women. The high dependency room had previously been located in a dismal and poorly decorated area without windows, but the team negotiated its relocation to a room with some natural light and did some fund raising to improve the decoration. Improvements have now been extended to the purchasing of a television, video and compact disc player which can be extremely helpful to women who are beginning to get better, but are not yet fit for transfer to the postnatal ward. There are also pictures on the walls and curtains at the windows, which make a difference to a woman who is feeling ill, frightened and in need of as 'homely' an atmosphere as possible.

Conclusion

In the UK it is a sad fact that approximately two-thirds of the maternal deaths that occur each year have avoidable factors (Lewis 2004). During the last decade some maternity units in the UK have developed different schemes to help reduce maternal mortality and morbidity, but there still appear to be many units who do little more than provide a room that is designated the 'high dependency room', where the care that women receive from midwives can be variable. A midwifery high dependency team, working in partnership with obstetricians, anaesthetists and other members of the multidisciplinary team, has made significant improvements to the way critically ill women are cared for at Queen Mary's Sidcup NHS Trust. Some of these improvements have been discussed in this chapter and it is hoped that the reader will recognise the vital role that midwives can play in reducing maternal morbidity and mortality by encouraging developments with similar aims in their own units.

References

Audit Commission (1997) *First Class Delivery: Improving maternity services in England and Wales*. Her Majesty's Stationery Office (HMSO), London.

Bradshaw, C., Lewis, P. and Steer, P. (1995) A midwifery team for high-risk pregnancies. *Modern Midwife*, **5** (5): 26–9.

Cordingley, J. and Rubin, A. (1997) A survey of facilities for high risk women in consultant obstetric units. *International Journal of Obstetric Anaesthesia*, **6**: 156–60.

Department of Health (1993) *Changing childbirth: Report of the Expert Maternity Group*. HMSO, London.

Department of Health (1996) *Report on Confidential Enquiries into Maternal Deaths in the United Kingdom 1991–1993*. HMSO, London.

Department of Health (1998) *Why mothers die: Report on Confidential Enquiries into Maternal Deaths in the United Kingdom 1994–1996*. HMSO, London.

Ennis, M. (1991) Training and supervision of obstetric senior house officers. *British Medical Journal*, **303**: 1442–3.

Gregson, S. (2003) Learning the lessons. *RCM Midwives Journal*, **6** (11): 476–9.

Hugman, R. and Hadley, R. (1993) Involvement, motivation and reorganisation in a social services department. *Human Relations*, **46** (11).

Lewis, G. (2001) *Why Mothers Die 1997–1999: The Confidential Enquiries into Maternal Deaths in the United Kingdom.* Royal College of Obstetricians and Gynaecologists (RCOG) Press, London.

Lewis, G. (2004) *Why Mothers Die 2000–2002: Report on Confidential Enquiries into Maternal Deaths in the United Kingdom.* RCOG Press, London.

Mackay, L. (1993) *Conflicts in Care: Medicine and nursing.* Chapman & Hall, London.

McLachlan, B., Yeadon, D. and Johanson R. (1996) Care of the critically ill woman *MIDIRS Midwifery Digest*, **6** (4): 449–50.

Oakley, A. (1994) *Essays on Women, Medicine and Health.* Edinburgh University Press, Edinburgh.

Royal College of Midwives and Royal College of Obstetricians and Gynaecologists (1999) *Towards safer childbirth. Minimum standards for the organisation of labour wards. Report of a joint working party.* RCOG Press, London.

Sauter, S. (1999) *Local Supervising Authority Audit 1998–1999.* Kent, Surrey and Sussex LSA, Aylesford, UK.

Strong, P. and Robinson, J. (1990) *The NHS: Under new management.* Open University Press, Milton Keynes, UK.

Wilson, D. (1990) *Managing Organisations, Text Readings and Cases.* McGraw Hill, London.

3 Autonomous Practice: a Critical Investigation

Angela Bromley

In this chapter, it is proposed to examine the ethical principle of autonomy, its characteristics, requirements and responsibilities. This will then be applied to the principles of autonomy of women when using the maternity services, with reference to consent and refusal of consent. This will include the professional and legal responsibility that midwives hold to promote the autonomy of pregnant women. Finally, the concept of professionalism and professional autonomy will be examined and its application to midwives in a high risk setting.

What is autonomy?

Autonomy is a familiar word to midwives but do we really understand what it means? Autonomy originates from two Greek words, *Autos*, meaning self, and *nomos*, meaning rule, self-rule or the right of self-government (Chambers 1992). Before the modern age, the principle of autonomy only applied to nations or states (Marshall & Kirkwood 2000), but now it is more often thought of as applying to individuals.

If we look at autonomy in this individualistic way, consider for a minute what the principle of *self-rule* might mean to you, not as a midwife, but as a human being. Some might consider that it is freedom, freedom to act according to self-interests or desires. A wider view of autonomy not only includes the freedom to act but also identifies other intrinsic principles. First, it is necessary to be able to make rational decisions (Jones 2000) and second, once the action has been taken, the individual is then accountable for the consequences of those actions (Pollard 2003).

To illustrate this difference consider the following situation. If you decided to drive your car at 70 mph down a crowded street without consideration for other people you would be exercising freedom because you wanted to do it and were able to. To be autonomous in this situation you would have to consider how many people you might run into during the drive, rationalise your decision and be prepared to stand accountable for the mayhem that you cause. Clearly, a rational person would not act in this way and would therefore decide to drive at a more reasonable speed.

An important feature of autonomy is that the decisions and actions are the result of internal values, not external constraints. In the example above, the driver who drives at 30 mph rather than 70 mph simply because there is a policeman standing on the corner of the street is not necessarily acting autonomously. There is a need for an internalisation of values that guide the rational decision. The person who decides to drive at 30 mph because they can avoid knocking over pedestrians at this speed is acting autonomously, although avoiding losing your driving licence might also be considered a rational response.

The following list suggests the necessary factors for an individual to exercise autonomy:

- The ability to think and reason
- The ability to take action or verbalise your desires
- Information and knowledge in order to make decisions
- An environment that allows individuals to act on decisions made
- Intrinsic moral values

Without even one of the above, an individual cannot be fully autonomous. Individuals who live either in an oppressive society or even face oppression in their own homes, as in the case of those experiencing domestic violence, may not be able to exercise their autonomy.

Individuals with severe physical and mental disability may be unable to take action or communicate their desires in order for another to act on their behalf. Jones (2000) suggests that autonomy is not an all or nothing situation. She suggests that in society, those able to demonstrate greater rational thought and deliberate action are given more choice. Also, individuals may be able to exercise autonomy in one situation because they are able to understand it, but in a more complex situation understanding may be limited and therefore the ability to make an autonomous decision less likely (Johnstone & Slowther 2003).

Our moral values, or what we consider reasonable behaviour, will vary according to our upbringing, social values and possibly religious beliefs. It is possible that the rational decision of one individual could be considered irrational by another (Johnstone & Slowther 2003). However, it is the internal rationality that is important in autonomy. In a health care setting, an inability to understand the beliefs or values of another may result in removal of that person's autonomy because they are considered incompetent to make a choice. It is our responsibility as midwives to not only promote the autonomy of women using the maternity services but to respect the decisions they make.

Promoting autonomy in maternity care

One of the major changes of the last 30 years has been the increasing voice of women in forming policies and patterns of service provision. Government papers such as *Changing Childbirth* (Department of Health 1993) drew on the opinions of user representative groups to form recommendations. It also highlighted the importance of enabling women to have choices in maternity care and more involvement in the decision-making process. Since 1993, further government reports have repeated the emphasis of user involvement in health care services. These include *The NHS Plan* (Department of Health 2000) and the *National Service Framework for Children* (Department of Health 2004). Whilst these reports have influenced the structures of maternity services, the focus of this discussion will be on a more individual basis for both mother and midwives.

Specific guidance is given to midwives in relation to facilitating the autonomy of women in the Midwives Rules:

> "A midwife: Should enable the woman to make decisions about her care based on her individual needs, by discussing matters fully with her." (Nursing and Midwifery Council (NMC) 2004a, rule 6, p. 16)

This rule identifies the need for midwives to provide women with the necessary information to make an informed choice about their care. This requirement is also found in the NMC Code of Professional Conduct:

> "All patients and clients have a right to receive information about their condition. You must be sensitive to their needs and respect the wishes of those who refuse or are unable to receive information about their condition. Information should be accurate, truthful and presented in such a way as to make it easily understood." (NMC 2004b, point 3.1)

As the promotion of the autonomy of those in our care is a professional responsibility, it is worth considering what may enable this process and what may cause a stumbling block. Table 3.1 shows suggested enhancers and hurdles to women's autonomy.

Table 3.1   Enhancers and hurdles to women's autonomy.

Enhancers	Hurdles
Ability to process the information provided	Difficulty understanding
Ability of the individual to recognise hypothetical situations	Overanxiety created by inability to understand the probability of complications occurring
Plenty of time to discuss issues	Busy workload
Individualised approach to care	Inaccurate stereotyping
Discussing all options but explaining fully why some options may be less beneficial	Concealing choices not considered appropriate
Flexible policies and procedures	Limited resources
Good communication between professional disciplines	Conflicting opinions among carers
An approach to care that promotes an individual's right to choose	Paternalistic attitude of carers

As the table shows, there are some variables that are outside the midwife's control. These need ingenuity on the part of the midwife to work around them to promote or protect a woman's autonomy. For others, such as the filtering of information, it is in the midwife's hands to decide what is appropriate and what is not. The one commodity, which is key in many of the factors identified above, is time and this is in short supply in most maternity units today. The reality of how midwives facilitate informed choice was examined in a qualitative research study carried out by Levy (1999). Levy believes that this is a highly complex activity and found that midwives acted in a way that she named 'protective steering'. This was likened to walking a tightrope. Midwives wanted to give unbiased information but needed to achieve a balance between giving enough information and not frightening women. They also did not wish to raise unrealistic expectations or step outside available resources or create conflict with other professionals.

The real skill of the midwife was found to be in assessing each individual woman to determine quickly the information needs of the women, the detail required and the ability of the individual to understand the information and assess the type of language to use and the speed at which the information could be delivered. In this way midwives were behaving as 'gatekeepers' of information. It is important to note that the midwives were not deliberately exerting power over the women in their care but were negotiating a difficult route to provide appropriate information for an individual woman, whilst at the same time trying to prevent harm to both the mother and baby. Their perception was that misjudging this situation could result in either the woman being frightened, or feeling patronised. Other hazards identified were creating unrealistic expectations for the women or causing conflict between themselves and other health care professionals.

These findings highlight an important issue – that the partnership between midwife and woman is not necessarily an equal relationship. The midwife possesses more detailed knowledge of childbirth than most women in her care. However, Cooke (2005) states that women contribute knowledge of their own bodies and their personal values and beliefs that are of equal contribution to the final decision they will make.

In the high risk/critical care setting, the autonomy of women may be more difficult to protect. Obstetric complications can be medically complex and therefore more difficult to discuss in a way that women will understand. It is the responsibility of the midwife to make her knowledge accessible to the woman in her care so that she can understand the information provided and therefore use it to inform the decisions she makes regarding her care.

When an emergency situation arises, it is particularly difficult to protect the autonomy of the woman. Providing clear explanations quickly is a difficult skill especially when the woman and her partner are highly anxious. There are several ways in which a midwife can be prepared for this situation. First, it is important to practice obstetric emergency drills regularly, ideally as a multidisciplinary team. This will mean that when the situation arises, the procedures carried out are familiar, the problem is dealt with more efficiently and as a result the anxiety of the team of midwives and obstetricians is reduced. In relation to autonomy and informed consent this has two effects. If you are calmer it is easier to think more clearly and therefore present information in a coherent and concise way.

This calm approach will be transmitted to the women and her partner and not only increases their confidence in those who are helping them, but increases their likelihood of making an informed choice.

Second, it is important to allocate one person in the team whose role is just to provide information and support. There is potential for women to be bombarded with information from many different directions, from the midwife, the obstetrician and the labour ward coordinator who comes into the room to assist. The result is a cacophony of sound which is difficult to gather information from, even when not overanxious. This role is ideally that of the midwife already caring for the couple because she has an existing relationship with them. This is more difficult when this midwife is directly providing emergency care, as in the case of a postpartum haemorrhage for example. Another midwife may then need to adopt this role.

Finally, if possible, it is important to be prepared for potential risks. Whilst we know that emergency situations can occur without warning, there are also known associated risks that should be familiar to practitioners (Symon 1998). These may be identified at any point from antenatal history taking onwards into labour. Some are more obvious than others. For example, a multiparous woman who says that during her last delivery the midwife had difficulty delivering the shoulders should start a process of antenatal discussion, observation and decision making between the woman and obstetrician. Accurate documentation will mean that the midwife providing care in labour (if this option is chosen) will not only be mentally prepared herself, but will be able to discuss with the woman the procedures which would facilitate delivery of the shoulders if necessary. Another example might be an associated risk between cholestasis and postpartum haemorrhage. Having discussed this possibility ahead of the birth may mean that, should it occur, the woman is more aware of what is going on and is therefore able to understand, make decisions and give or withhold consent.

Advocacy on behalf of individuals and groups

To act as an advocate for women has become accepted within the role of the midwife (Warriner 2003). This has been adapted from the law where an advocate is one who pleads for another (Chambers 1992). There is, however, a difference between the role of a legal advocate and a health care professional acting as an advocate. In the legal setting, the lawyer only has to act on behalf of the person or persons they are representing (Grace 2001). Unfortunately advocacy is not as straightforward in health care. The Code of Professional Conduct (NMC 2004b) requires nurses and midwives to act on behalf of individual patients and clients. In addition to this, it places the same requirement to act on behalf of the wider community. This duel role has the potential to place the midwife in a situation where needs are conflicting. For example, if an individual woman chooses a course of action that will have a negative impact on other women, it is not possible for the midwife to act as advocate for the individual. Grace (2001) suggests that 'professional advocacy' is the solution in which the health professional is expected to achieve a balance between the needs of the individual and that of the wider population.

In midwifery care, there are undoubtedly situations where the midwife needs to present the opinions or desires of the woman in her care. Some women will require an advocate more than others, such as those who have difficulty articulating their wishes either due to disability or language difficulties. Also, vulnerability increases with illness (Woodward 1998), therefore in the high risk setting the midwife may need to represent the views of a woman if her autonomy is compromised. Warriner (2003) suggests that often, instead of acting as advocates, midwives find themselves behaving as arbitrators. Again the picture is of tightrope walking with midwives negotiating a compromise between the wishes of the woman and the limitations of the organisation.

The autonomy of groups of women with specific conditions may also require midwives to act in a more strategic or political way to enhance their autonomy. An example of this might be the support of women who are HIV positive but desire a vaginal delivery because culturally a caesarean birth is either unacceptable or may, within their community, almost label them as being immunosuppressed. Presenting the views of women by midwives in the policy-making process may increase the available choices.

Refusal of care

There are occasionally situations in practice where women will make decisions that are not considered beneficial either to themselves, their babies or both. This situation is thankfully rare and most women will take decisions that benefit their unborn babies, sometimes at detriment to themselves. In most cases, the refusal of medical advice is the result of extreme fear or lack of understanding, which with careful discussion may be overcome. However, it is important that we under-stand our professional responsibilities and the legal position if this situation is encountered.

Aveyard (2000) states that, in English law, an adult is considered to have the capacity to consent to, or refuse, medical treatment if they understand and can retain the relevant information, believe it and can weigh up the information in order to make a choice. The NMC Code of Professional Conduct states that:

> "You must respect patients' and clients' autonomy – their right to decide whether or not to undergo any health care intervention – even where a refusal may result in harm or death to themselves or a fetus, unless a court of law orders to the contrary." (NMC 2004b, point 3.2, pp. 7–8)

Although as health professionals in this situation we may have a strong moral desire to defend the fetus' right to life, there is no legal right to overrule the auto-nomy of the mother (Burrows 2001). In this situation, the midwife must ensure that the woman is in possession of the necessary information regarding the range of options open to her and the consequences of the course of action she has chosen (NMC 2004a). Accepting the responsibility for the consequences of a decision is inherent in the ethical principle of autonomy.

This is extremely stressful, especially in an emergency situation that allows little time for detailed explanations. It is appropriate in this situation to call a supervisor of midwives (NMC 2004a). The supervisor's role is to ensure that all possible options have been considered and discussed and that all details have been accurately documented. The importance of documentation cannot be overstressed in these circumstances. It is possible that in the future, when faced with the long-term care of a disabled child, the parents may say that they did not fully understand the implications of their decisions. The Midwives Rules suggest that "the women should be offered the opportunity to read what has been documented about the advice she has been given" (NMC 2004a, p. 18) and to sign it if she wishes.

It is not our role as midwives to judge the decisions of the women in our care. We will have an opinion, but it is our professional duty to uphold the decisions of the woman (Burrows 2001), and even in situations where our advice has not been followed, midwives are required to continue care in the best way possible (NMC 2004a).

Whilst the legal position appears to be quite clear, there have been, and will be, situations where the woman's autonomy is overruled in favour of the fetus. These cases occur because the competence of a woman to make an autonomous decision has been questioned. In one case, a woman was sectioned under the Mental Health Act because she refused to be admitted to hospital after being diagnosed with pre-eclampsia (Dyer 1998). She later underwent a caesarean section, also against her will, after a court order was obtained. Despite being approved by a High Court Judge, this ruling was overturned at appeal and ruled as unlawful.

Rarely a situation may occur where there is no question that the individual is unable to give consent, for example if they are unconscious. In these circumstances, it is the health professionals' responsibility to as far as possible carry out the wishes of the woman as expressed prior to their unconsciousness (Burrows 2001). An example might be a woman who is a Jehovah's Witness who has previously stated that she would not accept a blood transfusion, but following a haemorrhage has lost consciousness. The team caring for her could not then give her a blood transfusion as she is no longer able to refuse because they are aware of her prior wishes. In situations where the woman has not expressed an opinion, health care professionals should resort to another ethical principle, beneficence. This means to do the most good to the most people.

The new Mental Capacity Act, likely to come into force in April 2007 (Johnstone & Slowther 2005), has two significant changes that may impact on situations where capacity is questioned. First, it will allow consent to be given or withheld by another person, usually a close relative, if an individual is shown to lack capacity to give consent themselves. This has only been possible for children up to now. Second, there is the capacity for advance directives to be made that allow people to state what their wishes would be in a given situation should they be unable to give or withhold consent in the future. In situations where a woman is unconscious, the partner may have the right to give or withhold consent. Where capacity is less clearly defined, recourse to the courts may still be necessary. The Mental Health Act currently defines what is required in order to give consent (Johnstone & Slowther 2005). An individual must be able to understand the relevant information and retain it for the necessary time needed to make a decision. They also have to be able to weigh up that information and communicate the decision they have reached.

Most midwives will not find themselves in these extreme situations during their careers, but many will find that not all women will agree with their professional opinions and may make alternative decisions or choices. In many cases, careful discussion and respect for the woman's right to autonomy will enable open discussion and compromise on both sides likely to increase the safety of the birth.

Professional autonomy

As we have already seen, personal autonomy is exercised within the boundaries of our society and personal beliefs, combined with the accountability of our actions. Before expanding this principle to encompass professional autonomy it is helpful to clarify what is a 'profession'.

Hunt and Symonds (1995) suggest that a profession or professional has traditionally had the following traits:

- Academic education
- A specific body of knowledge
- Responsibility for practice
- Ethical standards adhered to by members
- Independence
- Autonomy

One may consider these attributes to be present in midwifery practice based on the belief that:

- The sphere of midwifery has been identified as normal childbirth.
- Midwives are accountable for their practice to the governing body of the Nursing and Midwifery Council (NMC 2004b).
- Ethical codes and Midwives' Rules (NMC 2004a, 2004b) are applied to midwives when they register as a midwife.
- Acceptance onto the register confers on the midwife the right to make autonomous decisions in the care of women whilst they remain in the sphere of normality.

Sargent (2002) describes an autonomous midwife as one who is able to practice using her knowledge and skills to plan and execute the care of women for whom she is responsible. The autonomous midwife is free to adopt or reject the advice of others because she is accountable for the care she gives (Marshall 2005).

However, in reality, the degree of professional autonomy available to the midwife is rarely, if ever, absolute. Like personal autonomy, there are degrees of professional autonomy dependent on the environment in which the midwife works and the degree of autonomy she chooses to exercise. The degree of professional autonomy will depend on the authority given to the midwife by their employer and their own attitude to professional autonomy (Marshall 2005).

It might be argued that midwives who choose to work in the high risk setting have adopted an obstetric nursing role, relinquishing their autonomy to the obstetrician. There are two reasons why this is not the case. First, it is a requirement that when midwives detect a deviation from the normal they should refer to an obstetrician (NMC 2004a). This shows that the professional scope of the midwife has been breeched and therefore they are no longer able to exercise their professional autonomy. Whilst this is true, women who experience an obstetric complication continue to have other needs that remain in the scope of the midwives' professional role. For example, women with pregnancy-induced hypertension may be critically ill but they still need advice regarding infant feeding. Second, the NMC Code of Professional Conduct states that nurses and midwives are personally accountable for their practice (NMC 2004b). Earlier in this chapter we have seen that accountability for the results of decisions is inherent in both personal and professional autonomy. In the high risk setting, accountability for one's own actions still applies and this means that when a midwife decides to act, whether it be her own decision or on the instruction of another, she is making a decision about whether this action is appropriate or not and therefore, within the sphere of her professional activity, is acting autonomously. This is the key to the midwife as an autonomous practitioner.

Despite this assertion, there are factors that influence the autonomy of midwives. The history and regulation of midwifery have been well documented elsewhere (Donnison 1988; Sargent 2002) so it is proposed, before closing this chapter, to consider how individuals can enhance their autonomy when working with high risk women.

The first consideration is a *firm belief and grounding in normal midwifery*. Understanding the normal physiological process and recognising it even when obstetric complications occur enables midwives to exercise midwifery autonomy (Marshall 2005).

Second, *involvement in the production of unit policies and procedures*. This is not a new activity for midwives. However, it is likely that policies written by midwives are usually focused on low risk maternity care. Specialist midwives can be equally involved in this process for policies associated with obstetric complications either as author or as part of a guideline group.

Finally, *education*. When working in the high risk setting a thorough knowledge of obstetrics complications is necessary. This allows midwives to meet the information needs of the women in their care and also enhances communication and relationships with obstetric personnel. In her study of midwives' perceptions of autonomy, Pollard (2003) found that midwives felt their autonomy was enhanced by good relationships with obstetricians. This is not to suggest that midwives should engage in the 'doctor–nurse game', which is based on assuming a subservient role whilst subtlety putting forward one's own opinion or idea in such a way as to make the doctor think it was theirs (Marshall 2005). Alternatively, a confident, knowledgeable midwife who demonstrates advanced knowledge of obstetric complications and applies that knowledge to the care of women can earn the respect of obstetric colleagues. This increases the midwife's authority and autonomy.

Conclusion

This chapter has examined the ethical concept of autonomy in which individuals exercise the right to decide their own actions with reference to moral considerations and accepting the consequences of those actions. It has been suggested that autonomy is not absolute and that individuals are able to exercise different degrees of autonomy in different situations.

Promoting the autonomy of women in our care is a key role of the midwife, which is emphasised in statute and government policy. Midwives working with women experiencing obstetric complications need particular skills in order to provide relevant information in a form that is understood by women so that they can make informed choices. Advocacy to promote autonomy for vulnerable individuals and groups is also the role of the midwife. Difficulties can occur when women make choices that may not be seen as rational to the midwife. In these situations, as long as the individual is considered competent to make a decision, the midwife needs to respect their rights and continue to care for them in the best way possible without infringing their wishes. This situation has the potential to be very stressful for midwives and the support of a supervisor of midwives is recommended.

Midwives have been identified as autonomous practitioners in the context of normal midwifery. It is argued that professional autonomy is inseparable from accountability and therefore midwives also have an autonomous responsibility in the high risk environment. In addition to this, women experiencing obstetric complications continue to have normal midwifery needs that remain firmly in the scope of the midwife's role. Finally, midwives specialising in high risk maternity care need to gain a thorough education in obstetric complications in order to not only give a high standard of care but to gain the respect of their obstetric colleagues as skilled clinicians.

References

Aveyard, H. (2000) Is there a concept of autonomy that can usefully inform nursing practice? *Journal of Advanced Nursing*, **32** (2): 352–8.

Burrows, J. (2001) The parturient woman: can there be room for more than 'one person with full and equal rights inside a single human skin'? *Journal of Advanced Nursing*, **33** (5): 689–95.

Chambers (1992) *Chambers Concise Dictionary*. W. & R. Chambers, Edinburgh.

Cooke, P. (2005) Helping women to make their own decisions. In: M.D. Raynor, J.E. Marshall and A. Sullivan (Eds) *Decision Making in Midwifery Practice*. Elsevier/Churchill Livingstone, London.

Department of Health (1993) *Changing Childbirth, Part 1: Report of the Expert Maternity Group*. Her Majesty's Stationery Office (HMSO), London.

Department of Health (2000) *The NHS Plan*. HMSO, London.

Department of Health (2004) *National Service Framework for Children*. HMSO, London.

Donnison, J. (1988) *Midwives and Medical Men – A history of the struggle for the control of childbirth*. Historical Publications Ltd, London.

Dyer, C. (1998) Trusts face damages after forcing women to have caesareans, *British Medical Journal*, **316** (7143): 1480.

Grace, P.J. (2001) Professional advocacy: widening the scope of accountability, *Nursing Philosophy*, **2**: 151–62.

Hunt, S. and Symonds, A. (1995) *The Social Meaning of Midwifery*. Macmillan Press, London.

Johnstone, C. and Slowther, A. (2003) Ethical considerations. Respect for autonomy. www.ethics-network.org.uk/Ethics/econsent.htm

Johnstone, C. and Slowther, A. (2005) Medical ethics and law. Consent handout 5. www.ethox.org.uk/education/teach/Consent/consent5.htm

Jones, S. (2000) *Ethics in Midwifery.* Mosby, London.

Levy, V. (1999) Protective steering: a grounded theory study of the processes by which midwives facilitate informed choices during pregnancy. *Journal of Advanced Nursing,* **29** (1): 104–12.

Marshall, J.E. (2005) Autonomy and the midwife. In: M.D. Raynor, J.E. Marshall and A. Sullivan (Eds) *Decision Making in Midwifery Practice.* Churchill Livingstone, Edinburgh.

Marshall, J.E. and Kirkwood, S. (2000) Autonomy and teamwork. In: D. Fraser (Ed.) *Professional Studies for Midwifery Practice.* Churchill Livingstone, London.

Nursing and Midwifery Council (2004a) *Midwives Rules and Standards.* Nursing and Midwifery Council (NMC), London.

Nursing and Midwifery Council (2004b) *The NMC Code of Professional Conduct: Standards for conduct, performance and ethics.* NMC, London.

Pollard, K. (2003) Searching for autonomy. *Midwifery,* **19** (2): 113–24.

Sargent, L. (2002) Practice and autonomy. In: R. Mander and V. Fleming (Eds) *Failure to Progress.* Routledge, London.

Symon, A. (1998) Known complications and rare occurrences. *British Journal of Midwifery,* **6** (2): 114–17.

Warriner, S. (2003) Midwives: advocates or arbitrators? *British Journal of Midwifery,* **11** (9): 532–3.

Woodward, V.M. (1998) Caring, patient autonomy and the stigma of paternalism. *Journal of Advanced Nursing,* **28** (5): 1046–52.

4 Medical Disorders and the Critically Ill Woman

Mary Billington and Tina Heptinstall

This chapter provides an overview of critical illness caused by some of the more common medical conditions that may complicate, or be complicated by, childbearing.

Substandard care identified in the current Confidential Enquiry into Maternal Deaths (CEMD) includes failure of some obstetricians and midwives to recognise and act on medical conditions outside their immediate experience; a lack of communication and teamwork within obstetric and midwifery teams, and in multidisciplinary team working; and failure to appreciate the severity of illness (Lewis 2004). The CEMD recommends that protocols and local referral pathways should be developed for multidisciplinary management of women with pre-existing medical conditions, including cardiac disease, epilepsy and diabetes (Lewis 2004). This chapter should be read in conjunction with any such protocols available in the reader's place of practice.

In addition to recognising the importance of multiprofessional working, which may necessitate transfer of a woman to a specialist centre, the midwife should also remember the importance of record keeping, support, information and consent, and attention to comfort, hygiene, pressure areas, privacy and dignity. Intensive monitoring and possibly early delivery of a potentially sick baby may also be features of management and care.

Assumed prior knowledge

- Physiological changes of pregnancy affecting the cardiovascular, respiratory, renal, hepatic and endocrine systems.
- Basic understanding of cardiac, respiratory, renal, hepatic, thyroid and connective tissue disorders, and diabetes and epilepsy.

Cardiac disorders

Serious cardiac disease in pregnancy is relatively uncommon, affecting approximately 1% (Tomlinson & Cotton 1999), but it is significant in terms of maternal and fetal morbidity and mortality. Cardiac disease was the second most common cause of maternal death in the current CEMD, the number of deaths being 44 (Lewis 2004) compared with 35 in the previous triennium (Lewis 2001). Specific causes of death were pulmonary hypertension, cardiomyopathy, myocardial infarction, valvular disease, and aneurysm or dissection of the aorta or its branches (Lewis 2004). Infective endocarditis, arrhythmias and heart failure may also occur (Oakley 1996; Siu & Colman 2001).

There are two main physiological changes of the cardiovascular system in childbearing that can have serious implications for women with pre-existing disease:

- An increase in cardiac output by 20% at 8 weeks and up to 50% by the end of the second trimester of pregnancy (Oakley 1996; Williams 1999; Nelson-Piercy 2002). This increase is achieved mainly by an increase in stroke volume – the rise in heart rate is only 10–15 beats/min (Oakley 1996; Tomlinson & Cotton 1999).
- A further increase in cardiac output during labour of 15% in the first stage and 50% in the second stage due to pain and uterine activity, and 60–80% immediately following delivery due to relief of caval compression and autotranfusion of 300–500 ml of blood from the contracted uterus (Nelson-Piercy 2002).

To some extent, changes in cardiac output are balanced by changes in peripheral resistance as systemic and pulmonary vascular resistance fall by 25–30% during pregnancy (Nelson-Piercy 2002).

The physiological changes in the cardiovascular system, along with changes in the respiratory system (see below), may delay diagnosis of cardiac deterioration as dyspnoea, syncope, oedema, full, bounding peripheral pulses and a degree of valvular regurgitation, which are indicative of heart disease, are also features of normal pregnancy, as are premature atrial and ventricular ectopic beats (Williams 1999; Nelson-Piercy 2002). Furthermore, diagnosis may be further delayed if women (or family members used as interpreters) minimise or deny symptoms of heart disease due to strong desire or cultural pressure for motherhood (Lewis 2001, 2004).

Types of cardiac disorders

Rheumatic and congenital heart disease are the two most common causes of structural anomaly, with the former mainly being in recent immigrants to the UK, particularly from Asia, Africa and South America (Tomlinson & Cotton 1999; Lewis 2001). However, the incidence of *ischaemic heart disease* is rising due to its increased prevalence in the female population (particularly those who smoke) and the increasing age of motherhood.

Rheumatic heart disease is a complication of rheumatic fever, which is caused by the group A beta-haemolytic streptococcus. Chronic inflammation causes thickening, distortion and loss of elasticity of heart valves leading to stenosis (thickening) or incompetence (incomplete closure) with regurgitation of blood. Valvular stenosis and regurgitation may also be congenital in origin, although the most common congenital defects are atrial septal defect (ASD), ventricular septal defect (VSD) and patent ductus arteriosus (PDA), which together account for 60% of the congenital defects seen in pregnancy (Nelson-Piercy 2002). Other significant congenital defects are coarctation of the aorta, Marfan's syndrome and Fallot's tetralogy (Tomlinson & Cotton 1999).

Stenosed valves impede the flow of blood through the heart, causing back pressure which is aggravated by the haemodynamic changes of pregnancy and labour, and may result in tachyarrhythmias and heart failure. Mitral valve stenosis is the most common manifestation of rheumatic heart disease, and the associated back pressure causes pulmonary hypertension and pulmonary oedema (Williams 1999; Siu & Colman 2001; Nelson-Piercy 2002). This is signified by breathlessness (Williams 1999) and is aggravated by tachycardia caused, for example, by exertion or infection (Oakley 1996). Aortic valve stenosis is less common in childbearing as congenitally it is more common in males, and following rheumatic fever it progresses with age. However, when severe it can reduce cardiac output leading to inadequate coronary and cerebral perfusion, and sudden death in the event of hypovolaemia or hypotension (Tomlinson & Cotton 1999).

In the absence of stenosis, *valvular incompetence and regurgitation* tend to improve in pregnancy as decreased arterial resistance facilitates flow of blood through the valve. However, it worsens in the presence of hypertension and during the third stage of labour with the return of blood from the uterine to the general circulation (Tomlinson & Cotton 1999).

With *uncorrected ASD, VSD and PDA*, blood generally follows the normal path of circulation as pressure in the arterial system is less than in the opposite side of the heart. This continues in normal pregnancy as the increase in blood volume is balanced by the decrease in peripheral resistance (Siu & Colman 2001). However, systemic or pulmonary hypertension and hypotension may cause shunting of blood across the defect. Long-term left-to-right shunting is associated with development of pulmonary hypertension while a sudden left-to-right shunt may lead to reduced left ventricular output and reduced cardiac and cerebral perfusion. Right-to-left shunting is associated with cyanosis as deoxygenated blood bypasses the lungs.

Coarctation of the aorta, a marked narrowing of the aortic arch, may lead to hypertension and congestive heart failure, and can be associated with other defects such as aneurysms of the circle of Willis, intercostal arteries and distal aorta, and aortic valve defects. The cardiac features of *Marfan's syndrome*, an autosomal dominant connective tissue disorder, are mitral valve prolapse and aortic root dilatation. These abnormalities are associated with regurgitation, arrhythmias, syncope and aortic dissection or rupture, particularly when blood volume is increased. Lewis (2004) suggests that the possibility of dissection is often not considered in pregnant women despite the fact that all blood vessels are more likely to rupture during pregnancy due to arterial dilatation. Maternal mortality is between 5 and 50%, for both coarctation of the aorta and Marfan's syndrome, depending on the presence of associated complications (Tomlinson & Cotton 1999).

In *Fallot's tetralogy* there is VSD, an aorta that overrides the septum, pulmonary stenosis and right ventricular hypertrophy. Pregnancy rarely occurs if the defects are uncorrected as there is a short lifespan and subfertility, but if pregnancy does occur the increased blood volume leads to increased cyanosis (Siu & Colman 2001), and maternal mortality is up to 15% (Tomlinson & Cotton 1999).

Myocardial infarction (MI) may occur due to coronary spasm, thrombosis or dissection of the coronary arteries. It may also be associated with connective tissue disorders such as systemic lupus erythematosus (de Swiet 2002), and cocaine use (Nelson-Piercy 2002). The maternal mortality rate is 20%, the risk of death being higher if labour occurs within 2 weeks (Tomlinson & Cotton 1999). Onset is often unheralded and is more common in the third trimester of pregnancy and puerperium. Diagnosis may be delayed because MI is unexpected in relatively young women. However, between 2000 and 2002, three women died of ischaemic heart disease and a further five of MI due to coronary artery dissection (Lewis 2004). Thus Lewis (2004) suggests angiography when MI is suspected.

Peripartum cardiomyopathy is a dilated cardiomyopathy specific to childbearing, although some believe it may be pre-existing heart disease revealed by the physiological changes of pregnancy (Tomlinson & Cotton 1999). Its incidence is less than 1:5000 (de Swiet 2002) and onset is usually in the first month postpartum, but it may present in the last few weeks of pregnancy or first six months postnatally. The underlying cause may be immunological, nutritional or infective (de Swiet 2002), and it is more common in African women over the age of 30, women from lower socioeconomic groups and women who are hypertensive, obese or who have a multiple pregnancy (Tomlinson & Cotton 1999; Nelson-Piercy 2002; de Swiet 2002; Lewis 2004). There is high morbidity and mortality due to cardiac dysfunction, pulmonary oedema, arrhythmias and thromboembolism (Tomlinson & Cotton 1999; de Swiet 2002), with mortality in the range of 20–80% (Tomlinson & Cotton 1999). It accounted for four of the eight deaths from cardiomyopathy in the current CEMD (Lewis 2004).

Pregnancy outcome

Nelson-Piercy (2002) suggests that this is related to:

- Presence of cyanosis (i.e. arterial oxygen saturation < 80%)
- Presence of pulmonary hypertension (see below)
- Haemodynamic significance of any lesion
- Functional class (New York Heart Association classification), with poor outcome likely with class III or IV regardless of the specific lesion (Table 4.1).

Table 4.1   New York Heart Association functional classification.

Class I	No breathlessness/uncompromised
Class II	Breathless on severe exertion/slightly compromised
Class III	Breathless on mild exertion/moderately compromised
Class IV	Breathless at rest/severely compromised

Pulmonary hypertension, defined as a mean pulmonary artery pressure greater than 25 mmHg (Tomlinson & Cotton 1999), may be primary or secondary in origin. It has a maternal mortality rate of 30–50% as pulmonary vascular resistance is fixed – i.e. the fall in pulmonary vascular resistance that occurs in normal pregnancy does not take place and thus pulmonary blood flow cannot increase to match the increase in cardiac output (Tomlinson & Cotton 1999; Nelson-Piercy 2002). Labour and the early postpartum periods are the most dangerous periods as increased cardiac output and the postpartum fluid shift may lead to sudden right heart failure (Tomlinson & Cotton 1999; Siu & Colman 2001; de Swiet 2002).

Primary pulmonary hypertension is an idiopathic disorder which although rare, may be familial, and presents primarily in young women (de Swiet 2002). Secondary pulmonary hypertension results from a longstanding increase in pulmonary pressure from underlying cardiac disease, such as left-to-right shunting associated with ASD, VSD, PDA, mitral stenosis or lung disease, such as cystic fibrosis. It is known as Eisenmenger's syndrome when it is associated with uncorrected ASD, VSD or PDA. When pulmonary artery pressure exceeds systemic pressure, the shunt is reversed, leading to cyanosis as desaturated blood bypasses the lungs. The decrease in systemic resistance during pregnancy increases the likelihood of right-to-left shunting.

Investigations

- Chest X-ray: if the fetus is screened, the dose of radiation is less than 1 day of background radiation (Williams 1999).
- Echocardiography: a safe and accurate method of discriminating significant heart disease from the physiological changes of pregnancy (Williams 1999). It should be repeated through pregnancy in women at risk of pulmonary vascular disease (Lewis 2004).
- Electrocardiogram (ECG, see Chapter 10): this is vital to enable the likely effects of the cardiovascular changes of pregnancy to be determined (Oakley 1996).

Care and management

With careful management, many women with cardiac disorders have a satisfactory outcome to pregnancy. However, in addition to critical illness caused by cyanosis, heart failure and pulmonary oedema, bacterial endocarditis and thromboembolism may occur when there is damage to the cardiovascular system from any cause, including surgical correction of defects. Lewis (2001) suggests that about 10% of all cardiac deaths are due to endocarditis and that it should always be considered in pregnant women with obscure febrile illness.

Principles and considerations

- Termination of pregnancy is only beneficial under 16 weeks before significant increase in cardiac output has occurred.

- Avoid the supine position as associated caval compression reduces venous return and thus cardiac output by up to 25% in the second half of pregnancy (Kerr, cited by Jevon & Raby 2001).
- A rise in resting heart rate indicates reduced cardiovascular reserve and failure to increase stroke volume (Oakley 1996).
- Careful fluid management: avoid overload (which may precipitate aneurysm rupture or dissection) but also prompt replacement during haemorrhage, to avoid shunt reversal or reduced cardiac and cerebral perfusion.
- Correct tachyarrhythmias: beta-blockers and antiarrhythmics are safe (Tomlinson & Cotton 1999) with the exception of amiodarone, which can cause fetal thyroid dysfunction (Williams 1999). Successful cardioversion has also been reported (Tomlinson & Cotton 1999).
- Continuous ECG (see Chapter 10).
- Oxygen therapy and continuous oxygen saturation monitoring, with blood gas sampling as necessary.
- Invasive haemodynamic monitoring with a pulmonary artery catheter and arterial line for women at 'high risk' or deteriorating condition (see Chapter 10).
- Fetal wellbeing: use continuous electronic fetal monitoring (Edozien 2004).
- Antibiotic prophylaxis if there is any type of structural damage. Bacterial endocarditis is rare when labour and delivery is uncomplicated (Tomlinson & Cotton 1999), but it is difficult to predict when complications may occur (Williams 1999; Siu & Colman 2001). Williams (1999) suggests a regime of amoxycillin 1 g intramuscularly and gentamicin 120 mg intravenously (over 3 minutes) at the onset of labour (or anaesthesia), followed by intravenous amoxycillin 500 mg 6-hourly.
- Asepsis and minimisation of invasive procedures may also help reduce endocarditis.
- Thromboembolism prophylaxis in the presence of cardiac damage including artificial valves (see Chapter 5).
- Take care to reduce pain in labour to minimise hypertension and tachycardia. Consider using a 'low dose' continuous epidural to avoid swings in blood pressure.
- Consider operative vaginal delivery to avoid blood pressure changes associated with pushing and the Valsalva manoeuvre, but reserve caesarean section for obstetric indications (although Williams (1999) recommends the latter to avoid exertion).
- Exercise caution with oxytocic drugs for both induction/acceleration of labour and the third stage of labour. Syntocinon infusion is associated with fluid retention; Lewis (2001) suggests a maximum dose of 5 units/day. Ergometrine (including Syntometrine) is contraindicated due to its vasoconstrictive and hypertensive effects. When Syntocinon is used for active management of the third stage of labour, it should be administered slowly as rapid intravenous injection is associated with transient hypotension (British Medical Association & Royal Pharmaceutical Society of Great Britain 2005).
- Continue high dependency care for 24–72 hours after delivery as significant fluid shift can lead to congestive cardiac failure and, if spontaneous diuresis

does not occur, pulmonary oedema may develop (Tomlinson & Cotton 1999). Consider diuretics if pulmonary oedema develops.

* Women with Eisenmenger's syndrome need intensive care for at least 7 days after delivery (Edozien 2004).

Respiratory disorders

Anatomical, biochemical and hormonal adaptations in the respiratory system occur during pregnancy to enable the increased metabolic demands of the mother and the fetoplacental unit to be met (Knox 2001; Nelson-Piercy 2001). Many of the changes are due to progesterone, which has a stimulating effect of on the maternal respiratory centre, causing increased sensitivity to carbon dioxide (Knox 2001) and a relaxing effect on the muscles and cartilage of the thoracic cavity.

Oxygen consumption increases by 20% and this is met by a 20–50% increase in resting ventilation, which is apparent by the end of the first trimester and continues for the remainder of pregnancy (Knox 2001). It is achieved mainly by a 40% rise in tidal volume which, by term, has increased from 500 to 700 ml (Rankin 2005a), rather than a change in respiratory rate (Nelson-Piercy 2001). This is facilitated by anatomical changes in the thoracic cavity – by late pregnancy, the transverse diameter of the ribcage increases by 2 cm and the subcostal angle widens from 60 to 103° (de Swiet 1998).

In early pregnancy, the diaphragm rises by 4–7 cm, even before pressure is exerted by the uterus (Rankin 2005a) and this, combined with the increased tidal volume, leads to a reduction in functional residual capacity (lung volume at rest after passive expiration). This is due to reduction in both the expiratory reserve (the amount of air that can be forcibly expelled after normal expiration) and the residual volume (the amount of air remaining in the lungs after forceful expiration) (Coleman & Rund 1997; Knox 2001; Nelson-Piercy 2001). However, there is no change in peak expiratory flow rate which is normally 380–550 L/min (Coleman & Rund 1997) or forced expiratory volume in 1 second (FEV_1) (Nelson-Piercy 2001).

Changes in arterial oxygen tension (Pao_2) and arterial carbon dioxide tension ($Paco_2$) occur as there is less air remaining in the lungs after expiration to be mixed with air in the next inspiration. This results in a fall in $Paco_2$ from approximately 35–40 to 25–32 mmHg (Coleman & Rund 1997; de Swiet 1995), with a compensatory fall in serum bicarbonate from 22–26 mmol/L (Cox & Grady 1999) to 18–22 mmol/L (Nelson-Piercy 2001). There may be an associated increase in Pao_2 (Knox 2001; Nelson-Piercy 2001) although some suggest it remains unchanged at approximately 100 mmHg (Coleman & Rund 1997) or 104–108 mmHg (Cox & Grady 1999).

A mild respiratory alkalosis is normal in pregnancy with arterial pH increasing slightly to 7.4–7.45. These changes optimise fetal oxygen–carbon dioxide exchange (Coleman & Rund 1997; Nelson-Piercy 2001). However, minimal changes in maternal oxygenation may result in appreciable changes in fetal oxygenation – with a maternal Pao_2 of less than 60 mm Hg, an increasing arterial Pco_2 and acidosis being harmful (Coleman & Rund 1997).

The changes outlined above result in physiological hyperventilation that causes up to 75% of women to experience feelings of breathlessness and giddiness, especially in the third trimester. As this is not always related to exercise, and may occur while at rest, there is potential for over- or underdiagnosis of respiratory disorders (Coleman & Rund 1997; Nelson-Piercy 2002). However, for women with existing respiratory compromise the physiological changes of pregnancy can contribute to further deterioration (Knox 2001).

Hypoxia

Clinical features

Clinical features of mild to moderate hypoxia include irritability and restlessness. Extremities may be cool and pale as a sympathetic response shunts blood away from the peripheries. Confusion, disorientation, loss of consciousness, depressed myocardial contractility, and arrhythmias occur as the hypoxia worsens (Coleman & Rund 1997).

Investigations (Cox & Grady 1999; de Swiet 1999)

- Careful history and examination
- Peak expiratory flow
- Oxygen saturation (Sao_2): should be > 95%
- Arterial blood gasses in severe cases (e.g. $Sao_2 \leq 92\%$)
- Haemoglobin
- Chest X-ray: should not be withheld if clinically indicated
- Ventilation-perfusion scan
- Echocardiography (to differentiate from cardiac disease)
- ECG
- Continuous cardiotocography

Care and management (Coleman & Rund 1997)

- Supplemental oxygen to maintain Pao_2 at more than 60–70 mmHg, and oxygen saturation of haemoglobin at 90%.
- Intubation if blood gasses are borderline or poor (e.g. $Pao_2 < 70$ mmHg or $Paco_2 > 55$ mmHg), if there is respiratory compromise (e.g. respiratory rate of more than 35 breaths/min) or diminished consciousness.
- Intensive care may be required if the pH is below 7.35 or if arterial $Paco_2$ rises above 38 mmHg during the pregnancy.

Asthma

Asthma is a chronic inflammatory condition of the airways, defined as reversible airways obstruction (de Swiet 1999). The inflammation is associated with

---

Box 4.1   Features of severe acute asthma (Nelson-Piercy 2002; British Guideline on the Management of Asthma 2003b).

Features of acute severe asthma

Any one of:
- Peak expiratory flow (PEF) 33–50% of best or predicted
- Respiratory rate $\geq$ 25 breaths/min
- Heart rate > 110 beats/min
- Inability to complete sentences in one breath
- Use of accessory muscles of respiration

Life-threatening features

- PEF < 33% of predicted or best
- $Sao_2 < 92\%$
- $Pao_2 < 60$ mmHg
- Silent chest, cyanosis, or feeble respiratory effort
- Bradycardia, dysrhythmia or hypotension
- Exhaustion, confusion or coma

---

swelling and excessive production of mucus, while reversible bronchospasm occurs due to spasm of smooth muscle in the airway walls (Nelson-Piercy 2002). Asthma is the commonest respiratory disorder affecting women of childbearing age, with an incidence of up to 7% (Nelson-Piercy 2002). There were five deaths from asthma in both the current and previous CEMD (Lewis 2001, 2004).

Attacks may be triggered by allergens (e.g. pollen, dust, mould, animal dander), irritants (e.g. smoke, air pollution), drugs (e.g. aspirin, non-steroidal anti-inflammatory drugs (NSAIDs), beta-blockers), cold air, stress, exercise, upper respiratory infection, infestation with round worms and hypocarbia.

Clinical features

Clinical features include dyspnoea, tachypnoea, cough, thick sputum, chest tightness and expiratory wheeze. The condition is often worse at night and early morning. Features of a severe attack may be underestimated and deterioration can be sudden, as was the case for three of the five women who died in the triennium 1997–1999 (Lewis 2001). Box 4.1 lists the features of severe acute asthma.

Effects of pregnancy on asthma

There is no consistent trend to improvement or worsening of asthma for individual women in pregnancy (Nelson-Piercy 2001), although the 'rule of 1/3' suggests that it improves in 1/3, deteriorates in 1/3 and remains the same in 1/3 (Tan & Thomson 2000). Theoretically, physiological changes in pregnancy which have opposing effects are that progesterone and cortisol are bronchodilators while prostaglandins tend to be bronchoconstrictors (although prostaglandin E_2 is an exception) (de Swiet 1995).

Deterioration is more likely in women with more severe disease and is most prevalent between 24 and 36 weeks of pregnancy (de Swiet 1999; Tan & Thomson 2000; Nelson-Piercy 2002; British Guideline on the Management of Asthma 2003a).

Deterioration is also more likely if the fetus is male, but this is only of practical use when the sex of the fetus is known (Tan & Thomson 2000). For some women, deterioration in pregnancy is related to unsupervised reduction in medication due to concern about possible teratogenic effects on the fetus (de Swiet 1999; Nelson-Piercy 2002). The same drugs and doses as in the non-pregnant condition should be continued as the risks of severe asthma outweigh any small risk from medication (British Guideline on the Management of Asthma 2003a). Inhalational rather than oral preparations are used as these reduce systemic effects including placental transfer (de Swiet 1999; Nelson-Piercy 2002).

Asthma attacks rarely occur during labour, possibly because of increased secretion of cortisol (de Swiet 1995; British Guideline on the Management of Asthma 2003a), while women whose condition improves during the third trimester of pregnancy often experience deterioration postnatally (Nelson-Piercy 2002).

Effects of asthma on pregnancy

Outcome is generally good if the asthma is mild and/or well controlled, although severe or poorly controlled asthma, leading to chronic or intermittent hypoxaemia, may be associated with the following (de Swiet 1999; Tan & Thomson 2000; Nelson-Piercy 2002; British Guideline on the Management of Asthma 2003a):

- Preterm labour
- Maternal hypertension
- Pre-eclampsia
- Fetal growth restriction
- Hyperemesis gravidarum
- Antepartum haemorrhage

These complications may be due to a combination of the effects of hypoxia, drug therapy and an underlying predisposition to increased smooth muscle tone (Schatz 1999; de Swiet 1999).

Prevention of severe attacks

Midwives have an important role in helping prevent severe asthma attacks through providing education and support (including emotional support) about continuation of medication, avoidance of triggers, early recognition of chest infection and the importance of early admission in the event of deterioration because of the rapidity with which further deterioration may occur.

During labour, caution is advised with drugs such as pethidine, ergometrine and prostaglandin $F_{2\alpha}$ (carboprost/Hemabate), which are associated with bronchospasm (de Swiet 1999; Nelson-Piercy 2002). However, the British Guideline on the Management of Asthma (2003a) suggests that all forms of pain relief may safely be used, and that the bronchospasm associated with ergometrine does not occur with syntometrine. Regional anaesthesia is preferable to general anaesthetia due to the risk of chest infection and associated atelectasis with the latter (de Swiet 1999; Nelson-Piercy 2002; British Guideline on the Management of Asthma 2003a).

Care and management of acute severe asthma

Acute severe asthma (status asthmaticus) is an extremely dangerous condition, requiring care in an intensive care environment in conjunction with a respiratory physician.

Immediate treatment includes the following (Nelson-Piercy 2002; British Guideline on the Management of Asthma 2003b):

- Oxygen to maintain saturation above 95%
- Hydration (to restore volume and help liquefy sputum)
- Beta2-agonist (e.g. salbutamol 5 mg or terbutaline 10 mg) via an oxygen-driven nebuliser
- Ipratropium bromide 0.5 mg via an oxygen-driven nebuliser
- Prednisolone 40–50 mg orally or hydrocortisone 100 mg i.v. (or both)
- No sedatives of any kind
- Antibiotics for suspected infection
- Chest X-ray if pneumothorax is suspected
- Consideration of pulmonary embolism if there is sudden deterioration or failure to respond to treatment

In addition, if the condition is life-threatening, the following should be considered (de Swiet 1995; Cox & Grady 1999; British Guideline on the Management of Asthma 2003b):

- Magnesium sulphate 1.2–2 g i.v. infusion over 20 minutes
- More frequent nebulised beta2-antagonist (e.g. salbutamol 5 mg every 15–30 minutes or 10 mg continuously hourly)
- Aminophylline 250 mg i.v. over 20 minutes, or salbutamol or terbutaline 250 µg over 10 minutes. NB aminophylline should not be used if oral theophyllines have been given, and inform the paediatrician if it is given before delivery as it may cause neonatal irritability and apnoea
- Intubation
- Termination of pregnancy may be suggested if the condition fails to improve

Cystic fibrosis

Cystic fibrosis (CF) is an autosomal recessive inherited condition caused by abnormalities to genes on the long arm of chromosome 7 (Edenborough 2001). It has an incidence of approximately 1:2000 live births and, with improved care in childhood, more women are surviving to childbearing age (de Swiet 1999). Although CF is associated with a reduction in female fertility, this is minimal when overall health is good (Edenborough 2001; Gillet et al. 2002).

CF is a multisystem disease characterised by dysfunction of all exocrine glands with production of thickened and desiccated secretions (de Swiet 1999; Edenborough 2001; Nelson-Piercy 2002). The lungs are usually the most severely affected, leading to recurrent pneumonia, bronchitis and bronchospasm. Progressive lung destruction may result in respiratory failure.

Over 90% of all people with CF have pancreatic insufficiency, which is associated with malabsorption and undernourishment; 20% have diabetes; and a further 15% have impaired glucose tolerance, which increases the risk of gestational diabetes (de Swiet 1999; Edenborough 2001; Nelson-Piercy 2002).

Cystic fibrosis and pregnancy

Maternal mortality is significantly increased compared with pregnant women without CF, but risk of death is not increased when compared with non-pregnant women with CF. Most die in early adult life, the median age of death being approximately 30 years (Nelson-Piercy 2002). Factors associated with adverse outcome are moderate to severe lung disease ($FEV_1 < 60\%$ predicted), pulmonary hypertension, cyanosis and oxygen saturation $< 90\%$ (Nelson-Piercy 2002).

The commonest maternal complications are poor weight gain due to additional nutritional demands of the fetoplacental unit; deterioration in lung function, particularly from the mid third trimester, with worsening dyspnoea, exercise tolerance and oxygen saturation; exacerbation of pulmonary infection; and congestive cardiac failure. The main risks for the fetus are intrauterine growth restriction (due to maternal malnutrition and hypoxaemia) and induced preterm birth (de Swiet 1999; Edenborough 2001; Nelson-Piercy 2002).

Care and management

Principles of management are as for hypoxia, outlined above, as well as the following (de Swiet 1999; Nelson-Piercy 2002):

- Care should be at a specialist obstetric unit in conjunction with a CF centre.
- Aggressive control of pulmonary infection.
- Oxygen therapy, bronchodilators and corticosteroids as needed.
- Admission and possible delivery if respiratory condition and/or malnutrition worsen, particularly if there is associated fetal growth restriction. However, de Swiet (1999) suggests that women most at risk of death are those with a good-sized fetus due to the increased demand this places on maternal oxygen and nutrition.
- Parenteral nutrition may be required if malnutrition and emaciation occur.
- Regional analgesia and anaesthesia are preferable to opiate analgesia and general anaesthesia.
- Avoid prolonged pushing and the Valsalva manoeuvre during the second stage due to the increased risk of pneumothorax.

Pneumonia

Pneumonia is a rare complication of pregnancy, with an incidence of less than 1% (de Swiet 1999). However, it is the most frequent cause of fatal non-obstetric infection (Lim et al. 2001) and accounted for three deaths in the current CEMD (Lewis 2004). During pregnancy, alterations in cellular immunity predispose to infection, and anatomical changes such as elevation of the diaphragm and splaying of the ribcage predispose to pneumonia due to decreased ability to clear respiratory secretions (Lim et al. 2001).

Specific risk factors include smoking, anaemia, asthma, corticosteroid use and use of tocolytic agents, due to their association with pulmonary oedema (de Swiet 1995; Lim et al. 2001).

Types of pnuemonia

- Bacterial pneumonia is no more common than in the non-pregnant population. Causative organisms include *Streptococcus pneumoniae* (which accounts for more than 50% of cases), *Haemophilus influenzae, Staphylococcus* and *Legionella*.
- Viral pneumonia is more severe in pregnancy. Causative organisms include influenza A virus and varicella-zoster. Nelson-Piercy (2002) suggests that 10–20% of women who develop chicken pox in pregnancy will develop varicella pneumonia. It is associated with high maternal and fetal mortality, particularly in later pregnancy, possibly due to increased immunosuppression.
- Atypical pneumonia may be due to *Mycoplasma pneumoniae* or *Pneumocystis carinni*. The latter is the most common opportunistic infection in acquired immune deficiency syndrome (Nelson-Piercy 2002).

Clinical features

- Cough (often dry initially) and purulent sputum
- Fever and rigors
- Breathlessness and pleuritic pain
- Purulent sputum

It is important to exclude pulmonary embolism which mimics some of the features of pneumonia (de Swiet 1999).

Investigations

In addition to the investigations for hypoxia, listed above, specific investigations are:

- Chest X-ray
- Sputum culture

Care and management:

The principles of management are as for hypoxia, outlined above, with the addition of adequate hydration (especially if pyrexial) and physiotherapy to clear secretions. Specific aspects of management are:

- Bacterial pneumonia: give appropriate antibiotic therapy.
- Varicella pneumonia: give intravenous acyclovir.
- Non-immune women exposed to varicella in pregnancy should be offered zoster immunoglobulin (ZIG).
- *Pneumocystis carinni* pneumonia (PCP): give high dose trimethoprim-sulphamethoxazole (co-trimoxazole) with or without pentamidine.

Renal disorders

A range of complications can arise in pregnancy that may affect renal function; some occur in usually well women, such as urinary tract infections (asymptomatic bacteriuria, symptomatic bacteriuria, cystitis and pyelonephritis), while others are associated with other conditions such as diabetes, connective tissue disorders and acute or chronic renal failure/chronic renal insufficiency.

Functions of the renal system are:

- Elimination of waste products and toxins, and production of urine.
- Control of blood pressure, water and electrolyte balance.
- Endocrine: production of renin when blood flow and sodium levels fall, leading to vasoconstriction and retention of sodium and water; and production of erythropoietin which stimulates red cell production.

Urinary tract infections

While urinary tact infection is common in pregnancy, Nelson-Piercy (2002) cautions that it should not be assumed to be the cause of abdominal pain until the diagnosis is confirmed or refuted. The commonest urinary tract infection is asymptomatic bacteriuria (affecting 4–7% of pregnant women) which is defined as the persistent bacterial colonisation of the urinary tract in the absence of specific symptoms. This diagnosis is made when a midstream urine (MSU) specimen reveals more than 100 000 colonies of bacteria per millilitre of urine.

Most urinary infections are caused by the bacteria *Escherichia coli*. If left untreated asymptomatic bacteriuria can lead to cystitis (affecting 1% of pregnant women) and, more significantly, pyelonephritis (affecting 1–2% pregnant women), which in turn can lead to critical illness and even maternal death (Lewis 2004). Physiological changes of pregnancy that predispose to ascending infection include the effects of progesterone (reduced peristalsis and kinking of uteters) and pressure on the ureters at the pelvic brim as the uterus enlarges.

Clinical features

Features of cystitis and pyelonephritis are urgency, frequency, dysuria, loin pain, tachycardia, headache and pyrexia. Proteinuria and haematuria may also be present. With pyelonephritis the onset is often acute and the features more severe, possibly including rigors, nausea and vomiting and pyuria. However, diagnosis can be difficult based on the clinical picture – a common differential diagnosis is acute appendicitis.

Investigations

- MSU for culture and sensitivity
- Possibly blood cultures

Complications of pyelonephritis

- Permanent renal damage
- Spontaneous abortion or preterm labour
- Fetal growth restriction
- Sepsis and shock

Care and management

As pyelonephritis is a cause of critical illness the woman will be admitted to hospital. Management includes:

- Antibiotic therapy: usually penicillins or cephalosporins – possibly intravenously initially.
- Measures to reduce pyrexia (e.g. medication, tepid sponging)
- Analgesia (e.g. buscopan) and warmth to reduce pain (and neurogenic shock)
- Antiemetics
- Assessment of renal function: fluid balance
- Increased fluid intake: oral and intravenous
- Blood for haemoglobin, urea and electrolyte levels (Table 4.2).

Table 4.2   Normal values of renal function (Nelson-Piercy 2002).

	Non-pregnant	First trimester	Second trimester	Third trimester
Urea (mmol/L)	2.5–7.5	2.8–4.2	2.5–4.1	2.4–3.8
Creatinine (μmol/L)	65–101	52–68	44–64	55–73
24-hour creatinine clearance	70–100	140–162	139–169	119–139

Following the acute phase, monthly MSU is often recommended for the remainder of pregnancy to detect asymptomatic bacteriuria as antibiotic therapy reduces the risk of pyelonephritis (Smaill 2001). Investigations such as intravenous pyelograms (IVPs) and renal scans may be undertaken 6–10 weeks postnatally to exclude structural abnormalities of the renal tract that predispose to stasis and infection.

Chronic renal disease/chronic renal insufficiency

Chronic renal disease encompasses nephritis, nephrotic syndrome, diabetic nephropathy, connective tissue disorders, polycystic kidney disease and acute and chronic glomerulonephritis. Chronic renal insufficiency may be asymptomatic until the condition worsens – for example when the glomerular filtration rate is less than 25% of normal.

Clinical features

- Proteinuria
- Reduced creatinine clearance and increased urea
- Hypertension and oedema

Diagnosis

Asrat and Nageotte (1999, p. 838) state that "the diagnosis is based on decreased creatinine clearance, increased 24 h urine protein excretion and abnormal microscopic examination of the urine sediment with red blood cells."

Complications

Creatinine is a waste product of metabolism and the degree of renal function is usually determined by plasma creatinine levels. Women with chronic disease but normal or mildly decreased pre-pregnancy renal function (serum creatinine < 125 µmol/L) usually have successful pregnancy outcomes when there is no significant hypertension, proteinuria or overt renal insufficiency. Pregnancy does not usually unfavourably influence the progression of renal disease except for women with more serious renal impairment; they are more likely to have a permanent decline of renal function (Asrat & Nageotte1999; Nelson-Piercy 2002). For women with moderate (> 125 µmol/L) or severe (> 250 µmol/L) serum creatinine levels, pregnancy outcomes are likely to be less favourable and may result in:

- Impaired fertility
- Acceleration of renal disease
- Spontaneous abortion and preterm birth
- Pre-eclampsia
- Polyhydramnios
- Anaemia
- Intrauterine growth restriction

As Williams (2004) states, "pre-existing hypertension, proteinuria and recurrent urinary tract infections (and poor glycaemic control in women with diabetic nephropathy) are all independently but cumulatively detrimental to maternal and fetal outcome."

Care and management

- Ideally, there should be pre-pregnancy assessment of renal function, and advice against pregnancy if renal insufficiency is severe.
- Regular monitoring of renal function by serum urea (blood urea nitrogen, BUN) and creatinine levels, creatinine clearance and 24-hour protein excretion.
- Regular monitoring for development of pre-eclampsia, anaemia and asymptomatic bacteriuria.
- Use of low dose aspirin may be considered in light of an increased risk of pre-eclampsia (Nelson-Piercy 2002).

- Assessment of fetal growth and wellbeing.
- Possible admission for rest (to facilitate renal function).

In situations where women become critically ill, such as when hypertension becomes uncontrollable, pre-eclampsia worsens, renal function decreases and antenatal fetal testing is abnormal, delivery of the baby is indicated (Asrat & Nageotte 1999). In labour, for women with no complications, but with a condition such as pre-eclampsia, care may proceed normally. Epidural anaesthesia is not contraindicated but fluid administration must be carefully managed in order to avoid rapid changes in blood pressure or blood volume (Asrat & Nageotte 1999). Careful monitoring of fluid balance is vital, using appropriate urinary collection and recording methods. Also central venous pressure measurements may be required as "injudicious fluid replacement readily leads to pulmonary oedema, a major cause of maternal death" (Williams 2004, p. 166).

Acute renal failure

Acute renal failure is a rare complication of pregnancy affecting less than 0.005% of pregnancies. It is characterised by an unpredictable, sudden and marked decrease in glomerular filtration, as a result of reduced renal blood flow which may be due to:

- Hypovolaemic shock following placental abruption, placenta praevia, uterine rupture or operative trauma.
- Endotoxic shock (chorioamnionitis, pyelonephritis, puerperal sepsis, poisoning).
- Urinary obstruction (polyhydramnios and damage to ureters) (Gilbert & Harman 2003).
- Pre-eclampsia, particularly the HELLP syndrome ((*h*aemolysis, *e*levated *l*iver *e*nzymes, *l*ow *p*latelets; see Chapter 6).
- Mismatched blood transfusion (agglutination of red blood cells).

Tubular cell damage results in the inability of the kidneys to excrete creatinine and urea, leading to acidosis. Accurate measurements of glomerular filtration is difficult in acute situations so indirect measures are used, namely rising serum urea and creatinine levels and a decrease in urinary output to less than 400 ml in 24 hours (Davison & Baylis 1995).

Care and management

The management of acute renal failure is determined by the underlying cause, but in all situations, especially in pre-eclampsia, appropriate fluid management is essential in order to maintain circulating volume and blood pressure while avoiding fluid overload and resultant pulmonary oedema. Hourly measurements of central venous pressure, use of a urinary catheter and accurate measurements of fluid intake and output are essential.

Depending on severity, the condition may resolve completely or result in permanent renal damage requiring dialysis and transplant. See Chapter 8 for specific management of various causes of shock.

Hepatic disorders

Liver disease occurs in less than 1% of pregnancies (Sillender 2002), but a variety of acute and chronic disorders may disrupt the complex functioning of the liver and precipitate critical illness.

The functions of the liver are (Sillender 2002):

- *Transformation* of insoluble compounds into soluble forms that can be excreted by the kidneys (e.g. drugs, toxins, unconjugated bilirubin).
- *Excretion* of cholesterol and conjugated bilirubin.
- *Synthesis* of plasma proteins, such as albumin, coagulation factors, transferrin and specific binding proteins, including thyroid-binding globulin.
- *Metabolism* of amino acids, carbohydrates and lipids.

Investigations

Investigations for suspected liver dysfunction include:

- Ultrasonography
- Computed tomography (CT or CAT scan)
- Magnetic resonance cholangiopancreatography (MRCP)
- Endoscopic retrograde cholangiopancreatography (ERCP) – this is regarded as safe in pregnancy (Sillender 2002)
- Liver biopsy
- Serum liver function tests (LFTs)

Serum liver function tests

- *Liver enzymes.* Apart from alkaline phosphatase, liver enzyme levels fall during pregnancy (Ramsay et al. 2000; Nelson-Piercy 2002). Elevated levels occur when cellular damage allows enzymes to leak out of cells.
  - Aspartate (or aspartamine) transaminase (or aminotransferase) (AST): this is not a specific test for liver function as it is also found in the heart, muscle, kidney, pancreas and red blood cells (Sillender 2002).
  - Alanine transaminase (or aminotransferase) (ALT): this is a relatively specific test for liver function as it is only present in low levels in other tissues (McKay 1999).
  - Alkaline phosphatase: this is not a specific test for liver function as it is found in most tissues. Levels increase by 2–4 times during pregnancy, mainly due to placental production and increased bone production (Ramsay et al. 2000; Sillender 2002) and increase further when there is liver damage, particularly when the drainage of bile is blocked (McKay 1999).
  - Gamma glutamyl transferase (or transpeptidase) (GGT or GGTP): elevated levels are a more specific indication of liver damage.
- *Albumin.* Levels fall by 10–60% in pregnancy due to increased blood volume (Sillender 2002). Hepatic disorders result in reduced synthesis of albumin, but

Table 4.3   Liver function tests (Cox & Grady 1999; Nelson-Piercy 2002).

	Non-pregnant	Pregnant	First trimester	Second trimester	Third trimester
AST (iu/L)	5–40	10–40	10–28	11–29	11–30
ALT (iu/L)	0–40	6–35			
Alkaline phosphatase (iu/L)	30–200	90–600	32–100	43–135	133–418
Gamma-glutamyl transpeptidase (iu/L)	11–50		5–37	5–43	3–41
Albumin (g/L)	35–50	25–43			
Bilirubin (µmol/L)	0–20	4–20	4–16	3–13	3–14
Bile acids (µmol/L)	0–14	0–14			

levels are also reduced in conditions associated with proteinuria. Low albumin occurs in chronic rather than acute liver disease, as it takes at least 10 days for levels to fall significantly (Beckingham & Ryder 2001; Sillender 2002).

- *Bilirubin.* There is little change in pregnancy, but levels are elevated when there is increased destruction of red blood cells or reduced removal of bilirubin from the blood stream, such as with cholestasis and biliary tract obstuction (Nelson-Piercy 2002; Sillender 2002). Jaundice is apparent when levels exceed 40 µmol/L and concentrations of > 100 µmol/L require emergency referral (Beckingham & Ryder 2001).
- *Serum bile acids.* Changes in bile acid metabolism and excretion due to oestrogen and progesterone lead to a rise towards term (Ramsay et al. 2000).
- *Clotting factors.* Most are synthesised by the liver, and some require the presence of vitamin K. Levels of factors I (fibrinogen), VII, VIII and X increase as early as the end of the first trimester of pregnancy (Rankin 2005b) while factor XI falls (Ramsay et al. 2000). Obstructive and parenchymal liver disease are associated with coagulopathy because of reduced production of clotting factors and because lowered excretion of bile leads to reduced absorption of fat-soluble vitamin K (Sillender 2002).
- *Blood glucose.* Hypoglycaemia can be severe in fulminant liver disease due to the function of the liver in regulating blood sugar levels by glycogenolysis and gluconeogenesis (Nelson-Piercy 2002).

Table 4.3 shows the values for liver function tests. Note that any interpretation of results must be in the context of the overall clinical picture as specific values will vary according to the methods used in individual laboratories (Ramsay et al. 2000).

Liver disease

Liver disease may be chronic or acute, and whatever the cause it may result in:

- *Hepatic encephalopathy.* This is a reversible state of impaired cognitive function characterised by drowsiness, monotonous speech, tremor, muscular inco-ordination, hypo- or hyperactive reflexes, and possibly a characteristic odour of the breath (fetor hepaticus). Management includes identifying and treating the precipitating factors, emptying the bowels of blood, protein and stool, correcting the electrolyte imbalance and maintaining hydration. Liver transplant may be considered (Kreige & Beckingham 2001).
- *Hepatorenal syndrome.* This is an acute oliguric renal failure associated with intense intrarenal vasoconstriction. The diagnosis is one of exclusion of other causes of renal failure and prognosis is poor, with liver transplant being the only effective treatment (Kreige & Beckingham 2001).

Chronic liver disease

Chronic liver disease may be due to primary biliary cirrhosis or chronic hepatitis B or C infection and is associated with subfertility, spontaneous abortion, preterm labour and stillbirth, but the progress of pregnancy may be uncomplicated (Sillender 2002).

Acute liver disease

Non-obstetric causes of acute liver disease predominate in the first trimester of pregnancy and include acute viral hepatitis, immunological hepatitis, gallstones and deliberate or accidental drug overdose (e.g. paracetamol, aspirin and other NSAIDs, methyldopa, phenothiazines and sodium valproate).

The progress of *acute viral hepatitis* is generally not affected by pregnancy, except when it is due to hepatitis E (the enteric form of non-A, non-B hepatitis) or disseminated herpes simplex virus (HSV). Hepatitis E is associated with an increased incidence of hepatic encephalopathy and fulminant hepatic failure, especially during the third trimester (Nelson-Piercy 2002). Disseminated HSV is rare and generally due to primary HSV type 2 infection. Features are fever, abdominal pain and marked elevation of AST and ALT. There may be prolongation of prothrombin time, jaundice, pneumonitis or encephalitis (Nelson-Piercy 2002). Sillender (2002) suggests mortality is up to 50% in the absence of prompt antiviral therapy.

Gallstone formation is increased from 2.5 to 11% during pregnancy due to the changed composition of bile and slower emptying of the gall bladder (Nelson-Piercy 2002). However, acute cholestasis, characterised by colicky pain in the right upper quadrant, fever, jaundice, nausea, pale stools and dark urine, is found in only 0.1% of pregnant women (Nelson-Piercy 2002). In 75%, symptoms resolve with conservative management comprising withdrawal of oral intake, nasogastric aspiration, intravenous fluids, analgesics and antibiotics. A small number may require emergency cholecystectomy, which is relatively safe in the first and second trimesters of pregnancy, but difficult during the third trimester due to altered anatomy. Mortality is high if there is associated pancreatitis (Sillender 2002).

Obstetric causes of acute liver disease that may result in critical illness include hyperemesis gravidarum, intrahepatic cholestasis of pregnancy and acute fatty liver of pregnancy. Pre-eclampsia and HELLP syndrome are covered in Chapter 6.

Hyperemesis gravidarum

Hyperemesis gravidarum is a condition in which continuous, severe vomiting commences in the first trimester of pregnancy. It persists beyond 20 weeks in only a minority (Nelson-Piercy 2002). It results from a combination of hormonal, mechanical, psychological and social factors, with specific risk factors being over 25 years of age, obesity, a multiple or molar pregnancy, non-tolerance of oral contraception and social difficulties.

The incidence is 0.1–1% (Nelson-Piercy 2002) with a 50% risk of recurrence in subsequent pregnancies (Walters 1999).

Clinical features

Clinical features include dehydration, electrolyte disturbance, malnutrition, vitamin deficiency, weight loss and ketosis, and possible muscle wasting and ptyalism.

Transient hyperthyroidism occurs in 50% (Sillender 2002), possibly because human chorionic gonadotrophin acts on the TSH (thyroid-stimulating hormone) receptor, resulting in raised free T4 and/or suppressed TSH (Hill et al. 2002; Nelson-Piercy 2002). Assessing thyroid function in all women with hyperemesis (Chan 1999) or those with clinical features of thyrotoxicosis (Tan et al. 2002) enables antithyroid medication to commence. This can lead to rapid control of vomiting, and thus prevention of the complications that lead to critical illness.

Potential complications that may lead to critical illness include:

- Dehydration: this is indicated by raised haematocrit, postural hypotension and tachycardia, and may be severe enough to cause acute renal failure (Hill et al. 2002).
- Liver dysfunction: this occurs in 50%, and is indicated by raised AST and ALT in the region of 50–200 iu/L (Nelson-Piercy 2002) and raised bilirubin (Sillender 2002), although jaundice is uncommon (Nelson-Piercy 2002).
- Coagulopathy: this is secondary to vitamin K deficiency due to inadequate uptake and absorption (Robinson et al. 1998).
- Deficiency of cyanocobalamin (vitamin B_{12}) and pyridoxine (vitamin B_6), leading to anaemia and peripheral neuropathy.
- Deficiency of thiamine (vitamin B_1) leading to Wernike's encephalopathy. Features are diplopia, abnormal ocular movements, ataxia, confusion and coma (Nelson-Piercy 2002). The mortality rate is 10–20% (Spruill & Kuller 2002) and up to 50% may have persistent neurological deficits such as retrograde amnesia and confabulation (Korsakoff psychosis). Fetal loss is 40% (Nelson-Piercy 2002). Diagnosis is confirmed by low levels of red cell transketolase, a thiamine-dependent enzyme (Nelson-Piercy 2002).
- Hyponatraemia (i.e. plasma sodium < 120 mmol/L): this causes lethargy, seizures and respiratory arrest. Severe hyponatraemia and its rapid reversal may precipitate central pontine myelinolysis, which causes pyramidal tract signs, spastic quadraparesis, pseudobulbar palsy and impaired consciousness (Nelson-Piercy 2002).

- Aspiration of vomit, and possible Mendelson's syndrome.
- Mallory–Weiss tears of the oesophagus, and haematemasis, following prolonged vomiting.
- Thromboembolism, due to a combination of dehydration and bed rest.

Psychological factors, a possible cause of hyperemesis, may also result from the condition, and Nelson-Piercy (2002) suggests that requests for termination may indicate the degree of psychological morbidity caused by hyperemesis rather than being an indication that the pregnancy was not wanted.

Fetal effects of hyperemesis, particularly when there is malnutrition and excessive weight loss, are low birth weight, preterm delivery and fetal malformations, although spontaneous abortion is about 50% less than average (Walters 1999; Hill et al. 2002; Nelson-Piercy 2002; Sillender 2002).

Investigations

- Urea and electrolyte levels
- Liver function tests
- Thyroid function tests
- Haemoglobin and haematocrit
- Urinalysis (for ketones)
- Maternal weight
- Ultrasonography, to confirm gestation and multiple or molar pregnancy

Care and management:

A biopsychosocial approach should be taken.

- Admission for observation and treatment. This in itself may lead to rapid improvement due to removal from a stressful home environment (Nelson-Piercy 2002).
- Social and emotional support (Sillender 2002).
- Basic care, including oral and pressure area care, with respect for privacy and dignity.
- Early intravenous hydration with normal saline (sodium chloride 0.9%) or Hartmann's solution, with added potassium chloride as necessary, to correct dehydration and electrolyte imbalance.
- Dextrose-containing fluids are avoided as they may precipitate Wernicke's encephalopathy and do not correct hyponatraemia (Nelson-Piercy 2002).
- Fluid intake–output chart.
- Antiemetics administered on a regular basis rather than 'as required' – e.g. chlorpromazine, prochlorperazine, promethazine, cyclizine, metoclopramide or domperidone (Nelson-Piercy 2002).
- Parenteral nutrition via a central venous catheter (see Chapter 10) if rehydration and antiemetic therapy fails, or maternal weight loss exceeds 10%, which is associated with decreased birth weight (Van de Ven 1997). Complications are due to both catheter insertion and the hyperosmolar infusate, and include infection, metabolic complications, phlebitis and thrombosis.

Thiamine supplementation is mandatory due to the use of high concentrations of glucose.

- Continuous nasogastric enteral feeding (with regular aspiration of the stomach to prevent gastric retention and aspiration) is an alternative to parenteral nutrition. A small study by Hsu et al. (1996) found it to be less costly, less invasive and easier to administer.
- Thiamine supplementation to prevent Wernicke's encephalopathy may be advised for all women with hyperemesis (Tesfaye et al. 1998; Nelson-Piercy 2002) or only when vomiting persists for 3–4 weeks (Spruill & Kuller 2002). The intravenous regime is 100 mg diluted in 100 ml of normal saline, infused over 30–60 minutes on a weekly basis. If tablets can be tolerated, the dose is 25–50 mg three times daily (Nelson-Piercy 2002).
- Histamine 2 receptor blockers (e.g. ranitidine or cimetidine) if dyspeptic symptoms accompany vomiting (Nelson-Piercy 2002).
- Short courses of high dose steroids may be tried if other courses of treatment are ineffective – e.g. prednisolone 40–50 mg orally daily in divided doses or hydrocortisone 100 mg intravenously twice daily (Nelson-Piercy 2002; Sillender 2002).
- If all else fails and the mother's life or long-term health is threatened, termination of pregnancy may be suggested as it is the only definitive cure (Nelson-Piercy 2002).

Intrahepatic cholestasis of pregnancy (obstetric cholestasis)

Intrahepatic cholestasis of pregnancy (ICP) is an idiopathic condition that usually presents in the third trimester of pregnancy and resolves within a week of delivery, although it may occur as early as the first trimester (Walters 1999). Production of bile by the liver and flow of bile in the intestine are impaired, resulting in an accumulation of bile acids (which aid the digestion, absorption and excretion of fats) and bilirubin, which spill into the blood stream.

The aetiology of ICP is multifactorial involving geographical, environmental, genetic and hormonal factors. Liver dysfunction occurs in women with a genetic predisposition to sensitivity to raised oestrogen levels.

The incidence in the UK is 0.5–1% (Burroughs, cited by Coombes 2000) with a recurrence rate of up to 90% (Nelson-Piercy 2002), the onset being at a similar or earlier gestation. The highest incidence in Europe is in Scandinavia (2%), while up to 22% of pregnancies are affected in Bolivia and Chile (Nelson-Piercy 2002; Sillender 2002).

Incidence is increased with a multiple pregnancy, and in women who are hepatitis C positive or who have a history of gallstones (Locatelli et al. 1999; Walters 1999).

Clinical features

The most characteristic feature is diffuse, intractable itching, possibly due to raised bile salts, which tends to be worse at night and is particularly on the palms of the hands and soles of the feet. There is no rash but scratching stigmata may be present. Most women have dark urine and pale, fatty stools (steatorrhoea) and there may be nausea, vomiting or upper abdominal pain preceding the itching, and increased sweating (Walters 1999). Jaundice is present in approximately 20% (Sillender 2002) representing a more severe manifestation of the condition (Walters 1999; Milkiewicz et al. 2002).

Investigations

Diagnosis is mainly one of exclusion based on the clinical picture and serum liver function tests. Hepatitis serology, ultrasonography and autoantibody screen may be undertaken to exclude conditions such as hepatitis, gallstones and cirrhosis (Walters 1999), although these conditions may coexist with ICP.

Serum bile acids are generally 5–100 times higher than normal (Walters 1999; Nelson-Piercy 2002). More moderate rises are likely in alkaline phosphatase, GGT, AST and ALT. For example, raised AST and ALT levels are present in 60%, and may be up to four times normal levels (Sillender 2002), and GGT is raised in about 20% (Nelson-Piercy 2002). Approximately 25% will have raised serum bilirubin, although this is rarely greater than 80 μmol/L (Sillender 2002).

Complications

ICP is not inherently a life-threatening condition for the woman, although severe morbidity may result from the intense itching. However, critical illness may result from malabsorption of fat and fat-soluble vitamins, leading to nutritional deficiency and hypoprothrombinaemia. Reduced absorption of fat-soluble vitamin K is associated with a 10–22% risk of obstetric haemorrhage (Walters 1999; Sillender 2002).

ICP has more serious implications for the fetus as increased levels of bile salts are associated with increases in prostaglandin, vasoconstriction and stimulation of the fetal bowel. The stillbirth rate is up to 2% (Milkiewicz et al. 2002), the risk increasing towards term but not correlating with maternal symptoms or transaminase levels (Nelson-Piercy 2002). Overall, perinatal mortality may be up to 3% (Sillender 2002) due to low birth weight, preterm delivery (in up to 60%), fetal distress and meconium-stained liquor in labour (in up to 33%) or anoxia (Milkiewicz et al. 2002; Burrows et al. 2005).

Care and management

- Assessment of fetal growth and wellbeing.
- Elective delivery at 37–40 weeks' gestation (Sillender 2002).
- Drugs to reduce bile acid levels (e.g. activated charcoal, guar gum and ursodeoxycholic acid 1000–1500 mg daily in 2–3 divided doses, either alone or in combination with S-adenosylmethionine) may help relieve pruritis (Nicastri et al. 1998) although a Cochrane review of nine randomised, controlled trials concluded that there is insufficient evidence to recommend their use (Burrows et al. 2005).

- Oral dexamethasone 12 mg daily may help reduce bile and oestrogen production (Nelson-Piercy 2002).
- The use of antihistamines such as chlorpheniramine (Piriton) 4 mg tds or promethazine (Phenergan) 25 mg at night is debatable. Sillender (2002) states that they are not beneficial, although Walters (1999) suggests they may allow sleep and brief respite, and they are recommended by Nelson-Piercy (2002). Measures such as cool bathing and application of calamine lotion may also help.
- Vitamin K 10 mg orally per day, to reduce the risk of obstetric haemorrhage, either from 36 weeks' gestation (Walters 1999) or 32 weeks in view of possible preterm delivery (Nelson-Piercy 2002).

Acute fatty liver of pregnancy

Acute fatty liver (AFL) of pregnancy is a rare metabolic disorder that occurs mainly in the third trimester, although cases have been reported as early as 23 weeks (Suzuki et al. 2001). Its onset never occurs after delivery (Bird 1997). Aetiology is unknown although it may be an abnormal reaction to the normal hormonal changes of pregnancy (Brooks et al. 2002), and incidence is increased with obesity, a male fetus, multiple pregnancy and first pregnancy (Nelson-Piercy 2002). It has high mortality associated with acute liver failure and coagulopathy, and is very difficult to prevent or treat (Lewis 2004). Thus AFL is one of the first conditions to be studied by the UK Obstetric Surveillance System (UKOSS), an initiative to gather information about a variety of uncommon disorders of pregnancy which was launched in February 2005 with the aim of developing knowledge on prevention and management of rare conditions (Knight et al. 2005).

The incidence rate is 1:9000 to 1:13 000 pregnancies, with maternal and perinatal mortality rates being 10–20% and 20–30%, respectively (Nelson-Piercy 2002). There is a recurrence risk of 20% (Walters 1999).

Clinical features

Although there is overlap with clinical features of HELLP syndrome, the underlying physiopathology is different (Bird 1997). Histologically, in HELLP syndrome there is necrosis which is predominantly periportal, whereas in AFL the characteristic change is fatty infiltration of hepatocytes mainly in the central zone (Fraser & Caunt 1996; Nelson-Piercy 2002).

There is gradual onset of nausea, anorexia and malaise. Other features include epigastric pain, vomiting, hypertension, proteinuria, oedema, ascites, elevated liver enzymes, jaundice (although bilirubin levels rarely exceed 167 µmol/L (Sillender 2002)), hyperuricaemia and disseminated intravascular coagulopathy (DIC). However, in AFL, hypertension and proteinuria tend to be milder than in HELLP syndrome, while liver enzymes tend to be more elevated, hyperuricaemia more marked and DIC more severe. Furthermore, severe hypoglycaemia is more common with AFL, although hypoglycaemia is not invariably present with either condition.

Investigations

Diagnosis is based on clinical features as there is no specific diagnostic test (Brooks et al. 2002). Fatty infiltration may be apparent on ultrasound, CT scan or magnetic resonance imaging (MRI) studies, but liver biopsy is often contraindicated due to severe coagulopathy (Walters 1999). It is also a difficult procedure to perform during pregnancy.

Complications

Renal impairment and fulminant liver failure with hepatic encephalopathy may develop. These are associated with poor outcome, with coagulopathy being the main cause of morbidity and mortality. However, women who survive the initial episode generally experience complete recovery, with liver function returning to normal 7–9 days after delivery (Brooks et al. 2002; Nelson-Piercy 2002). Thus Castro et al. (1999) suggest that liver transplant is not indicated as AFL is due to functional failure rather than a destructive cause of hepatic insufficiency.

Care and management

As the cause of AFL is unknown, management is supportive therapy.

- Early recognition and prompt delivery following correction of coagulopathy (see Chapter 7) and hypoglycaemia improves maternal and fetal outcomes (Brooks et al. 2002).
- Intravenous dextrose is essential to avoid rapid onset of hypoglycaemic coma and death (Castro et al. 1999).
- Monitor glucose levels until normal liver function returns (Castro et al. 1999).
- Referral should be made to a specialist liver unit in the event of fulminant hepatic failure and encephalopathy (Lewis 2001).
- Pain relief is challenging as epidural analgesia may be contraindicated in the presence of coagulopathy and narcotics may worsen hepatic encephalopathy (Walters 1999).
- Avoid episiotomy; perineal repair should be done by experienced personnel as vulval and perineal haematomas may develop (Walters 1999).
- There is no consensus about the mode of delivery – caesarean section may be advantageous for the baby but vaginal delivery is generally preferable for the mother due to the bleeding tendency (Walters 1999). In the event of caesarean section, wound drains should be inserted in anticipation of problems with haemostasis.
- Be alert to postpartum haemorrhage.

Diabetes mellitus

Diabetes is a condition affecting the metabolism of carbohydrate, fat and protein, which occurs either because of inadequate insulin production or the presence of factors that oppose the action of insulin.

In *Type 1 diabetes* there is total or near total lack of insulin production. The onset is usually acute, under the age of 25 and insulin therapy is required.

Type 2 diabetes usually has a more gradual onset in the older age group and occurs if there is reduced secretion of, or increased resistance to, insulin. Control is generally by diet or oral hypoglycaemic agents. However, the incidence of Type 2 diabetes in the under 25 age group is increasing in association with the increase in childhood obesity. It is more prevalent in women and typically has an onset at puberty. With Type 2 diabetes there is usually sufficient insulin for some glucose to be used and breakdown of fat and ketosis is rare.

Type 2 diabetes in the younger age group is often confused with *maturity-onset diabetes of the young* (MODY), which is due to a mutation of one gene from a group of at least six, resulting in beta-cell dysfunction or poor recognition of hyperglycaemia (Diabetes UK 2003). It is not normally associated with insulin dependence initially or ketoacidosis, but insulin dependence may occur due to ageing and during pregnancy (Dalton & Shepherd 2004; Ehtisham et al. 2004).

Incidence

The incidence of Type 1 and Type 2 diabetes is 0.5 and 2%, respectively (Nelson-Piercy 2002), with MODY accounting for 1–2% of people with diabetes (Dalton & Shepherd 2004).

Physiological changes of pregnancy

There is a tendency for hypoglycaemia to occur in the first trimester and hyper-glycaemia in the second and third trimesters.

During the first trimester, oestrogen and progesterone cause beta-cell hyper-plasia and increased insulin secretion (Landon & Gabbe 1999) at a time when insulin requirements are likely to be reduced due to haemodilution (Jordan 2002). Nausea and vomiting may also interfere with carbohydrate intake and, further-more, there is relative hypoglycaemic unawareness (Nelson-Piercy 2002).

As pregnancy progresses, glucose tolerance decreases, largely due to the anti-insulin action of hormones secreted by the placenta, especially placental lactogen, glucagons and cortisol (Nelson-Piercy 2002). Furthermore, progesterone decreases gastrointestinal motility resulting in increased absorption of carbohydrates, thereby promoting hyperglycaemia (Kamalakannan et al. 2003). These physio-logical changes lead to doubling of insulin production by the end of the third trimester and increased needs for insulin in women with impaired carbohydrate metabolism (Nelson-Piercy 2002).

Effect of diabetes on pregnancy

There is an increased risk of miscarriage, pre-eclampsia (particularly if there is pre-existing hypertension or renal disease) and infection, especially vaginal candidasis and urinary tract, respiratory, uterine and wound infections. Fetal risks are increased mainly as a result of maternal hyperglycaemia, which may result in congenital anomalies, sudden unexplained intrauterine death, macrosomia (and shoulder dystocia), polycythaemia and respiratory distress syndrome (Nelson-Piercy 2002).

Critical illness

Critical illness associated with childbearing may occur due to deterioration of micro- and macrovascular function, which is linked to the duration of the disease and with the level of control, or development of hyper- or hypoglycaemia, both of which are potentially life threatening.

Deterioration of vascular function

Blood vessels are damaged by prolonged exposure to hyperglycaemia.

- Atheroma and arteriosclerosis in large blood vessels cause cardiovascular disease, which increases the risk of stroke and myocardial infarction (Nelson-Piercy 2002). Mortality rates exceed 50% in pregnancy if there is a history of myocardial infarction (Landon & Gabbe 1999).
- Nephropathy is present in 5% of women with Type 1 diabetes (Stables 2005a). There may be severe oedema, related to proteinuria and hypoalbuminaemia, anaemia, increased risk of pre-eclampsia and fetal growth restriction (Landon & Gabbe 1999). Renal function may deteriorate during pregnancy, particularly if pre-pregnancy impairment was moderate to severe and/or there was hypertension, while deterioration of mild impairment is usually reversed post-natally (Nelson-Piercy 2002). Proteinuria > 3.0 g/24 h and serum creatinine above 1.5 mg/dl are associated with particularly poor outcomes (Landon & Gabbe 1999).
- Diabetic retinopathy progresses two-fold during pregnancy (Landon & Gabbe 1999). It is often associated with the improvement in glycaemic control that occurs in early pregnancy, and with the increased retinal blood flow caused by the increased blood volume of pregnancy (Nelson-Piercy 2002). Laser photocoagulopathy may be required during pregnancy (Landon & Gabbe 1999) and the Valsalva manoeuvre should be avoided during labour because of the risk of haemorrhage (Stables 2005a).
- Neuropathy leading to sensory deficits often deteriorates during pregnancy (Nelson-Piercy 2002).

Diabetic ketoacidosis

Ketoacidosis is a serious complication of diabetes, with a maternal mortality rate of 4–15% and a fetal mortality rate of up to 50%, as fetal death from acidosis may occur before the mother is seriously ill (Jordan 2002; Kamalakannan et al. 2003). However, none of the deaths from diabetes in recent CEMDs have been from ketoacidosis (Lewis 2004).

Ketoacidosis occurs when fats are burned to provide energy when relative or absolute lack of insulin prevents utilisation of glucose. It is rare in pregnancy, possibly due to closer supervision, but is a risk in association with hyperemesis, infection, trauma, tocolytic or cortiocosteriod therapy, or inadequate insulin intake (Cox & Grady 1999; Nelson-Piercy 2002).

Clinical features (Charalambos et al. 1999; Cox & Grady 1999; Stables 2005a)

- Gradual onset of polyuria (osmotic diuresis), polydipsia and drowsiness
- Ketonuria and glycosuria
- Dehydration, tachycardia, postural dizziness and hypotension
- Anorexia, nausea and abdominal pain
- Tachypnoea, deep sighing respirations/hyperventilation and smell of ketones on the breath
- Severe metabolic acidosis
- Coma due to ketosis and electrolyte imbalance. Serum sodium may be low as hyperglycaemia induces water movement from the intracellular to extra-cellular space, thus diluting sodium. However, if the osmotic diuresis causes a greater loss of water as compared to sodium, the result is hypernatraemia. Total body potassium stores are depleted, but serum potassium is usually elevated as metabolic acidosis induces the exchange of extracellular hydrogen for intracellular potassium. However, there may be hypokalaemia if there is high loss via the kidneys or with severe vomiting.

Care and management

Management involves correcting the glucose, fluid and elecrolyte disturbance; identifying and treating the precipitating factors; and resuscitation (Charalambos et al. 1999; Cox & Grady 1999; Jordan 2002; Kamalakannan et al. 2003; Edozien 2004).

- Cardiopulmonary resuscitation.
- Pulse oximetry.
- ECG.
- Catheterise: urinalysis for ketones and measure output every 15 minutes, and specimen for bacteriology.
- Blood for glucose, electrolytes, full blood count, arterial blood gasses and blood cultures.
- Aggressive rehydration with normal saline (0.9%) 1–2 L in the first hour then 300–500 ml/h. Replace with dextrose saline or 0.5% dextrose when blood glucose is 11–12 mmol/L.
- Possible central venous pressure monitoring.

- Insulin infusion to correct hyperglycaemia, which may be continued for up to 24 hours after the urine is free from ketones.
- Correct electrolyte imbalance. Monitor potassium 2-hourly during insulin infusion as insulin causes potassium to enter the cells – many need 20–40 mmol in each litre of saline.
- Stop potassium if there is anuria, potassium level > 6.0 mmol/L or peaked T-waves or widening of the QRS complex on the ECG.
- Sodium levels and acidosis are usually corrected by correcting dehydration and hyperglycaemia.
- Fetal wellbeing: use continuous electronic fetal monitoring. Correction of maternal metabolic abnormalities generally improves the fetal condition.

Hypoglycaemia

Hypoglycaemia is more likely to occur during pregnancy, largely due to tighter control of blood sugar (Walkinshaw 2005). Nelson-Piercy (2002) suggests that for every 1% fall in $HbA1_C$ there is a 33% increase in hypoglycaemic attacks. All of the deaths from diabetes in the current CEMD were associated with hypoglycaemia (Lewis 2004).

Clinical features

Early features of hypoglycaemia are shaking/tremor, palpitations, tachycardia, sweating and pallor, hunger, headache and irritability. Later features include double vision, slurred speech, confusion, aggression, convulsions and coma. Loss of consciousness can be rapid and is immediately life threatening – it is more rapid than with ketoacidosis (Cox & Grady 1999). The features are mainly caused by adrenaline, which is released when blood sugar levels fall.

Care and management (Cox & Grady 1999; Jordan 2002; Edozien 2004)

- Cardiopulmonary resuscitation.
- Pulse oximetry.
- ECG.
- BMstix: treat if glucose < 2.3 mmol/L without waiting for laboratory tests. Check half hourly; level should be 4–9 mmol/L.
- Blood for glucose, electrolyte levels and full blood count.
- Dextrose 50% 50 ml i.v. or 20% glucose 50 ml.
- Glucagon 1 mg i.v. (or i.m. if i.v. is not possible.)
- Start glucose, potassium and insulin regime. May need dextrose 10% infusion for 24–48 hours if long-acting insulin or large doses of insulin have been taken, to prevent hypoglycaemia recurring.
- Fetal wellbeing: use continuous electronic fetal monitoring and anticipate rebound neonatal hypoglycaemia.

Thyroid disease

Thyroid function

The thyroid gland is regulated by the hypothalamus and the pituitary gland through a negative feedback mechanism. The hypothalamus produces thyrotrophin-releasing hormone (TRH) which then stimulates the pituitary gland to produce thyroid-stimulating hormone (TSH). Subsequently, TSH stimulates the thyroid gland to produce two hormones – thyroxine (T3) and tri-iodothyronine (T4). Additionally, sufficient dietary iodine is essential for the production of these hormones.

When thyroid function is abnormal and hormone (T3 and T4) levels are low, there are increased amounts of TSH, as in hypothyroidism. On the other hand, when T3 and T4 levels are high, as in hyperthyroidism, there are decreased amounts of TSH (Ramsey 1995).

Although there are some changes to the structure and function of the thyroid gland in pregnancy, a balanced thyroid function is achieved by the alterations in the metabolism of iodine (Stables 2005b). Pregnant women may have abnormal thyroid function which responds well to treatment. However, others could become critically ill as a result of thyroid disease and midwives need to be aware of the rare but significant complications that may arise.

Hyperthyroidism (thyrotoxicosis)

Hyperthyroidism occurs in 1:500 pregnancies; 95% of cases are due to autoimmune disease (Graves' disease) (Nelson-Piercy 2002). In most instances a diagnosis is made before pregnancy and women will be taking antithyroid medication. For women whose condition is well controlled, or they are in remission from previously treated Graves' disease, maternal and fetal outcomes are usually good. If the thyrotoxicosis is poorly controlled, women may have difficulty in becoming pregnant. Those who do become pregnant have an increased risk of spontaneous abortion, preterm labour, fetal growth restriction and perinatal mortality. Furthermore, women who are poorly treated may develop two rare but serious complications: heart failure and thyroid crisis or 'storm' (Major & Nageotte 1999; Nelson-Piercy 2002).

Care and management

Hyperthyroid disease is managed by drug therapy, the commonest drugs being carbimazole and propylthiouracil. These drugs are safe in pregnancy, except if high doses are used which then may cause fetal hypothyroidism and goitre. Fetal umbilical blood should be tested for thyroid function and, later, cord blood should be tested if the mother is taking high doses of antithyroid drugs and is breast feeding.

Beta-blockers such as propanolol may be used to improve sympathetic symptoms of tachycardia, sweating and tremor (Nelson-Piercy 2002). In pregnancy, aside from taking the appropriate drugs, and during labour there are no special interventions. If there are complications they are more likely to arise in the post-partum period when a thyroid crisis may occur.

Heart failure

Heart failure is rare in untreated hyperthyroidism. In some women, heart failure may be triggered by the increased blood volume of pregnancy, haemorrhage, anaemia, sepsis or pre-eclampsia. The heart failure must be treated immediately and the other conditions need to be managed appropriately (Sheffield & Cunningham 2004).

Thyroid crisis or 'storm'

A thyroid crisis occurs when hyperthyroidism is uncontrolled and is usually triggered by infection or stress, for example following a caesarean section. Although it is rare, Major and Nagoette (1999, p. 710) emphasise that "it is a medical emergency associated with a maternal mortality rate of 25% even with appropriate management."

Clinical features

There is rapid worsening of features of thyrotoxicosis including:

- Tachycardia
- Hyperpyrexia
- Rapid atrial fibrillation, which may lead to heart failure
- Nervousness and restlessness – the woman may appear psychotic
- Vomiting and diarrhoea may occur
- Coma may develop

Care and management

Intensive care is needed during the acute phase.

- Drug therapy involves the use of large doses of propylthiouracil followed by sodium or potassium iodide, or dexamethasone to decrease the release of T3 and T4.
- Beta-blockers (e.g. propanolol), antiarrhythmics (e.g. digoxin) and diuretics to control cardiac features.
- Phenobarbitone (to reduce restlessness and agitation).
- Antipyretics, but avoiding aspirin as it displaces T3 and T4 from thyroid-binding globulin.
- Supportive therapies including intravenous fluid, electrolyte replacement, glucose (for energy) and oxygen therapy.

Hypothyroidism (myxoedema)

Hypothyroidism, usually an autoimmune disorder, is more common than hyper-thyroidism and occurs in 1:100 pregnant women (Nelson-Piercy 2002). Untreated hypothyroidism is likely to result in infertility because an increase in TSH leads to an increase in prolactin, which in turn inhibits ovulation. It is likely, therefore, that most pregnant women who have hypothyroidism will be taking thyroxine medication, for example 0.1–0.2 mg thyroxine daily, and pregnancy outcomes are usually good. The fetus is not at risk as very little thyroxine crosses the placenta; nevertheless umbilical blood is usually tested for thyroid function.

Some clinical features of hypothyroidism are similar to those of pregnancy; these include weight gain, lethargy and tiredness, constipation, dry skin, carpel tunnel syndrome and fluid retention. A diagnosis is made by measurement of T4 which will be below normal values for that trimester (Ramsey 1995). It is important to diagnose hypothyroidism because while there are few effects of pregnancy on hypothyroidism there are some deleterious effects of untreated hypothyroidism on pregnancy, such as anaemia, pre-eclampsia, spontaneous abortion and growth restriction (Nelson-Piercy 2002).

Connective tissue disorders

The main connective tissue disorders that may be associated with critical illness in childbearing are systemic lupus erythematosus (SLE) and antiphospholipid syndrome (APS). Rheumatoid arthritis is the commonest disorder of connective tissue but it tends to go into remission during pregnancy so will not be discussed further as women are unlikely to become critically ill.

Systemic lupus erythematosus

SLE is an autoimmune rheumatic disease in which overproduction of antibodies leads to inflammation of virtually any system of the body. It is more common in women than men (ratio 9:1) and more common in African-Caribbean and Asian people that in Caucasian people (ratio 9:1) (Hay & Snaith 1995; Nelson-Piercy 2002). The incidence is approximately 1:1000 women and, like other autoimmune diseases, SLE is characterised by periods of disease activity ('flares') and remis-sion (Branch & Porter 1999; Nelson-Piercy 2002). The cause of SLE is unknown but involves a genetic predisposition and environmental triggers such as ultraviolet light or viral infections (Nelson-Piercy 2002). SLE is treated with immunosuppres-sive medication such as azathioprine (Imuran) or cyclophosphamide (Endoxana) (St Thomas Lupus Trust 2005).

Clinical features

Clinical features can be variable in severity and presentation (Nelson-Piercy 2002):

- Joint involvement: 90% have arthritis.
- Skin involvement in 80%: malar rash, photosensitivity, Reynaud's syndrome and hair loss.
- Serositis: pleuritis and pericarditis.
- Renal involvement: proteinuria and renal failure.
- Neurological involvement: fatigue, depression and chorea.
- Haematological involvement: anaemia, thrombocytopenia and leukopenia.
- Infection is a major cause of mortality.

Diagnosis

Diagnosis is made based on both the clinical picture and laboratory findings. The erythrocyte sedimentation rate (ESR) is raised and antinuclear antibody (ANA) will be found in 95% of women with SLE.

Complications

For women in remission there is little effect of SLE on pregnancy. However, SLE in pregnancy may become complicated if there is renal involvement, hypertension, antiphospholipid antibodies or disease activity at the time of conception (Nelson-Piercy 2002). The risks are therefore increased for spontaneous abortion, fetal death, preterm delivery, fetal growth restriction, pre-eclampsia and renal failure.

Care and management

During disease flares corticosteroids can be used, although pregnant women taking steroids are at an increased risk of developing gestational diabetes (Nelson-Piercy 2002). Aspirin, NSAIDS and azathioprine may be used safely. One of the most challenging aspects of managing SLE is that is difficult to distinguish between an exacerbation of SLE, involving active nephritis, and pre-eclampsia. In both situations women have proteinuria, hypertension and thrombocytopaenia. Furthermore, the two conditions may be superimposed on one another. Laboratory tests may help to distinguish between the two, such as a rising anti-DNA antibody titre and red blood cells or cellular casts in the urinary sediment (Nelson-Piercy 2002). Renal biopsy is the only definitive method to make the distinction, but this is unlikely to be undertaken in pregnancy.

If a woman becomes more unwell and the fetus is viable, delivery is the most appropriate option as it will address pre-eclampsia, minimise the risk of fetal hypoxia and allow for the administration of drugs to treat a renal flare (Branch & Porter 1999; Nelson-Piercy 2002).

Antiphospholipid syndrome/Hughes' syndrome

APS has similarities to SLE but in APS there is venous or arterial thrombosis ('sticky blood') rather than inflammation. It has an incidence of 1:500 (Hughes

Syndrome Foundation 2005) and approximately 30% of those with SLE also have APS (Hay & Snaith 1995).

Clinical features

Clinical features are mainly due to thrombosis in veins and arteries of all sizes and include the following (Nelson-Piercy 2002; Hughes Syndrome Foundation 2005):

- A lacy, net-like, red rash known as livedo reticularis, particularly over the wrists and knees.
- Thrombocytopaenia and haemolytic anaemia
- Venous leg ulcers
- Cerebral involvement (epilepsy, cerebral infarction, chorea and migraine)
- Heart valve disease, particularly of the mitral valve

Investigations

Diagnosis is made on an individual's history, examination and blood tests. Specialised blood tests reveal anticardiolipin antibodies or lupus anticoagulant – the latter is a misnomer as it is not a test for lupus, nor is it an anticoagulant! Diagnosis is made if the tests are positive on two occasions 6–8 weeks apart as antibodies can be present for short periods in the presence of infection or antibiotic therapy.

Complications

The complications that may arise in pregnancy relate primarily to the hypercoagulable state of both pregnancy and APS; the risk of thrombosis is therefore increased. Women with APS may also become ill when their pregnancy is complicated by recurrent miscarriage, early-onset pre-eclampsia, intrauterine growth restriction, placental abruption and second and third trimester fetal death. These factors are attributed to abnormal placentation and placental failure (Nelson-Piercy 2002).

Care and management

- Anticoagulation with low dose aspirin (if there is no history of thrombosis), heparin or warfarin, aiming for an international normalised ration (INR) of 3 (Sheehan 2003).
- Immunosuprressive therapy may be required.
- Monitor for development of pre-eclampsia, and for fetal wellbeing.

Epilepsy

Epilepsy is a condition of the central nervous system that is characterised by recurrent seizures; most cases are idiopathic and no cause is known. It is the commonest neurological condition to complicate pregnancy and affects about

Table 4.4 Classification and characteristics of seizures.

Classification of seizures	Characteristics of seizure
Tonic-clonic seizures (grand mal)	Occur in 1–2% of women with epilepsy. During tonic phase respiratory muscles contract and impair adequate maternal oxygenation; there is a sudden loss of muscle tone, cyanosis, tonic stiffening and clonic jerking of limbs. Reflex emptying of the bladder and bowel may occur (National Society for Epilepsy 2002). Fetal hypoxia and bradycardia can occur, leading to asphyxia
Status epilepticus	An on-going seizure activity lasting greater than 30 minutes or recurrent seizures without full recovery of consciousness between episodes (Carhuapoma et al. 1999). The risk is low, at about 1% (Nelson-Piercy 2002) but fetal loss rate is approximately 50% (Donaldson 1995)

0.5% of women of childbearing age (Nelson-Piercy 2002). The types of seizure that have potential to cause critical illness are generalised tonic-clonic seizures and status epilepticus, the features of which are outlined in Table 4.4.

In the absence of prolonged seizures, women with epilepsy are not at increased risk for obstetric complications when appropriate care is available throughout pregnancy, labour and in the postnatal period (Royal College of Midwives 1997; Richmond et al. 2004). Most babies will be born without anomalies, especially with appropriate prenatal management including folic acid supplementation (5 mg daily) and the use of single antiepileptic drugs (Royal College of Midwives 1997).

Carhuapoma et al. (1999) suggest that one-third of women will have an increase in frequency of seizures and the remainder will have no change or a decrease. Poor control before pregnancy and poor use of medication is associated with an increased risk of seizures. Physiological changes of pregnancy that may reduce medication to below therapeutic levels are the increased blood volume, increased metabolism, increased serum binding and reduced absorption from the intestines. Furthermore, some women will more frequently experience triggers for seizures such as lack of sleep, hyperventilation and physical or emotional stress during the childbearing period. Carhuapoma et al. (1999, p. 806) conclude that 'as a rule the fewer the number of seizures occurring in the 9 months before conception, the less the risk of worsening epilepsy during pregnancy' and only 1–2% of women with uncontrolled epilepsy will have a tonic-clonic seizure during labour (Royal College of Midwives 1997).

Clinical presentation and investigation

It is rare for a first seizure to occur in pregnancy without obvious cause and usually there is a previous history of idiopathic epilepsy. Differential diagnoses include eclampsia, cerebral tumour, encephalitis, electrolyte imbalance, drug toxicity or withdrawal, and cerebral hypoxia or haemorrhage.

A seizure should be investigated, including the following (Nelson-Piercy 2002):

- Blood pressure, urinalysis, uric acid, platelet count and clotting screen blood film
- Blood glucose, serum calcium, serum sodium and liver function tests
- CT or MRI of the brain, and an electroencephalogram (EEG)

Complications

Complications of seizures mainly relate to the hypoxia caused by ineffective action of the respiration muscles during both the tonic and clonic phases. Regurgitation and inhalation of the stomach contents is another risk, particularly in the immediate post-seizure period of semiconsciousness, which led the CEMD for the triennium 1994–1996 to the recommendation that relatives are taught the use of the recovery position (Department of Health 1998). Postpartum haemorrhage is a potential risk as antiepileptic drugs reduce the level of vitamin K-dependent clotting factors. This risk is reduced by the use of prophylactic vitamin K supplements of 10–20 mg orally daily in the last 4 weeks of pregnancy, which also reduces the risk of haemorrhagic disease of the newborn (Crawford 2002; Nelson-Piercy 2002).

Care and management

Prevention of tonic-clonic seizures and status epilepticus

This is an important principle of care, and includes ensuring that women continue with prescribed medication as the risks of teratogenesis are less than the risks associated with seizures, which may be detrimental to both maternal and fetal wellbeing. Monthly assessment of drug levels is only recommended if seizures increase or for women who have regular seizures (National Institute for Clinical Excellence 2002; Nelson-Piercy 2002). During labour, medication must be taken as usual; intravenous medication may be necessary in labour if vomiting occurs. Midwives have an important role in helping women to identify and avoid trigger factors such as sleep deprivation and stress as mentioned above. Hot steamy environments may also act as a trigger, and three of the nine deaths associated with epilepsy reported in the CEMD for 1997–1999 were due to drowning in the bath – hence the recommendation to bathe only in shallow water with someone else in the house (Lewis 2001). During labour, trigger factors such as bright lights, loud noises and hyperventilation should be minimised. Women need constant attendance and support from midwives, and oxygen and suction apparatus must be available.

Care during and following a seizure

Care and management during and after a tonic-clonic seizure is summarised in Table 4.5, and further measures in the management of status epilepticus are given in Table 4.6. Prompt recognition and action is vital to minimise further complications.

Table 4.5   Care and management during and after a tonic-clonic seizure.

Action	Rationale
Call for help: midwife, obstetrician and paediatrician	Multidisciplinary assistance is required for optimum management
During the seizure: remove nearby objects (e.g. chairs, tables) and do not restrain	To avoid injury
Immediately following seizure: assess airway and breathing. Oxygen via face mask at 6–10 L/min	To maintain maternal (and fetal) oxygenation
Left lateral or recovery position	To maintain airway, and prevent supine hypotension and inhalation of regurgitated stomach contents
Medication such as Diazemuls 5–10 mg i.v.	To prevent further seizures
Maternal vital signs	To assess maternal wellbeing
Continuous cardiotocography	To assess fetal wellbeing There may be transient fetal bradycardia, reduced baseline variability and decelerations for 30 minutes after a seizure (Crawford 2002)

Table 4.6   Management of status epilepticus.

Further measures in treatment of status epilepticus	Interventions
Monitor maternal and fetal condition	Maternal pulse, respiration and blood pressure, fetal heart rate/use of cardiotocography (CTG). A 30-minute CTG should be undertaken if a major convulsion associated with cyanosis occurs (Royal College of Midwives 1997). Pulse oximetry should be used to monitor oxygen saturation
Measures to control seizures	Intravenous anticonvulsant drugs should be administered, e.g. benzodiazepine and phenytoin. If seizures continue despite glucose, oxygen, fluids and anticonvulsants, endotracheal intubation and ventilation may be required (Carhuapoma et al. 1999)
Further investigations	Blood glucose, serum calcium, serum sodium and liver function tests

References

Asrat, T. and Nageotte, M. (1999) Renal disease. In: D. James, P. Steer, C. Weiner and B. Gonik (Eds) *High Risk Pregnancy: Management options*. W.B. Saunders, London.

Beckingham, I. and Ryder, S. (2001) ABC of diseases of liver, pancreas, and biliary system: investigation of liver and biliary disease. *British Medical Journal*, **322**: 33–6.

Bird, J. (1997) Intensive care problems in obstetric patients. *Care of the Critically Ill*, **13** (6): 241–4.

Branch, W. and Porter, F. (1999) Autoimmune disease. In: D. James, P. Steer, C. Weiner and B. Gonik (Eds) *High Risk Pregnancy: Management options*. W.B. Saunders, London.

British Guideline on the Management of Asthma (2003a) Asthma in pregnancy. *Thorax*, **58** (Suppl. 1): i47–i50.

British Guideline on the Management of Asthma (2003b) Management of acute asthma. *Thorax*, **58** (Suppl. 1): i32–i46.

British Medical Association and Royal Pharmaceutical Society of Great Britain (2005) *British National Formulary*, No. 49 (March). British Medical Association and Royal Pharmaceutical Society of Great Britain, London.

Brooks, R., Feller, C. and Mayne, J. (2002) Acute fatty liver of pregnancy: a case report. *Journal of the American Association of Nurse Anesthetists*, **70** (3): 215–17.

Burrows, R., Clavisi, O. and Burrows, E. (2005) Interventions for treating cholestasis in pregnancy. *Cochrane Library*, Issue 1. John Wiley & Sons, Chichester.

Carhuapoma, J., Tomlinson, M. and Levine, S. (1999) Neurological diseases. In: D. James, P. Steer, C. Weiner and B. Gonik (Eds) *High Risk Pregnancy: Management options* W.B. Saunders, London.

Castro, M., Fassett, M., Reynolds, T., Shaw, K. and Goodwin, M. (1999) Reversible peri-partum liver failure: a new perspective on diagnosis, treatment, and cause of acute fatty liver of pregnancy, based on 28 consecutive cases. *American Journal of Obstetrics and Gynecology*, **181** (2): 389–95.

Chan, N. (1999) Thyroid function in hyperemesis gravidarum. *Lancet*, **353** (9171): 2243.

Charalambos, C., Schofield, I. and Malik, R. (1999) Acute diabetic emergencies and their management. *Care of the Critically Ill*, **15** (4): 132–5.

Coleman, M. and Rund, D. (1997) Non-obstetric conditions causing hypoxia during pregnancy: asthma and epilepsy. *American Journal of Obstetrics and Gynecology*, **177** (1): 1–7.

Coombes, J. (2000) Cholestasis in pregnancy: a challenging disorder. *British Journal of Midwifery*, **8** (9): 565–70.

Cox, C. and Grady, K. (1999) *Managing Obstetric Emergencies*. BIOS Scientific Publishers, Oxford.

Crawford, P. (2002) Epilepsy and pregnancy. *MIDIRS Midwifery Digest*, **12** (3): 327–31.

Dalton, J. and Shepherd, M. (2004) Identification of MODY: the implications for Holly. *Journal of Diabetes Nursing*, **8** (1): 19–21.

Davison, J. and Baylis, C. (1995) Renal disease. In: M. de Swiet (Ed.) *Medical Disorders in Obstetric Practice*. Blackwell Science, Oxford.

Department of Health (1998) *Report on Confidential Enquiries into Maternal Deaths in the United Kingdom 1994–1996*. Her Majesty's Stationery Office (HMSO), London.

Diabetes UK (2003) Information: MODY Q & A. www.diabetes.org.uk

Donaldson, J. (1995) Neurological disorders. In: M. de Swiet (Ed.) *Medical Disorders in Obstetric Practice*. Blackwell Science, Oxford.

Edenborough, F. (2001) Women with cystic fibrosis and their potential for reproduction. *Thorax*, **56**: 649–55.

Edozien, L. (2004) The Labour Ward Handbook. London, Royal Society of Medicine.

Ehtisham, S., Hattersley, A., Dunger, D. and Barrett, T. (2004) First UK survey of paediatric type 2 diabetes and MODY. *Archives of Disease in Childhood*, **89**: 526–9.

Fraser, R. and Caunt, A. (1996) The HELLP syndrome. *Care of the Critically Ill*, **12** (6): 188–9.

Gilbert, E. and Harmon, J. (2003) *Manual of High Risk Pregnancy and Delivery*. Mosby, St Louis.

Gillet, D., de Braekeleer, M., Bellis, G., and Durieu, I. (2002) Cystic fibrosis and pregnancy: report from French data (1980–1999). *British Journal of Obstetrics and Gynaecology*, **109**: 912–18.

Hay, E. and Snaith, M. (1995) ABC of rheumatology: systemic lupus erythematosus and lupus-like syndromes. *British Medical Journal*, **310**: 1257–61.

Hill, J., Yost, N. and Wendel, G. (2002) Acute renal failure in association with severe hyperemesis gravidarum. *Obstetrics and Gynecology*, **100** (5), Part 2: 1119–21.

Hsu, J., Clark-Glena, R., Nelson, D. and Kim, C. (1996) Nasogastric enteral feeding in the management of hyperemesis gravidarum. *Obstetrics and Gynecology*, **88** (3): 343–6.

Hughes Syndrome Foundation (2005) What is Hughes syndrome? http://www.hughes-syndrome.org (last accessed 22/12/2005)

Jevon, P. and Raby, M. (2001) *Resuscitation in Pregnancy: A practical approach*. Books for Midwives, Oxford.

Jordan, S. (2002) *Pharmacology for Midwives: The evidence base for safe practice*. Palgrove, Houndmills, UK.

Kamalakannan, D., Baskar, V., Barton, D. and Abdu, T. (2003) Diabetic ketoacidosis in pregnancy. *Postgraduate Medical Journal*, **79**: 454–7.

Knight, M., Kurinczuk, J. and Brocklehurst, P. (2005) UK obstetric surveillance system uncovered. *Midwives*, **8** (1): 38–9.

Knox, A. (2001) Respiratory disease in pregnancy: introduction. *Thorax*, **56**: 324.

Kreige, J. and Beckingham, I. (2001) ABC of diseases of liver, pancreas, and biliary system: portal hypertension – 2. Ascites, encephalopathy, and other conditions. *British Medical Journal*, **322**: 416–18.

Landon, M. and Gabbe, S. (1999) Diabetes in pregnancy. In: D. James, P. Steer, C. Weiner and B. Gonik (Eds) *High Risk Pregnancy: Management options*. W.B. Saunders, London.

Lewis, G. (2001) *Why Mothers Die 1997–1999: The Confidential Enquiries into Maternal Deaths in the United Kingdom*. Royal College of Obstetricians and Gynaecologists (RCOG) Press, London.

Lewis, G. (2004) *Why Mothers Die 2000–2002: Report on Confidential Enquiries into Maternal Deaths in the United Kingdom*. RCOG Press, London.

Lim, W., Macfarlane, J. and Colthorpe, C. (2001) Pneumonia in pregnancy. *Thorax*, **56**: 398–405.

Locatelli, A., Roncaglia, N., Arreghini, A., Bellini, P., Vergani, P. and Ghidini, A. (1999) Hepatitis C infection is associated with a higher incidence of cholestasis in pregnancy. *British Journal of Obstetrics and Gynaecology*, **106**: 498–500.

Major, C. and Nageotte, M. (1999) Thyroid disease. In: D. James, P. Steer, C. Weiner and B. Gonik (Eds) *High Risk Pregnancy: Management options*. W.B. Saunders, London.

McKay, K. (1999) Biochemical and blood tests in midwifery practice (1): pre-eclampsia. *Practising Midwife*, **2** (8): 28–31.

Milkiewicz, P., Elias, E., Williamson, C. and Weaver, J. (2002) Obstetric cholestasis. *British Medical Journal*, **324** (7330): 123–4.

National Institute for Clinical Excellence (2002) The epilepsies: the diagnosis and management of the epilepsies in adults and children in primary and secondary care. www.nice.org.uk

National Society for Epilepsy (2002) *Epilepsy: Information on seizures*. http://www.epilepsynse.org.uk (last accessed 14/11/2005)

Nelson-Piercy, C. (2001) Asthma in pregnancy. *Thorax*, **56**: 325–8.

Nelson-Piercy, C. (2002) *Handbook of Obstetric Medicine*. Martin Dunitz, London.

Nicastri, P., Diaferia, A., Tartagni, M., Loizzi, P. and Fanelli, M. (1998) A randomised placebo-controlled trial of ursodeoxycholic acid and S-adenosylmethionine in the treatment of intrahepatic cholestasis of pregnancy. *British Journal of Obstetrics and Gynaecology*, **105**: 1205–7.

Oakley, C. (1996) Pregnancy and heart disease. *British Journal of Hospital Medicine*, **55** (7): 423–6.

Ramsay, M., James, D., Steer, P., Weiner, C. and Gonik, B. (2000) *Normal Values in Pregnancy*. W.B. Saunders, London.

Ramsey, I. (1995) Thyroid disease. In: M. de Swiet (Ed.) *Medical Disorders in Obstetric Practice*. Blackwell Science, Oxford.

Rankin, J. (2005a) Respiration. In: D. Stables and J. Rankin (Eds) *Physiology in Childbearing*. Elsevier, Edinburgh.

Rankin, J. (2005b) The haematological system – physiology of the blood. In: D. Stables and J. Rankin (Eds) *Physiology in Childbearing*. Elsevier, Edinburgh.

Richmond, J., Krishnamoorthy, P. and Benjamin, A. (2004) Epilepsy and pregnancy: an obstetric perspective. *American Journal of Obstetrics and Gynecology*, **190** (2): 371–9.

Robinson, J., Banerjee, R. and Thiet, M. (1998) Coagulopathy secondary to vitamin K deficiency in hyperemesis gravidarum. *Obstetrics and Gynecology*, **92** (4), Part 2: 673–5.

Royal College of Midwives (1997) *The Care of Women with Epilepsy: Guidelines for midwives*. Royal College of Midwives (RCM), London.

St Thomas Lupus Trust (2005) What is lupus? http://www.lupus.org.uk (last accessed 14/11/2005)

Schatz, M. (1999) Asthma and pregnancy. *Lancet*, **353**: 1202–4.

Sheehan, T. (2003) A guide to Hughes syndrome. *Nursing Times*, **26 Aug**: 24–5.

Sheffield, J. and Cunningham, F. (2004) Thyrotoxicosis and heart failure that complicate pregnancy. *American Journal of Obstetrics and Gynecology*, **190** (1): 211–17.

Sillender, M. (2002) The liver and pregnancy. *Care of the Critically Ill*, **18** (6): 181–6.

Siu, S. and Colman, J. (2001) Congenital heart disease: heart disease and pregnancy. *Heart*, **85**: 710–15.

Smaill, F. (2001) Antibiotics foe asymptomatic bacteriuria in pregnancy. *Cochrane Database of Systematic Reviews*, Issue 2. John Wiley & Sons, Chichester.

Spruill, S. and Kuller, J. (2002) Hyperemesis gravidarum complicated by Wernike's encephalopathy. *Obstetrics and Gynecology*, **99** (5), Part 2: 875–7.

Stables, D. (2005a) Diabetes mellitus and other metabolic disorders in pregnancy. In: D. Stables and J. Rankin (Eds) *Physiology in Childbearing*. Elsevier, Edinburgh.

Stables, D. (2005b) The endocrine system. In: D. Stables and J. Rankin (Eds) *Physiology in Childbearing*. Elsevier, Edinburgh.

Suzuki, S., Watanabe, S. and Araki, T. (2001) Acute fatty liver of pregnancy at 23 weeks of gestation. *British Journal of Obstetrics and Gynaecology*, **108**: 223–4.

de Swiet, M. (1995) Diseases of the respiratory system. In: M. de Swiet (Ed.) *Medical Disorders in Obstetric Practice*. Blackwell Science, Oxford.

de Swiet, M. (1998) The respiratory system. In: G. Chamberlain and F. Broughton Pipkin (Eds) *Clinical Physiology in Obstetrics*. Blackwell Science, Oxford.

de Swiet, M. (1999) Respiratory disorders. In: D. James, P. Steer, C. Weiner and B. Gonik (Eds) *High Risk Pregnancy: Management options*. W.B. Saunders, London.

de Swiet, M. (2002) Cardiac disease. In: A. MacLean and J. Neilson (Eds) *Maternal Mortality and Morbidity*. RCOG Press, London.

Tan, J., Loh, K., Yeo, G. and Chee, Y. (2002) Transient hyperthyroidism of hyperemesis gravidarum. *British Journal of Obstetrics and Gynaecology*, **109** (6): 683–8.

Tan, K. and Thomson, N. (2000) Asthma in pregnancy. *American Journal of Medicine*, **109**: 727–33.

Tesfaye, S., Achari, V., Yang, Y., Harding, S., Bowden, A. and Vora, J. (1998) Pregnant, vomiting and going blind. *Lancet*, **352** (9140): 1594.

Tomlinson, M. and Cotton, D. (1999) Cardiac disease. In: D. James, P. Steer, C. Weiner and B. Gonik (Eds) *High Risk Pregnancy: Management options*. W.B. Saunders, London.

Van de Ven (1997) Nasogastric enteral feeding in hyperemesis gravidarum. *Lancet*, **349** (9050): 445–6.

Walkinshaw, S. (2005) Very tight versus tight control for diabetes in pregnancy. *The Cochrane Library*, Issue 1. John Wiley & Sons, Chichester.

Walters, B. (1999) Hepatic and gastrointestinal disease. In: D. James, P. Steer, C. Weiner and B. Gonik (Eds) *High Risk Pregnancy: Management options*. W.B. Saunders, London.

Williams, D. (1999) Pregnancy and the heart. *Hospital Medicine*, **60** (2): 100–104.

Williams, D. (2004) Renal disease in pregnancy. *Current Obstetrics and Gynaecology*, **14** (3): 166–74.

5 Haematological Disorders and the Critically Ill Woman

Priscilla Dike

This chapter is divided into two parts. Part 1 considers critical illness associated with haemoglobinopathies in childbearing, while Part 2 considers critical illness relating to thromboembolism.

Assumed prior knowledge

- Basic understanding of sickle cell disorder and thalassaemia
- Physiological changes in the coagulation system in pregnancy

Part 1: Haemoglobinopathies

Haemoglobinopathies arise when there are alterations in the structure (sickle haemoglobin), quantity (thalassaemia) or function of alpha- or beta-polypeptide chains in the production of haemoglobin. Haemoglobinopathy is a term used to describe any one of a group of hereditary disorders where there is abnormality of haemoglobin, which during deoxygenation of the red blood cells creates shape distortion, thus blocking the microcirculation and causing severe pain and infarction to surrounding tissues (Adams 1996; Rust & Morrison 1996, cited in Hall 2002).

There are four protein chains in normal haemoglobin, which take up shapes that allow for maximum uptake and delivery/release of oxygen into body tissues. Abnormal genes produce abnormal proteins which cannot carry oxygen around the body systems efficiently. Three forms of inherited haemoglobinopathies exist:

- Structural haemoglobin variant, where there is a fault in either the alpha-globin or beta-globin chains
- The thalassaemias, where there is reduced production of either the alpha-globin or beta-globin chains

• Failure to switch from the production of fetal haemoglobin (HbF) to adult haemoglobin (HbA)

Pregnancy in a client with sickle cell disease or thalassaemia major is hazardous for both the mother and the baby. During pregnancy, women with major haemo-globinopathies are susceptible to exacerbations of their disease, and have an over-all increase in fetal and maternal morbidity and mortality. Therefore, adequate pregnancy care involving the efficient collaboration of relevant members of the multidisciplinary team ensures improved pregnancy outcome. Nonetheless, such pregnancies are considered high risk and demand highly skilled management. Two types of haemoglobinopathies are pertinent in pregnancy and childbirth: sickle cell disease and beta-thalassaemia major. Each may be associated with critical illness, and is discussed in relation to its pathophysiology, potential com-plications and management in pregnancy.

Sickle cell disease

Sickle cell disease (SCD) is a family of haemoglobin disorders in which sickle beta-globin is inherited. Many definitions and terms have been used to describe this condition. At times, the nature of the condition is confused in the sophistication of terms of definition. The term *sickle cell anaemia* is restrictive and has a tendency to portray the pathology of the condition, while *sickle cell disease* tends to denote illness and/or infectivity. Even terms such as *sickle cell disorder* are a misrepresentation of the condition as a minor ailment and hence do not make explicit the variable nature of this condition. Presented below is a proposed definition that encapsulates the vital realms of the condition:

> Sickle cell condition is a family of genetically inherited recessive haemoglobin disorders, in which beta-globin (a protein that aids oxygen transportation in the blood) creates sickle-shaped sticky abnormal versions of haemoglobin, which have low lifespan and carry less oxygen and block blood flow thereby causing painful crises, anaemia, tissue/organ damage and stroke.

There have been more than 325 different structural abnormalities of the haemo-globin molecule identified (Rust & Perry 1995) but the homozygous (HBSS) is said to be the most common type (Davies & Oni 1997), while the sickle cell thalassaemia and E thalassaemia remain the 'most important types' (Weatheral 1997a).

Background and prevalence

There are estimated to be 6000–10 000 people with sickle cell conditions in the United Kingdom (Laird et al. 1996; Streetly et al. 1997; Atkin & Ahmad 1998). Davies et al. (2000) estimate that per year, 171 infants are born with sickle cell disease in England alone. Globally, it is estimated that at least 5% of the world popu-lation are carriers for one or other form of the most serious types of sickle cell; among these, one person in four in West Africa is a carrier (Anionwu & Atkin 2001). Over 300 000 infants are born each year with the major sickle cell and thalassaemia syndromes, and a majority die undiagnosed, untreated or under-treated (Anagastiniotis & Modell 1998).

Sickle cell conditions mainly affect people who are descended from families where one or more members originate from parts of the world where falciparum malaria was, or still is, endemic (Anionwu & Atkin 2001). Hence, the sickle gene is spread widely throughout Africa, the Caribbean and the Middle East and Far Mediterranean (including south Italy, northern Greece and southern Turkey), and South East Asia (Sergeant 1992; Davies & Oni 1997; Anionwu & Atkins 2001). Inadvertently it is often controversially portrayed as 'black disease' in an attempt to categorise the client groups affected (Dyson 1999).

Migration of at-risk populations to different parts of the world has caused an unintended redistribution of the condition (Gelbart 1998) to Western countries including Europe and America. Racial intermixing through marriages and repro-ductive relationships invariably increase the prevalence rates of sickle cell among Caucasians. For example, the United States' national screening programmes have noted mean prevalence rates of 242–258 in 100 000 for sickle cell trait in white people and 1.72 in 100 000 for sickle cell disease (Sickle Cell Disease Guideline Panel 1993).

Pathophysiology, complications and management of sickle cell disease

During deoxygenation, molecular changes take place that affect the structure of the red blood cell giving it the classic 'sickle shape'. Repetitive clumping together of red blood corpuscles in serum (agglutination) and synthetic compounds formed through chemical reaction (polymerisation) lead to membrane rigidity and eventually an irreversible 'sickle-shaped' haemoglobin. Cells with sickle haemo-globin have an altered motion through the blood vessels due to their deformed erythrocyte membrane, which causes obstruction, hypoxia and tissue damage to affected areas. The sickle-shaped haemoglobin has an average lifespan of 17 days instead of the usual 120 days. This results in a chronic compensated anaemia that occurs as the rate of erythrocyte destruction exceeds the rate of formation of new red cells by the bone marrow. The clinical problems encountered in pregnancy complicated by sickle cell disease relate to haemolysis, vaso-occlusive crises result-ing from the blockage of blood vessels and increased susceptibility to infection, which in turn lead to the following complications.

Anaemia

The expansion in plasma volume associated with pregnancy results in physio-logical anaemia. For the pregnant mother with a sickle cell condition and chronic anaemia, this physiological process may turn pathological. The role of prophy-lactic transfusion in pregnancy is controversial as haematocrits of 30 and over can be dangerous due to the risk of increased blood viscosity at this level (Kaul et al. 1983). The primary goal of blood transfusion is to reduce the percentage of sickle haemoglobin. Iron supplementation may not be of much benefit, and blood transfusion is only indicated when the mother or fetus is clinically compromised (i.e. in crisis). Folic acid supplementation is needed in pregnancy and can be for a lifetime for people with SCD.

Infection

People with SCD are prone to infections particularly by *Pneumococcus*, *Salmonella* species and *Haemophilus*. Infection with human parvovirus B19, which infects developing erythroblasts, causes cessation of production of mature red cells for a period of 1–2 weeks, so the haemoglobin concentration falls catastrophically (hypoplastic crisis). This could result in congestive cardiac failure. The most common causes of death in the UK are pulmonary complications, cerebrovascular accidents, causes related to infection, acute splenic sequestration and chronic organ failure. Infections should be treated appropriately and promptly.

Infection is more frequent and more serious in pregnant women with sickle cell disease because of a number of secondary phenomena such as *hyposplenism* resulting from red cells causing autosplenectomy. Urinary tract infection (UTI) is a particularly important problem in pregnancy, occurring in 18% of women with SCD compared with 12% of controls, and with 10% suffering from recurring attacks as compared with 4% of controls. This is due to a high frequency of microscopic haematuria associated with renal papillary damage caused by sickling (Davies 1998), and obstruction of urinary flow by the fetal mass (Adams 1996). Increased white cell count (*leucocytosis*) is not indicative of infection as it is commonly raised in crises as a result of tissue damage (Adams 1996). Poor wound healing is not uncommon in people with SCD because of iron and zinc deficiency.

Avoidance (wherever/whenever possible) of infection and factors that predispose to infection is imperative. Prophylalactic antibiotic therapy (*penicillin V prophylaxis*) needs medical review in the presence of an infection. Pneumococcal vaccine should be standard practice in the fight against recurrent infections.

Abortion and stillbirth

These are considerably more common in sickle cell disease and are related to placental infarction/insufficiency. Davies (1998) suggests incidences of 12.5% for mothers with HBSC disease, 17.5% for sickle beta-thalassaemia and 20% in sickle cell disease (HBSS), compared with 10.5% for women without haemoglobinopathy.

Pre-eclampsia

In an observational study by Smith et al. (1996), hypertension was the most common complication during pregnancy for women with SCD. Davies (1998) reported a frequency of 5% for severe cases and 6.5% for mild cases in the UK. Multiple factors such as placental ischaemia and endothelial injury have been indicated as possible causative factors as well as a history of renal diseases, essential hypertension, multiple gestation and diabetes (Repke 1996). According to the Harvard Institute, the blood pressure in non-pregnant individuals with SCD tends to be in a lower range than that of their counterparts without SCD, ranging between 90/50 mmHg to 110/70 mmHg. Therefore, a systolic blood pressure rise of 30 mmHg, or a diastolic rise of 15 mmHg in association with oedema and proteinuria in the second trimester should, as in normal pregnancy care, be treated as pregnancy-induced hypertension.

Cerebrovascular accident (CVA)

There is an increased incidence of sudden CVA (stroke) due to subrachnoid haemorrhage, especially in the young woman (Davies 1998). In some hospitals, limits of about 1 hour of bearing-down efforts are permitted in second stage of labour for women with SCD in order to abate subrachnoid pressure.

Painful vaso-occlusive crises

Painful vaso-occlusive crises complicate 30% of pregnancies in women with SCD. Those particularly affecting bones are caused by the blockage of small blood vessels by sickle cells resulting in oxygen deprivation of the surrounding tissues. Pain, tenderness and swelling occur in the muscles or internal organs. Painful splenic infarcts may occur in women with HBSC disease or a thalassaemia interaction.

Sickling crises in the brain cause *neuropsychological damage* leading to about a five-point decrease in intellectual ability in people with sickle cell disease (Davies & Oni 1997). Sickling in the capillary bed of the lungs results in *'chest syndrome'* where there is thoracic cage bone pain, sometimes with pleuretic pain. Cardiac function may be compromised because of chronic hypoxemia and anaemia. Tachycardia, tachypnoea and cyanosis are initial signs prior to physical signs. If Po_2 falls below 60 mmHg on air, death may ensue. However, emergency exchange transfusion can be life saving. Exchange transfusion is used as an emergency treatment for chest syndrome, central nervous system problems, placental insufficiency, and in some cases of protracted and very severe vaso-occlusive crisis (Davies 1998). Elective exchange transfusion is usually used before a long-term hypertransfusion regime, which is done to maintain haemoglobin between 10 and 14 g/dl. Caution is exercised to avoid alloimmunisation, infection, iron overload and volume fluxes.

Repeated sickling in the bones can lead to avascular necrosis, particularly of the head of the femur and humerus. The weight of the gravid uterus, as well as the softening effects of oestrogen, can worsen this in pregnancy. The resultant static circulation predisposes the mother with SCD to venous thromboembolic problems, especially in the postnatal period.

Vaso-occlusive crisis should be treated routinely with oxygen therapy, hydration, antibiotics, and analgesia until bacteriological cultures are known to be negative. In severe crisis, subcutaneous infusion of morphine with patient-controlled boosts is most effective. Great caution is exercised with long-term use of morphine in pregnancy.

Retinopathy

The proliferative retinopathy (degenerative changes in the retinal blood vessels leading to loss of vision) of sickle cell disease deteriorates rapidly during pregnancy in some women with SCD. Therefore, regular ophthalmic (at least annual) review is desirable. The retinal vessel proliferation can be controlled with laser treatment (Weatheral 1997b).

Renal papillary necrosis

Death of the nipple-shaped protuberance of the kidney (renal papillary necrosis) may cause a drop in haemoglobin and therefore may exacerbate anaemia in women with SCD or sickle trait. Sequestration of red blood cells in the liver predisposes the pregnant woman with SCD to liver dysfunction, which may settle spontaneously following delivery.

Intra-uterine growth restriction

Intra-uterine growth restriction affects 24–65% of infants of SCD mothers (Davies 1998). Prematurity is also common and perinatal mortality is four times that of comparable pregnancies. Fetal wellbeing could be assessed through regular ultrasound assessment of fetal growth parameters and umbilical artery Doppler blood-flow assessment from viability to full term.

Antenatal management

Screening

All women at risk should be screened by haemoglobin electrophoresis at booking. Where sickle cell trait/disease is confirmed in the mother, the partner is offered screening, and subsequent counselling and diagnosis. The objective of preconceptional and antenatal screening is to maximise reproductive choice for parents and to enhance early detection and treatment of infants with SCD in order to reduce childhood morbidity and mortality associated with the condition. Davies et al. (2000) recommend that where there are more than five cases of SCD per 10 000 births or 15:1000 cases of sickle cell trait, it is cost effective to introduce universal screening for neonates. Universal screening is also recommended in areas where the proportion of people at risk is greater than 15% (Streetly 2000). All policies, whether for universal or selective screening must involve a protocol for informing women and their partners of the results and for counselling. Although antenatal screening and counselling are standard practice in the UK, this service is delivered inadequately. An explicit national policy is needed to improve screening service and prenatal diagnosis with on-going national audit (Modell et al. 2000).

Monitoring

Antenatal care should be at frequent intervals in collaboration with the obstetrician and haematologist, with the support of a haemoglobinopathy counsellor and liaison with the paediatrician and obstetric anaesthetist wherever necessary. This should be the gold standard.

Treatment of anaemia

Folic acid is given routinely while iron therapy is avoided. The nature and frequency of pregnancy complications dictate the frequency of blood transfusions. Packed red cells are transfused directly or as exchange transfusions to treat severe anaemia under the direction of the haematologist.

Action plan

An action plan for labour management should be discussed as the pregnancy approaches the thirtieth week and management strategies documented in the case notes.

Management of sickling crises

It is vital to maintain adequate rest, hydration (intravenous fluids 2–4 L/24 h), regular pain relief, vital signs monitoring including oxygen saturation, oxygen therapy via nasal cannula or mask, and antibiotics if required.

Intrapartum management

- As soon as labour is confirmed, the relevant multidisciplinary team should be notified. This will include the midwife, senior obstetrician/anaesthetist, paediatrician and haematologist.
- Aim for routine intrapartum care and vaginal delivery unless clear obstetric reasons dictate otherwise. Where operative delivery becomes necessary, combined spinal anaesthesia is preferred to general anaesthesia, and high dependency care should be implemented.
- Blood should be crossed-matched in readiness for caesarean section, and haemoglobin levels should be checked at least once daily.
- Avoid dehydration, acidosis and infection. Where oral hydration fails, an intravenous infusion of saline at 3 L/24 h is administered with a fluid balance chart to monitor fluid input and output throughout labour. Facial oxygen administration and the use of pulse oximetry to detect hypoxia in the mother is necessary. Some clinicians advocate the use of continuous oxygen therapy throughout labour while others suggest oxygen therapy with dropping Sao_2 levels ($\leq 97\%$). Oxygenation should be continued for at least six hours after operative delivery. The use of prophylactic antibiotics in labour is advocated.
- Avoid hypothermia. The use of electric blankets during surgery and at recovery ensures adequate temperature control. Regular observations of the vital signs, including temperature measurement, are vital.
- Stronger analgesia may be required. Pain relief occurs more slowly with intramuscular injections; consequently intravenous administration of analgesia is preferred. Pethidine should not be used, especially in clients who have suffered seizures or renal impairment (Adams 1996) because pethidine is poorly excreted due to early damage to the kidneys and the consequent poor kidney

function. Morphine is presently the drug of choice because it does not appear to have the same adverse effects as pethidine.

- Continuous cardiotocography is necessary because of increased rates of meconium-stained liquor and fetal distress, which may lead to emergency caesarean section.
- Antiembolic stockings and prophylactic anticoagulation therapy may be necessary to prevent thromboembolic disorders, especially with operative delivery or prolonged immobility.
- Cord blood is sent for neonatal sickle cell testing soon after delivery in some hospital trusts, while others adopt universal blood spot testing. Positive results should be referred and be followed up by the haematologist.

Postnatal care

- Routine postnatal care is advocated for women who had uncomplicated vaginal deliveries, and high dependency care for those who had caesarean section or assisted deliveries.
- Close monitoring of vital signs for signs of crisis.
- Antiembolic therapy should be continued until full mobility is regained.
- Antibiotic therapy is continued to avoid puerperal sepsis.
- Anaemia should be treated.
- Contraceptive advice is vital although IUCDs are avoided due to predisposition to intrauterine infection. Barrier methods are encouraged and progesterone-only pills preferred to combined pills in order to avoid thromboembolic events.
- The mother should be encouraged to stay in hospital for at least the first 24 hours for recuperation and stabilisation of her condition.

Summary of effects of sickle cell disease on pregnancy

- Generally, fertility is reduced.
- Pregnancy may be complicated by chronic ill health, severe anaemia, vaso-occlusive crisis, miscarriage, preterm labour and renal disease.
- There is increased risk of infection, particularly urinary tract infection, pneumonia and puerperal sepsis as well as venous thromboembolisms. Thromboembolic risk is a contributory factor to increased maternal morbidity and mortality, estimated at 2.5%.
- There is increased incidence of intrauterine growth restriction, pre-eclampsia, fetal distress and caesarean section.

Thalassaemia condition

Thalassaemia condition is also an inherited autosomal recessive haemoglobin disorder in which there is partial or no production of either the alpha- or beta-globin

Table 5.1 Types of thalassaemia and their implications.

Thalassaemia type	Description and implications
HbA beta-thalassaemia (β-thal trait)	The inheritance of HbA and Hb beta-thalassaemia from either parent. This results in carrier state of the gene
HbS beta-thalassaemia (sickle beta-thalassaemia)	The inheritance of HbS from one parent and beta-thal from the other parent. The severity of the condition varies according to the amount of globin produced by the beta-globin gene. The condition is almost identical to sickle cell disease. Common among Africans, Caribbeans, Greeks, Italians, Mediterraneans and Turks
HbA2/HbF	Beta-thalassaemia trait with increased presence of fetal haemoglobin. This has a protective measure against sickling crisis
α^+ (α-thal-2: non-deletional α^+-thal)	Refers to a condition when one of the two alpha-globin genes is inactivated due to a defective gene
$\alpha°$ (α-thal-1)	Refers to the condition in which both alpha-globin genes on the same chromosome are deleted
β^+	A condition where some residual beta-globin chain is produced, but less than normal
$\beta°$	Neither gene produces beta-globin chains, but there is production of HbF and alpha-globin excess, which is destroyed by the immune system, leading to ineffective erythropoiesis (Yerby 2005)
HbH disease	Occurs when only one of four alpha-thalassaemia genes is inherited, which means that three of the four alpha-genes are non-functional. Affected individuals suffer severe anaemia, bone deformities and chronic fatigue and are prone to splenomegaly particularly during infection. They are usually not transfusion dependent
Alpha-thalassaemia major (hydrops fetalis)	There are no alpha-genes in the individual's DNA, which causes the gamma-globins produced to form haemoglobin Bart's. This results in miscarriage or stillbirth (Anionwu & Atkin 2001) or death soon after birth without *in utero* blood transfusions
Beta-thalassaemia major (Cooley's anaemia)	This is the most severe form of beta-thalassaemia in which the complete lack of beta-globin in the haemoglobin causes a life-threatening anaemia that requires blood transfusions and extensive medical care. Iron overload is a complication of life-long blood transfusion, which is corrected by chelation therapy to prevent early death from organ failure
Beta-thalassaemia intermedia	In this condition, there is a lack of beta-globin in the haemoglobin, which causes severe anaemia and significant health problems, including bone deformities and splenomegaly. Generally, blood transfusion is needed to improve quality of life, but not for survival
E beta-thalassaemia	This causes moderately severe anaemia that has similar symptoms to beta-thalassaemia intermedia. The affected person may still experience anaemia, bone changes, leg ulcers and delayed development (Weatherall 1997b) as well as psychological consequences approaching those for beta-thalassaemia major

chains which form part of the structure of haemoglobin in the red blood cell (Weatheral 1997b).

Background and prevalence

There are no reliable figures for the prevalence of thalassaemia but it is estimated that there are around 600 people with thalassaemia major in the UK (Laird et al. 1996; Streetly et al. 1997; Atkin & Ahmad 1998). According to Davies et al. (2000), 17 infants are born with thalassaemia each year in England alone. The carrier rate in the UK for beta-thalassaemia is about 1:10 000 of the entire population (Kean et al. 2000). Globally, it is estimated that 1:30 Chinese, 1:7 Cypriot, 1:20 Asian, 1:50 African-Caribbean and 1:1000 white people carry the beta-thalassaemia trait (Department of Health 1993).

Four genes, two on each strand of chromosome 16, make alpha-globin. People who do not produce enough alpha-globin protein chains have alpha-thalassaemia. An individual with one abnormal alpha-globin is said to be a *silent carrier* of alpha-thalassaemia. Individuals who have one or two abnormal alpha-globin genes have *alpha-thalassaemia trait*. The alpha-thalassaemia traits combine in different ways to produce blood disorders that range from mild to severe in their effect on the human body. Some of these conditions and their implications for pregnancy are described in Table 5.1.

Pathology and complications

A mean cell haemoglobin (MCH) concentration of < 27 pg suggests a thalassaemia (Modell et al. 1997). Diagnosis of alpha- or beta-thalassaemia trait is by the presence of low mean corpuscular volume (MCV), low MCH and a normal mean cell haemoglobin concentration (MCHC) level. Diagnosis is confirmed by globin chain synthesis studies and DNA analysis (Weatheral 1997a).

Pregnancy is very rare in women with beta-thalassaemia major (Kean et al. 2000), mainly because they barely survive to childbearing years. α° (α-thal-1) is associated with anaemia and pregnancy complications such as antepartum haemorrhage, heart failure, hydrops fetalis, postpartum haemorrhage and renal failure, as well as convulsions (Oteng-Ntim et al. 2003). Without treatment, people with homozygous beta-thalassaemia would die in childhood but treatment increases the likelihood of a woman with homozygous beta-thalassaemia becoming pregnant. In infants, failure to thrive, poor weight gain, feeding problems and irritability are common (Newland & Evans 1997).

Iron overload is caused by repeated blood transfusions resulting in hepatic, endocrine and cardiac dysfunction and bone marrow deformities, from expansion of bone marrow, especially in those not transfused regularly (Weatheral 1997b; Kean et al. 2000). Iron overload becomes toxic to tissues and organs, particularly the liver and heart, resulting in the patient's early death from organ failure. Advancement in medical technology now enables the use of magnetic resonance imaging (MRI) to estimate iron levels within the heart and liver in beta-thalassaemia management.

Care and management

- *Screening and diagnosis*. Once a woman has been diagnosed as a carrier for one or other form of thalassaemia, her partner should be offered testing and the couple referred for expert genetic counselling and prenatal diagnosis. Each district health authority needs a policy promoting screening for carriers early in pregnancy, and before pregnancy. There should be immediate expert counselling in couples' own language, as well as appropriate fast track referral.
- *Pre-preganancy assessment* includes partner testing (haemoglobin electrophoresis), subsequent genetic counselling, pre-implantation investigations and semen analysis of the partner.
- *Blood transfusion*. People with thalassaemia are only short of red blood cells; they make the other components of blood quite normally. Some doctors recommend blood transfusion at about 6 g/dl and raise the haemoglobin only to about 10 g/dl (low transfusion scheme). The management of severe forms of beta-thalassaemia entails regular blood transfusion backed up by chelating therapy (using oral deferiprone or subcutaneous desferrioxamine 12–24 hours for 5–7 days or a combination of these) to prevent the effects of iron accumulation. Deferiprone is usually stopped three months prior to conception to avert its tetragenic effect. Chelating in effect causes neutropenia and a transient arthritis in about 5% of patients.
- *Bone marrow transplant* is particularly effective if carried out before complications arise. The main controversy revolves around the safety and efficacy of transplantation in older patients who already have iron overload, as they have a potential mortality up to 30%.
- *Iron deficiency* is not usually a problem; therefore, iron therapy is inappropriate unless deficiency is proven. Folic acid supplementation is needed in pregnancy to maintain the generation of blood within the bone marrow.
- *Experimental treatments*:
  - Pharmacological stimulation of fetal haemoglobin and the development of somatic gene therapy to replace defective globin genes (Olivieri 1995).
  - The administration of hydroxyurea, which reduces the frequency of painful crises in sickle cell anaemia, also seems to be of value in managing sickle cell thalassaemia. The role of gene therapy is still uncertain (Weatheral 1997a).
- Fetal blood is tested for abnormal haemoglobin at birth in some hospital trusts, while a majority have adopted universal blood test screening within the first week of life.

The midwife's role in the management of haemoglobinopathies

The midwife needs a basic knowledge of: genetic inheritance, clinical manifestation, care of carriers, care of pregnant women with sickle cell and thalassaemia disorders, knowledge of antenatal screening programmes, knowledge of neonatal screening programmes, identification of clients and/or partners at risk and appropriate referral systems as well as awareness of available services.

Health education involves educating the woman and her family about her condition, which is essential in enhancing her coping strategies. Emphasis should be placed on measures to prevent crises and to report symptoms of ill health as early as possible.

The midwife's health education role incorporates but is not limited to:

- Preconception care and screening
- Clinical/social care of the woman and her family, especially during hospitalisation
- Genetic counselling
- Involvement and liaison with relevant health care team members
- Agreed management guidelines should be made accessible to all health care professionals involved in the woman's care and to the client and family

Pregnancies complicated by haemoglobinopathies can prove challenging to manage. Such pregnancies are associated with an increased frequency of complications and impending morbidity and mortality. However, this can be averted by multiprofessional collaboration of relevant health care staff, thereby enhancing an optimum pregnancy outcome for both mother and baby.

Part 2: Thromboembolism in pregnancy

Pregnancy is an important risk factor for venous thrombosis, and venous thromboembolism is a leading cause of preventable death in pregnancy. Thromboembolism is the obstruction of a blood vessel with thrombotic material carried by the blood from the site of origin to plug another vessel (Tiran 2003). Thromboembolic disorders are a group of disorders characterised by inflammation of the veins and the formation of blood clots (thrombus) that obstruct blood flow beyond the affected site. Although deep venous thrombosis and pulmonary embolism are two separate manifestations of the pathophysiological process known as venous thromboembolism, other terms/descriptions of the embolic disorders abound:

- *Pulmonary embolism* (PE). This occurs when an embolus reaches the lungs and blocks an artery. This can be life threatening and remains a major cause of maternal mortality and morbidity and is currently the most common direct cause of maternal death in the UK (Lewis 2004).
- *Deep vein thrombosis* (DVT). This involves the formation of a blood clot in the deep veins of the calves, legs or pelvis. If part of the blood clot breaks away and passes into the blood stream, it may cause damage elsewhere in the body. Interestingly, almost 90% of instances of DVT in pregnancy affect the left side, in contrast to only 55% in non-pregnant situations (Greer & Thomson 2001). DVT of a lower limb is a common precursor to PE. In untreated cases with DVT, 24% will have a PE, with a mortality rate of 15%. If treated with anticoagulants, embolisation will occur in only 4.5%.
- *Superficial thrombophlebitis*. This is the inflammation of the wall of a superficial vein. It may be accompanied by blood clot formation and may be uncomfortable, but it is not as dangerous as other forms of thromboembolism.
- *Phlebothrombosis*. This involves blood clot formation without vein inflammation.

Incidence

Thromboembolism is up to ten times more common in pregnant women than in non-pregnant women of comparable age (Rodger et al. 2003). It is estimated that a thrombolic event occurs in 1:1000 to 1:1500 pregnancies and accounts for about 15 maternal deaths a year in the UK (Greer 1999, 2001; Bothamley 2002; Bates 2003). In the triennium 2000–2004, thromboembolism caused 1.2 deaths per 100 000 women and accounted for almost 30% of direct deaths (Lewis 2004). In a study to determine the incidence of pregnancy-related venous thromboembolism, Lindqvist et al. (1999) reported a ratio of 13 per 10 000 cases.

Pathophysiology

Virchow's classic triad of factors underlying venous thrombosis occur in the course of normal pregnancy and involve hypercoagulability, venous stasis and vascular damage (Greer 2001). The factors contribute differently depending on the site of thrombosis: hypercoagulability and sluggish flow occur in the venous system while endothelial defects and thrombocyte activation and apposition occur in the arteries.

Hypercoagulability results from alterations in the proteins of the coagulation and fibrinolytic systems, which act to control bleeding in the third stage of labour. This is compounded by impaired fibrinolysis, through an increase in plasminogen-activator inhibitors (Greer 1999), which aids the coagulation of blood. Pregnancy-associated changes in coagulation are related to: an increase in clotting factors (I, VII, VIII, IX and X), a decrease in protein S, venous stasis, vascular injury associated with delivery, increased activation of platelets and resistance to activated protein C (Women's Health and Education Centre 2004). Venous stasis results from wide venous lumina, the reduction of muscle tone caused by progesterone, and the weight of the growing uterus compressing the inferior vena cava. Blood remains within the vessels for longer and may predispose to DVT. Vascular damage is caused by trauma to the blood vessel walls, which precipitates chemical reactions that allow platelet aggregation at the site of injury and fibrin formation that results in the development of a clot (Bothamley 2002).

Additional risk factors to thromboembolism

According to Brenner and Kupferminc (2003), combinations of inherited or acquired thrombophilic states increase the risk for venous thrombosis. These result from alteration in the balance between the coagulation and fibrinolytic systems and may include the presence of Leiden factor V, and deficiencies of protein C, protein S and antithrombin III (Bothamley 2002). This occurs in about 5% of the general population and in 20–60% of patients with a venous thrombosis (Tutschek et al. 2002). The risks for miscarriage, intrauterine fetal death, placental abruption and severe intrauterine growth restriction are increased in women with inherited thrombophilia in pregnancy (Brenner & Kupferminc 2003); therefore such women need close obstetric monitoring.

In a study by Tutschek et al. (2002), the only pre-conceptional risk factors were a positive family history for DVT or PE and the only post-conceptional risk factor was immobilisation due to bed rest in about one in four of cases. The following have also been identified as risk factors for thrombembolic disorders: age over 35 years, acquired or inherited thrombophilia, history of thrombosis, obesity and varicosis (Tutschek et al. 2002) and associated factors such as operative delivery (caesarean section), immobilisation, placental abruption, intrauterine growth restriction, pregnancy-induced hypertension and pre-eclampsia (Greer 1999, 2000). Bothamley (2002) listed some of the aforementioned and the following as additional factors for thromboembolism in pregnancy: anticardiolipin antibodies, blood group other than O, Caucasian, combined oral contraceptive pill, current infection, dehydration, major pelvic surgery, major current illness (e.g. heart or lung disease, cancer, inflammatory bowel disease or nephrotic syndrome), multi-parity, oestrogen treatment to suppress lactation, paralysis of the lower limbs, sickle cell anaemia and smoking.

Diagnosis

The Confidential Enquiries into Maternal Deaths (CEMD) in the UK has highlighted the need for adequate diagnosis and treatment of thromboembolic diseases in pregnancy (Lewis 2004).

Pulmonary embolism

The diagnosis of PE remains one of the most difficult problems confronting clinicians caring for pregnant women. However, given the high mortality rate of PE, timely diagnosis is fundamental to enable the initiation of antithrombotic therapy for women proven to have this condition, while avoiding the risks of unnecessary anticoagulation therapy when this diagnosis is excluded. PE most frequently presents with dyspnoea and tachypnoea, while cough, haemoptysis and pleuritic chest pain may also sometimes be present. Physical examination may reveal only tachycardia or a few 'crackles'. Severe PE may present with hypotension, syncope (loss of consciousness), right-sided heart failure with distension of the jugular vein, an enlarged liver, left parasternal heave and fixed splitting of the second heart sound sometimes combined with signs of DVT (Greer & Thomson 2001).

Laboratory studies

Electrocardiography is abnormal in 90% of cases with PE. Non-specific T-wave inversion is common in 40% of cases. Almost 12% of cases with PE have a Pao_2 of 80–90 mmHg on arterial blood gases. Almost all patients with pulmonary embolism have abnormal ventilation-perfusion (V/Q) scan results. Ventilation-perfusion lung scanning is the first-line diagnostic tool for PE and should ideally be combined with bilateral duplex venography (Greer 2001). Pulmonary angiography is recommended for cases where clinical suspicion fails to match lung scan results.

Deep vein thrombosis

DVT may be completely asymptomatic or commonly manifest as pain and swelling in the calves. Physical examination of the affected area may reveal tenderness, a difference in leg circumference, redness, a positive Homan's test (pain in a dorsiflexed/extended foot), increased body temperature, oedema, lower abdominal pain and elevated white cell count (Greer & Thomson 2001). Duplex ultrasound is the first-line diagnosis for DVT (Greer 2001). DVT is confirmed when venous ultrasound imaging demonstrates a non-compressible segment in a proximal leg vein (Rodger et al. 2003). Venography is useful when other studies are ambiguous. Measuring venous return in the lower extremities (impedance plethysmography: estimation of blood flow in the vessels) is an alternative technique for DVT diagnosis. Any obstruction of the proximal veins diminishes the volume change, which is detected by measuring changes in the electrical resistance (impendance) over the calf.

Treatment and management

Midwifery/medical care

- A personal or family history of thromboembolism should be established at booking and referral to the obstetric/medical team completed.
- A specialist doctor and midwife can be appointed by each obstetric unit to ensure that personnel with an active interest are involved in the care of the woman.
- Locally agreed policy/guidelines for the management of venous thrombo-embolism should be adhered to.
- Women on heparin prophylaxis for more than 6 weeks should be fully informed of the signs of complications to report to the midwife or doctor. Such signs include signs of heparin-induced osteoporosis and heparin-induced thrombocytopenia.
- Skills in active resuscitation are vital in the event of PE, as well as other routine measures in an emergency, including: alerting the emergency response team and summoning appropriate help, assessing and recording vital signs, administration of oxygen, heparin and other prescribed drugs, attaching an oxymeter and recording an electrocardiogram, administering and maintaining accurate fluid balance, assisting with/participating in endotrachial intubations, initiating intravenous access, monitoring fetal wellbeing and supporting the family.
- Health promotion strategies such as measures to avoid DVT and obesity, smoking cessation, exercise and the wearing of Ted stockings should be advocated at every opportunity.

Prophylaxis

- The British Society for Haematology guidelines recommend that all women with previous venous thromboembolism or a thrombophilia should be encouraged to wear class II graduated elastic compression below-knee stockings throughout their pregnancy and for 6–8 weeks after delivery. This reduces the risk of post-thrombotic syndrome from 23 to 11% if worn for 2 years (Girling 2004). Class 1 thromboembolic stockings are recommended for inpatients and pregnant women travelling by air (Walker et al. 2001).

- Aspirin has been found in a meta-analysis to have a beneficial effect in the prevention of DVT. Low doses (60–75 mg daily) are recommended, as aspirin is not associated with adverse pregnancy outcome in the second and third trimester (Rodger et al. 2003).
- Women with previous venous thromboembolism and no thrombophilia should be offered prophylaxis with low molecular weight heparin (LMWH) during pregnancy and for 6 weeks after delivery or until the international normalised ratio (INR) is greater than 2.0 (Royal College of Obstetricians and Gynaecologists 2004).
- Warfarin derivatives cross the placenta and as a result should be avoided during pregnancy, especially between 6 and 12 weeks' gestation because of its teratogenic effects. However, both warfarin and heparin are safe during lactation (Royal College of Obstetricians and Gynaecologists 2004).

Acute care

- The aim of care in the acute phase is to boost anticoagulation level without putting the woman at risk of bleeding.
- A woman with PE will need oxygen therapy, adequate analgesia and may require resuscitation.
- Before anticoagulation treatment is commenced, thrombophilia screening should be completed as well as full blood count, urea, electrolytes, liver function test and coagulation screen to exclude renal or hepatic dysfunction (Royal College of Obstetricians and Gynaecologists 2001).
- Acute thromboembolism in pregnancy should be treated with an intravenous heparin bolus of 5000 U (80 iu/kg) followed by continuous infusion of 2000 iu/h adjusted by at least daily laboratory results. This is followed by an infusion of 1000 iu/ml and a partial thromboplastin time (PTT) level check (Royal College of Obstetricians and Gynaecologists 2001). Heparin treatment should be continued until the INR is > 2.0 on two successive days (Greer & Thomson 2001).
- Warfarin should not be used in the management of thromboembolic disorder in pregnant women both because of its teratogenic effect and its anticoagulant effect on the fetus, as it increases the risk of spontaneous brain haemorrhage.

Treatment in labour

It is recommended that LMWH be continued in labour for women receiving antenatal thromboprophylaxis with LMWH. Women receiving high prophylactic or therapeutic doses should have their LMWH withheld or reduced to its thromboprophylactic dose at induction or spontaneous onset of labour or caesarean section. This dose should be continued throughout labour: 5000 U of unfractionated heparin are recommended every 12 hours or dalteparin 5000 iu, enoxparin 40 mg or tinzaparin 50 iu/kg (Royal College of Obstetricians and Gynaecologists 2004).

A regional epidural should be avoided within 12–24 hours following injection of LMWH, and should only be considered if platelets and clotting are normal after this to minimise the risk of haematoma formation (Girling 2004). An elevated APTT at delivery probably increases the risk of bleeding and makes epidural anaesthesia problematic (Bates 2003). Therefore, LMWH should not be given 3 hours after the epidural catheter has been removed, and the cannula should not be removed within 10–12 hours of the most recent injection (Checketts & Wildsmith 1999).

The treatment of women in whom a venous thromboembolism develops post-partum is similar to that of non-pregnant women.

Conclusion

Pregnancy is an important risk factor for venous thromboembolism, and thromboembolism is an avoidable leading cause of death in pregnancy. The midwife, mother and medical team play a vital role in the early detection, screening, treatment and management of this condition to avert morbidity and mortality associated with it.

References

Adams, S. (1996) Sickle cell disease in pregnancy: caring for the pregnant woman with sickle cell crisis. *Professional Care of Mother and Child*, **6** (2): 34–6.

Angastiniotis, M. and Modell, B. (1998) Global epidemiology of haemoglobin disorders. *Annals of New York Academy of Sciences*, **850**: 250–69.

Anionwu, E. and Atkin, K. (2001) *The Politics of Sickle Cell and Thalassaemia.* Open University Press, Milton Keynes, UK.

Atkin, K. and Ahmad, W. (1998) Genetic screening and haemoglobinopathies: ethics, politics and practice. *Social Science and Medicine*, **46** (3):445–58.

Bates, S. (2003) Treatment and prophylaxis of venous thromboembolism during pregnancy. *Thrombosis Research*, **108**: 97–106.

Bothamley, J. (2002) Thromboembolism in pregnancy. In: M. Boyle (Ed.) *Emergencies around Childbirth: A handbook for midwives.* Radcliffe Medical Press, Oxford.

Brenner, B. and Kupferminc, M. (2003) Inherited thrombophilia and poor pregnancy outcome. *Best Practice and Research in Clinical Obstetrics and Gynaecology*, **17** (3): 427–39.

Checketts, M. and Wildsmith, J. (1999) Central nerve block and thromboprophylaxis – is there a problem? *British Journal of Anaesthesiology*, **9** (82): 164–7.

Davies, S. (1998) Obstetric implications of sickle cell disease. *Health Visitor and Community Nurse*, **24** (9): 361–3.

Davies, S., Cronin, E., Gill, M., Greengross, P., Hickman, M. and Normand, C. (2000) Screening for sickle cell disease and thalassaemia – a systematic review with supplementary research. *Health Technology Assessment*, **4** (3): 1–101.

Davies, S. and Oni, L. (1997) Fortnightly review: management of patients with sickle cell disease. *British Medical Journal*, **315**: 656–60.

Department of Health (1993) *Report of Working Party of the Standing Medical Advisory Committee on sickle cell, thalassaemia, and other haemoglobinopathies.* Her Majesty's Stationery Office (HMSO), London.

Dyson, S. (1999) Genetic screening and ethnic minorities. *Critical Social Policy*, **19** (2): 195–215.

Gelbart, M. (1998) In our parents' shadow: thalassaemia. *Nursing Times*, **94** (24): 39.

Girling, J. (2004) Thromboembolism and thrombophilia. *Current Obstetrics and Gynaecology*, **14**: 11–22.

Greer, I. (1999) Thrombosis in pregnancy: maternal and foetal issues. *Lancet*, **353** (9160): 1258–65.

Greer, I. (2000) The challenges of thrombophilia in maternal–foetal medicine. *New England Journal of Medicine*, **342**: 424.

Greer, I. (2001) Acute management of venous thromboembolism in pregnancy. *Current Opinion in Obstetric and Gynaecology*, **13**: 569–75.

Greer, I. and Thomson, A. (2001) Management of venous thromboembolism in pregnancy. *Best Practice and Research in Clinical Obstetric and Gynaecology*, **15** (4): 583–603.

Hall, F. (2002) Screening for sickle cell disorders: part 1. *British Journal of Midwifery*, **10** (4): 223–37.

Kaul, D., Fabry, M., Windisch, P., Baez, S. and Nagel, R. (1983) Erythrocytes in sickle cell anaemia are heterogeneous in their rheological and haemodynamic characteristics. *Journal of Clinical Investigation*, **72**: 22–31.

Kean, L., Baker, P. and Edelstone, D. (2000) *Best Practice in Labour Ward Management*. W.B. Saunders, London.

Laird, L., Dezateux, C. and Anionwu, E. (1996) Fortnightly review: neonatal screening for sickle cell disorders: what about the carrier infants? *British Medical Journal*, **313**: 407–11.

Lewis, G. (2004) *Why Mothers Die 2000–2002: Report on Confidential Enquiries into Maternal Deaths in the United Kingdom*. Royal College of Obstetricians and Gynaecologists (RCOG), London.

Lindqvist, P., Dahlback, B. and Marsal, K. (1999) Thrombotic risk during pregnancy: a population study. *American College of Obstetrics and Gynaecology*, **94**: 595–9.

Modell, B., Harris, R., Lane, B. et al. (2000) Informed choice in genetic screening for thalassaemia during pregnancy: audit from a national confidential inquiry. *British Medical Journal*, **320**: 337–41.

Modell, B., Petrou, M., Layton, M. et al. (1997) Audit of prenatal diagnosis for haemoglobin disorders in the United Kingdom: the first 20 years. *British Medical Journal*, **315**: 779–84.

Newland, C. and Evans, T. (1997) ABC of clinical haematology: haematological disorders at the extremes of life. *British Medical Journal*, **314**: 2262.

Olivieri, N. (1995) Clinical experiences with reactivation of fetal haemoglobin in the beta haemoglobinopathies. *Seminars in Haematology*, **33**: 24–42.

Oteng-Ntim, E., Okpala, I. and Anionwu, E. (2003) Sickle disease in pregnancy. *Current Obstetrics and Gynaecology*, **13**: 362–8.

Repke, J. (1996) Intrapartum pre-eclampsia and hypertension. In: J. Repke (Ed.) *Intrapartum Obstetrics*. Churchill Livingston, London.

Rodger, M., Walker, M. and Wells, P. (2003) Diagnosis and treatment of venous thromboembolism in pregnancy. *Best Practice and Research Clinical Haematology*, **16** (2): 279–96.

Royal College of Obstetricians and Gynaecologists (2001) *Thromboembolic Disease in Pregnancy and the Puerperium: Acute management*. RCOG Guidelines No. 28. RCOG, London.

Royal College of Obstetricians and Gynaecologists (2004) *Thromboprophylaxis During Pregnancy, Labour and after Vaginal Delivery*. RCOG Guidelines No. 37. RCOG, London.

Rust, O. and Perry, K. (1995) Pregnancy complicated by sickle haemoglobinopathy. *Clinical Obstetrics and Gynaecology*, **38**: 472–84.

Sergeant, G. (1992) *Sickle Cell Disease*. Oxford University Press, Oxford.

Sickle Cell Disease Guideline Panel (1993) *Sickle Cell Disease: Screening, diagnosis, management and counselling in newborn infants*. Agency for Healthcare Policy and Research, US Department of Human Services, Rockville, MD.

Smith, J., Espeland, M., Bellevue, R., Bonds, D., Brown, A. and Koshy, M. (1996) Pregnancy in sickle cell disease: experience of the cooperation study of sickle cell disease. *Obstetrics and Gynecology*, **87**: 199–204.

Streetly, A. (2000) A national screening policy for sickle cell disease and thalassaemia major for the United Kingdom. *British Medical Journal*, **320**: 1353–4.

Streetly, A., Maxwell, K. and Mejia, A. (1997) *Sickle Cell Disorders in Greater London: A needs assessment of screening and care services*. Bexley and Greenwich Health Authority, London.

Tiran, D. (2003) *Bailliere's Midwives' Dictionary* (10th edn). Bailliere Tindall, London.

Tutschek, B., Truve, S., Goecke, T. et al. (2002) Clinical risk factors for deep venous thrombosis in pregnancy and the puerperium. *Journal of Perinatal Medicine*, **30**: 367–70.

Walker, I., Greaves, M. and Preston, F. (2001) British Society for Haematology Guideline. Investigation and management of heritable thrombophilia. *British Journal of Haematology*, **114**: 512–28.

Weatheral, D. (1997a) ABC of clinical haematology: the hereditary anaemias. *British Medical Journal*, **314**: 492–513.

Weatheral, D. (1997b) Fortnightly review: the thalassaemias. *British Medical Journal*, **314**: 1675–82.

Women's Health and Education Centre (2004) Thromboembolism in pregnancy. http://www.womenshealthsection.com (last accessed 10/06/2004)

Yerby, M. (2005) Anaemia and clotting disorders. In: D. Stables and J. Rankin (Eds) *Physiology in Childbearing*. Elsevier, Edinburgh.

Further reading

American Academy of Paediatrics (2002) Health supervision for children with sickle cell disease. *Paediatrics*, **109** (3): 526–35.

Anionwu, E., Patel, N., Kanji, G. et al. (1998) Counselling for prenatal diagnosis of sickle cell disease and β-thalassaemia major: a four year experience. *Journal of Medical Genetics*, **25**: 769–72.

Claster, S. and Elliot, P. (2003) Managing sickle cell disease. *British Medical Journal*, **327**: 1151–5.

Davies, S. and Roberts, I. (1996) Bone marrow transplant for sickle cell disease – an update. *Archives of Disease of Childhood*, **75**: 3–6.

Modell, B., Ward, R. and Fairweather, D. (1980) Effects of introducing antenatal diagnosis on the reproductive behaviour of families at risk for thalassaemia major. *British Medical Journal*, **280** (6228): 1347–50.

Neile, E. (1998) Who suffers when ignorance prevails? Stories about thalassaemia. *Practising Midwife*, **1** (6): 36–9.

Orion, A., Rust, M. and Kenneth, G. (1995) Pregnancy complicated by sickle cell haemoglobinopathy. *Clinical Obstetrics and Gynaecology*, **38** (3): 472–84.

Platt, O., Brambilla, D., Rosse, W. et al. (1994) Mortality in sickle cell disease: life expectancy and risk factors for early death. *North England Journal of Medicine*, **330**: 163–4.

Sears, D. (1994) Sickle cell trait. In: S. Embury, R. Hebbel, N. Mohandas and M.H. Steinberg (Eds) *Sickle Cell Disease: Basic principles and clinical practice*. Raven Press, New York.

Yost, N. (2001) Diagnosing and managing sickle cell disease in pregnancy. *Contemporary Obstetrics and Gynaecology Online*. www.contemporyobgyn.net

Zenner, D., Ades, A.E., Karnon, J., Brown, J., Dezateux, C. and Anionwu, E.N. (1999) Antenatal and neonatal haemoglobinopathy screening in the UK: review and economic analysis. *Health Technology Assessment*, **3**: 1–186.

6 Hypertensive Disorders and the Critically Ill Woman

Mandy Stevenson and Mary Billington

Hypertensive disorders of pregnancy are a major cause of critical illness and mortality (Lewis 2001, 2004; Robson 2002; Duley 2003). In the current Confidential Enquiry into Maternal Deaths (CEMD), 14 deaths were confirmed as a result of pre-eclampsia (Lewis 2004) which included nine deaths from intracranial haemorrhage. Substandard care was recognised in 46% of the cases reviewed. Such deaths may have been avoidable by prompt recognition of a deteriorating situation and by improving the clinical care and management provided by all the involved parties.

This chapter will focus on pre-eclampsia, eclampsia and HELLP syndrome (*h*aemolysis, *e*levated *l*iver *e*nzymes, *l*ow *p*latelets), as these are the hypertensive disorders most likely to progress to critical illness.

Assumed prior knowledge

- Physiological changes of pregnancy affecting the cardiovascular system
- Basic understanding of hypertensive disorders in childbearing

Classification

Although there is no universal agreement on precise definitions, hypertensive disorders in pregnancy can be divided into two main groups:

- *Hypertensive disorders that are unique to pregnancy*, which affect approximately 12% of pregnancies (Walker 2000); these include:
  - Pre eclampsia and eclampsia.
  - Pregnancy-induced hypertension/gestational hypertension, which are defined as raised blood pressure (BP) in the second half of the pregnancy

or the third trimester of the pregnancy without other features of pre-eclampsia (Higgins & de Swiet 2001; Nelson-Piercy 2002).
- HELLP syndrome.
- *Hypertension that pre-exists the pregnancy*. Chronic hypertension is estimated to affect between 3 and 5% of childbearing women (Walker 2000), and may be due to an underlying disease process such as renal disease or phaeochromocytoma or, more commonly, essential hypertension.

Hypertension may also occur during pregnancy due to a new medical problem coinciding with pregnancy by chance, and can also be a mixed syndrome, for example pre-eclampsia superimposed on essential hypertension.

Pre-eclampsia

Incidence

Pre-eclampsia is the commonest hypertensive disorder of pregnancy. It is widely estimated to affect 3–5% of pregnancies (Roberts & Cooper 2001), or one in ten pregnancies (Action on Pre-eclampsia (APEC) 2005a) with the incidence of severe pre-eclampsia being approximately 1% (Nelson-Piercy, 2002) or one in 50 pregnancies (APEC 2005a). However, it is difficult to give a precise incidence due to the wide spectrum of presenting factors that can range from mild to life threatening, and the lack of universally accepted diagnostic criteria.

Factors that predispose to pre-eclampsia are presented in Box 6.1.

Classic description and definitions

Traditionally, pre-eclampsia has been defined as a disorder of the second half of pregnancy which regresses after delivery, and in which at least two of the three cardinal signs of hypertension, oedema and proteinuria are present. Most current definitions no longer include oedema, as its assessment is subjective and it is not felt to have diagnostic or prognostic value (North et al. 1999; Higgins & de Swiet 2001), although Higgins and de Swiet (2001) suggest that rapid development of severe oedema should always be investigated as it may signify development of pre-eclampsia or other pathological conditions, such renal or cardiac disease.

Pre-eclampsia is generally regarded as a syndrome (a group of signs and symptoms that can be recognised as an entity) rather than a disease (which can be diagnosed by a specific test demonstrating specific causative factors) (Redman 1994; Robson 2002). It has also been referred to as a 'disease of theories' as the underlying cause and precise physiopathology are still unknown (Roberts & Cooper 2001).

It is increasingly recognised that the disorder is more than hypertension and proteinuria. There is multiorgan and system involvement due to maternal endothelial cell dysfunction which appears to be part of a more generalised maternal intravascular inflammatory response (Robson 2002) associated with vasospasm

---

Box 6.1   Factors that predispose to pre-eclampsia (Walker 2000; Dekker & Sibai 2001; Roberts & Cooper 2001).

Primigravid (increases the risk × 2)
Change of partner/primipaternity/limited sperm exposure/donor sperm
Partner who fathered a pre-eclamptic pregnancy in another woman
History of previous pre-eclampsia
Increasing maternal age/increasing interval between pregnancies/teenagers
Family history (up to 25% chance if mother had pre-eclampsia and up to 40% chance if sister had it (Nelson-Piercy 2002))
Donor eggs
Chronic hypertension and renal disease
Sickle cell disorder and sickle cell trait (Larrabee & Monga 1997)
Obesity, diabetes (including gestational diabetes) and low maternal birthweight
Activated protein C resistance (factor V Leiden) and protein S deficiency
Antiphospholipid antibodies
Hyperhomocysteinaemia (defined as elevated plasma homocysteine (tHcy) concentrations. This can be caused by genetic mutations, vitamin deficiencies, renal and other diseases, numerous drugs and increasing age (Hankey et al. 2004))
Stress; work-related psychosocial strain
Multiple pregnancy
Urinary tract infection
Structural congenital anomalies
Hydrops fetalis
Chromosome anomalies (e.g. triploidy – particularly associated with early onset of pre-eclampsia (Nelson-Piercy 2002))
Hydatidiform mole

---

and underperfusion (Roberts & Cooper 2001). However, assessment of BP and urinalysis remain the first line in screening because they are easy and relatively cheap to assess, even though they are not central to the pathogenesis of the condition (Robson 2002) and the accuracy of their assessment is questioned (Rubin 1996; Shennan et al. 1996; Saudan et al. 1997; Brown et al. 1998; Davies et al. 2002).

Early diagnosis is not always easy as presentation and progression can be extremely variable. Typically, hypertension occurs before proteinuria but some women may have a severe manifestation of the condition without the presence of proteinuria (Higgins & de Swiet 2001), while others may exhibit proteinuria before there is a marked increase in BP (Redman 1994).

Physiopathology

Many authorities currently suggest a two-stage model consisting of a placental trigger followed by a maternal systemic response. Differences in presentation and progression of the disorder are explained as being due to differences in the nature of the maternal response (Walker 2000; Briley et al. 2001).

It is suggested that the placental trigger is a state of absolute or relative ischaemia due to:

- Poor placentation which occurs when there is failure of trophoblastic invasion of the uterine spiral arteries. In normal pregnancy, the muscle walls of these arteries are stripped as far as the inner third of the myometrium (Roberts & Cooper 2001) resulting in greater perfusion of the intervillous spaces. Placental insufficiency is also associated with deposition of fibrin and thrombosis in the spiral arterioles (Walker 2000).
- An abnormally large placenta, which 'outgrows' its blood supply (Roberts & Cooper 2001) as in a multiple pregnancy or hydatidiform mole.
- Other factors which reduce placental perfusion, such as cardiovascular changes associated with diabetes, or essential hypertension.

It may be that placental ischaemia directly or indirectly triggers an abnormal maternal inflammatory response (part of which is generalised endothelial dysfunction) in women who develop pre-eclampsia and related disorders (Redman et al. 1999). However, not all women who have a potential placental trigger develop pre-eclampsia. Thus Walker (2000) argues that the maternal response may be influenced by genetic, behavioural or environmental factors. These may include the maternal or fetal genotype or an interaction between the two (Redman et al. 1999; Roberts & Cooper 2001). The immunological theory suggests that an excessive maternal response occurs when there has been minimal exposure to paternal antigen, for example in a first pregnancy, with a new partner or with the use of donor sperm (Roberts & Cooper 2001). Another theory is that of oxidative stress. This occurs when there is an imbalance between free radicals and antioxidants. Free radicals are generated by metabolism. They have the potential to damage cell membranes, proteins and DNA, and are produced in greater quantities when there is ischaemia.

It appears that there is no specific cause for pre-eclampsia and it may be that multiple routes, involving placental and maternal factors, lead to endothelial dysfunction which is part of a more extensive maternal intravascular inflammatory reaction (Redman et al. 1999; Higgins & de Swiet 2001). The concept of generalised endothelial cell dysfunction allows most of the clinical features of pre-eclampsia, which are used as a basis for diagnosis, to be explained.

Hypertension

Disturbed endothelial control of vascular tone, associated with altered rennin–angiotensin function, results in vasospasm, increased peripheral resistance and hence raised blood pressure.

Proteinuria

This occurs due to glomeruloendotheliosis, which resolves after delivery (Walker 2000). It is a later feature of pre-eclampsia but is associated with poorer outcome.

It is the presence of proteinuria once it exceeds 0.3 g in 24 hours that is significant, rather than its absolute amount (Schiff et al., cited in Walker 2000).

Oedema

Pathological oedema results from increased endothelial permeability compounded by loss of protein from the serum (signified by proteinuria), which alters the direction of osmotic pressure once serum albumin levels fall below 20 g/L (McKay 1999). As a consequence, there is reduced circulating volume and cardiac output, which further reduce organ perfusion, and increased haemoglobin and haematocrit, which are associated with poorer perinatal outcome. Pathological oedema gives rise to several features of severe pre-eclampsia, such as epigastric or back pain (liver oedema), headache and convulsions (cerebral oedema), and breathlessness (pulmonary oedema) (Walker 2000).

Coagulopathy

Vascular endothelial damage leads to activation of the coagulation system and platelet aggregation. Formation of microemboli in the smaller vessels further reduces organ perfusion.

Impaired renal function

Renal function is generally maintained until a late stage, but is impaired in severe pre-eclampsia due to vasoconstriction and reduced perfusion. Raised serum creatinine levels (and proteinuria) indicate impaired glomerular function while raised serum uric acid levels indicate impaired tubular function. There is also increased production of uric acid secondary to tissue ischaemia and oxidative stress. Tubular function is impaired before glomerular function, hence raised serum uric acid levels and hypertension generally precede proteinuria (Dekker & Sibai 2001).

Most cases of renal failure are due to acute tubular necrosis, which generally recovers with no long-term impairment. However, acute cortical necrosis, which occurs in less than 4% of cases of renal failure associated with pre-eclampsia (Naqvi et al., cited in Walker 2000), leads to permanent renal failure.

Liver dysfunction

This results from underperfusion due to vasoconstriction and local oedema. Raised levels of serum alanine aminotransferase (ALT), aspartate aminotransferase (AST) and alkaline phosphatase signify leakage across cell membranes. Raised levels of AST may also indicate damage to the heart, muscles, kidney, pancreas and red blood cells as it is involved in tissue metabolism and is found in high levels in these areas (McKay 1999). Liver involvement is also associated with reduced plasma albumin and clotting factors, which are synthesised by the liver.

Haemorhage within the liver capsule may lead to capsular rupture, which is rare but can produce a mortality rate of 60% (Bird 1997; Lewis 2001).

Box 6.2   Crises in pre-eclampsia (Redman 1994; Nelson-Piercy 2002).

Eclampsia
Cerebral haemorrhage (the largest single cause of death (Lewis 2004))
Retinal detachment
Cortical blindness (rare and usually reversible)
Pulmonary oedema and acute respiratory distress syndrome (ARDS)
Laryngeal oedema
HELLP syndrome
Hepatic infarction or rupture (two cases in the 1997–1999 CEMD (Lewis 2001))
Retroplacental haemorrhage/placental abruption
Intrauterine asphyxia and death
Disseminated intravascular coagulation
Renal failure/cortical and tubal necrosis

And in addition with eclampsia:
Aspiration
Pneumonia
Cardiopulmonary arrest (Mattar & Sibai 2000)

Box 6.2 provides a summary of crises that may occur in association with pre-eclampsia.

Care and management

The role of the midwife in the detection of any degree of hypertensive disorders is important. A through understanding of the pathophysiology relating to the disorder should ensure that any abnormal clinical signs are promptly recognised (Bennett 1994). This detection, followed by prompt appropriate management and referral, will ensure that the health and wellbeing of the mother and fetus are not unnecessarily compromised. Once a diagnosis has been made, the midwife will then continue to provide suitable continuing care in partnership with the multidisciplinary team (Bennett 1995). Care and management will greatly depend upon the degree of intervention required. Expectant management may be pertinent with medication in the form of an antihypertensive being administered.

Accurate diagnosis should prevent inappropriate treatment being implemented either prematurely or behind schedule with the aim of reducing the risk of maternal and fetal/neonatal mortality. The CEMD reports (Lewis 2001, 2004) continue to indicate the disproportionate maternal mortalities related to hypertensive disorders in pregnancy.

Expectant management for lesser degrees of the disorder will include regular monitoring of blood pressure, and the presence of proteinuria and oedema. Nevertheless our role as practitioners can be constantly challenged as the woman's disorder profile starts to deteriorate and intervention in the form of medication, regular blood profile testing, fluid monitoring, intensive monitoring and continuing fetal assessment is required.

Once pre-eclampsia has been considered or confirmed, the main objectives are:

- To prevent any detrimental deterioration of the woman's condition and also the development of any complications. The latter may arise from continuing deterioration such as a cerebral vascular haemorrhage due to uncontrolled blood pressure or pulmonary oedema due to inappropriate fluid overload/ management.
- To prevent convulsions.
- To preserve the mother's life, with the safe delivery of the fetus at a fitting time.
- Effective communication with the multidisciplinary team as well as the woman and her family.

Detection of the severe hypertensive disorders of pregnancy should be prompt and accurate, thus ensuring that suitable management plans are prepared and implemented. The principle signs, which indicate the presence of pre-eclampsia, are both hypertension and significant proteinuria. The National High Blood Pressure Education Program Working Group (1990) reported that the following criteria should to be considered when diagnosing pre-eclampsia:

An elevated blood pressure ≥ 140 mmHg systolic pressure or ≥ 90 mmHg diastolic pressure as opposed to a change in blood pressure

An absolute requirement of proteinuria defined as urinary excretion of 0.3 g of protein or higher in a 24-hour urine sample

Levine et al. (2000) propose that increases greater then 30 mmHg systolic or 15 mmHg diastolic above the booking baseline should not be utilised as the standard for the diagnosis of women having developed pre-eclampsia.

Clinical assessments for signs of physiological deterioration also need to be carefully considered and undertaken alongside measurements of blood pressure. These should include assessment for:

- Varying degrees of *oedema*: mild to severe amounts from the lower extremities rising to generalised overall oedema including the abdomen. This variant of oedema may pit with the application of digital pressure and is an indicator of altering cardiovascular stability.
- Regular *urinalysis* can provide variable evidence relating to an altering renal function as well as the presence of infection. Once a urinary tract infection has been excluded by laboratory testing, the degree of protein being excreted into the urine may be considered suggestive of glomerular endotheliosis and is often viewed as an indicator of the severity of the disorder. Chernecky and Berger (2001) provide comparisons of the urine dipstick recordings against total protein in milligrams found in excreted urine. It is proposed that 3+ equates to 300 mg of protein per litre of urine excreted and 4+ equates to more than 1 g protein/L urine being excreted. If the dipstick protein is found to be more than 1+ on more than one occasion in conjunction with the presence of other suggestive factors relating to the disorder, a 24-hour urine collection for

total protein and creatinine clearance may be demanded to provide an accurate quantitative result of protein excreted. A consensus of opinions concur that a protein excretion of more than 3 g in 24 hours is suggestive of mild to moderate pre-eclampsia, and of more than 5 g in such a period to be indicative of severe pre-eclampsia (Saudan et al. 1997; Warden & Earle 2005).

A reducing urine output may be indicative of the progression of the disorder and one needs to remain vigilant in relation to the development of *oliguria*. This is defined as an output of less than 120 ml urine excreted in a 4-hour period; regular (1–4-hourly), accurate measurements of intake and output should be undertaken to allow appropriate referrals and management to take place. This reducing urine output has been hypothesized as the result of renal artery vasospasm for which accurate fluid replacement should enable the constriction to be reversed.

Other components measured in the diagnosis and/or the presence of pre-elampsia are:

- *Epigastric pain, right upper quadrant discomfort and vomiting*. These may indicate hepatic dysfunction and should be considered with an altering blood picture that may highlight the presence of HELLP syndrome. The pain is considered to be due to the distension of the liver capsule by either oedema or haemorrhage and is liable to be present with severe pre-eclampsia.
- *Headaches or visual disturbances*. A headache that cannot be alleviated with medication such as paracetomol must be considered to be a sign that the woman's condition is worsening. Such deterioration may be an indicator of central nervous system impairment, and may also be suggestive of poor cerebral perfusion.
- *Deep tendon reflex response*. This should be assessed as its presence indicates the presence of hyperreflexia and/or the presence of *clonus*. However, one may choose to question the validity of undertaking such assessments if a 'normal' response has not been obtained at any stage during the pregnancy. Sibai et al. (1981) proposed that 'normal' women may have increased reactions; they, conversely, have viewed eclamptic seizures occurring in the absence of such increased neurological responses, and therefore deem that hyperreflexia should not be viewed as a sign of pre-eclampsia. However, if a marker is required to work from to measure any deterioration, a baseline response should be obtained when an altering physiological state is questioned in relation to pre-eclampsia. Many clinicians consider that increased neurological responses and the presence of clonus is an indicator that the woman's physiological condition is deteriorating. The reflex commonly challenged is the patella. The results expected from such intervention range from no response elicited through to brisk responses with the presence of clonus (Seidel 2002). Clonus is defined as an abnormal pattern of neuromuscular activity, characterised by rapidly alternating involuntary contraction and relaxation of skeletal muscles (Mosby 1986). Dorsiflexion of the foot is undertaken and resulting spasms of the muscle may be seen immediately upon relaxation. This presence of clonus implies neuromuscular irritability and the impending degeneration of the disorder.

To summarise, the clinical features of severe pre-eclampsia are:

- Severe hypertension: BP ≥ 160 mmHg systolic or ≥ 110 mmHg diastolic on at least two occasions more than 6 hours apart (Robson 2002)
- Proteinuria: ≥ 5 g/24 h (Robson 2002)
- Oligouria: ≥ 400 ml/24 h (Robson 2002)
- Cerebral or visual disturbance
- Epigastric pain
- Pulmonary oedema or cyanosis
- Thrombocytopenia
- Impaired liver function
- Hyperreflexia and clonus

Management of moderate to severe pre-eclampsia in the antenatal/intrapartum period

Decisions surrounding pertinent management often depend upon the severity of the maternal condition versus the maturity of the fetus. The woman's overall condition should be considered with a complete haematological/biochemical result profile. A deteriorating blood profile may confirm a diagnosis of pre-eclampsia and validate further aggressive management to protect the wellbeing of both the mother and fetus, whilst results within a normal range will allow expectant management to be undertaken. The frequency of sampling for diagnostic testing may vary between maternity units. However, guidance on the regularity of testing should be confirmed within the multidisciplinary team.

Dekker and Walker (1997) concur that serial measurements will indicate the evolution of the disorder. Proposals that plasma uric acid levels may be a fair indicator of the disorder have been refuted by the fact that the results only have a predictive value in one-third of all cases and should therefore not be used as a single confirmation (Lim et al. 1998). Stamilio et al. (2000) consider that no single screening test has to date been found to be reliable and cost effective. Hence a complete up to date blood profile should be available when a decision regarding expectant versus aggressive management of a woman's condition is made.

Blood diagnostic tests to confirm or refute the diagnosis should be used in conjunction with clinical assessment.

Maternal care and management

Once a decision has been made to deliver the woman on the grounds of her condition deteriorating, the following principles of management should be efficiently implemented.

Provision of holistic care for the woman and her family

Apprehension will probably be a key feature that will require consideration and management. This can normally be dispelled by encouraging the woman to consider her anxieties, doubts and resentment of the situation which may have developed. Information giving should be in the form of a comprehensible explanation of both the disorder and the actions involved in its management.

Physiological monitoring

- *Blood pressure measurements* need to be obtained and accurately documented on high dependency charts which will allow more frequent recordings to be charted. If using an automated sphygmomanometer, a comparison should be made of manual recordings against the automated recordings every hour to ensure consistency of results. Timing of recordings will depend upon the severity of the disorder and the involvement of pharmacological interventions such as anticonvulsive or antihypertensive therapy.
- *Pulse oximetry* should be undertaken to measure the oxygen saturation of haemoglobin in the arterial blood. (Pulse oximetry is a measure of the average amount of oxygen bound to each haemoglobin molecule.) The percentage saturation is given as a digital readout together with an audible signal varying in pitch depending on the oxygen saturation. This measurement can be considered as an indicator of maternal hypoxia.
- The *pulse rate* in beats per minute can also be measured.
- *Respiratory assessment* will be required to assess for the presence of pulmonary oedema (wheezes, crackles, signs of dysnoea, shallow respiration), magnesium sulphate toxicity or simply a chest infection.

Blood profile

A current blood profile with results for liver and renal function should be available in the form of urea, electrolytes and urate levels. A clotting screen should be maintained as well as blood group and 'save serum'. A decreasing platelet count may indicate that the woman's clotting mechanisms have been affected and attention needs to be paid to the clotting times and fibrin degradation to ascertain if disseminated intravascular coagulation (DIC) has begun.

Fluid balance and management

Strict fluid balance records need to be maintained, which include oral and intravenous maintenance, volume expanding fluids, blood products and any drugs being administered such as hydralazine or magnesium sulphate, as well as urine and gastrointestinal output. An indwelling urinary catheter attached to a urometer may be the most accurate method of obtaining a precise urine output, for detecting hypovolaemia or the presence of acute renal failure, and to enable a diagnosis of oliguria (< 100 ml urine) to be made, based on a 4-hour period of time. Using such a timeframe may enable women to resume a normal urinary output without any form of intervention.

Conversely, if after 4 hours, diuresis has not taken place, a fluid challenge of 500 ml colloid solution (such as Gelofusine) will be required. Colloid solutions have the benefit of having a higher molecular weight, hence having a 'pulling effect' on the fluids, pulling them back into circulation for a longer period of time, and thus reducing the risk of oedema occurring. If little or no response is obtained from the fluid challenge, it may be appropriate for a central venous pressure (CVP) catheter to be placed and utilised to ensure that fluid replacement is accurately managed. Repetitive unmonitored fluid administration should be avoided at all costs as this will lead to pulmonary oedema. Oliguria and a low CVP reading (< 5 cm) will point towards hypovolaemia, which will require correction. Conversely, oliguria and a high CVP reading (> 10 cm) may necessitate treatment with a diuretic such as frusemide 40 mg i.v. Nevertheless, diuretics should not be used until hypovolaemia has been substantiated and treated or excluded.

Care needs to be taken that appropriate fluids are administered and monitored, such as employing the use of CVP recordings when increasing doses of colloid fluids are utilised and the woman's urinary output fails to respond to the fluid challenge. CVP recordings reflect the volume of blood returning to the heart, but do not necessarily reflect intravascular volume status. Hence continuing fluid replacement without close attention and monitoring can easily encourage fluid transference into the inappropriate spaces and encourage pulmonary oedema to develop.

Cautious fluid management should be attempted to combat dehydration but with the aim of not being the causative factor of fluid overload and any resulting pulmonary oedema. Maternal plasma volume is reduced in pre-eclampsia in relation to a normal pregnancy; with the fluid retention in pre-eclampsia being associated with renal retention of both sodium and potassium. Pulmonary oedema is a significant problem of pre-eclampsia and transpires as a consequence of intravascular depletion due to reduced oncotic pressure, increased intravascular hydrostatic pressure and capillary permeability with the leakage of albumin into the interstitial spaces. This maldistribution of fluid from the vascular space into the interstitial space causes a hypovolaemic state and a resulting oedema. This may allow the potential for inappropriate management to take place with diuretics and the further depletion of the vascular space. Crystalloid fluid is recommended for fluid level maintenance (85 ml/h or urine output in preceding hour plus 30 ml) (Royal College of Obstetricians and Gynaecologists 1999). Any other intravenous fluids administered such as magnesium sulphate should be included in the 85 ml/h total. Additional fluid (colloid) may be required prior to drug-induced vasodilatation to prevent maternal hypotension and possible subsequent fetal compromise. Fluid overload has been recognised as a compounding factor in maternal deaths (Lewis 2001).

Protocols should be present in the clinical area to ensure consistent approaches to safe and effective fluid management. An example of a fluid management flow chart to guide therapy is presented in Figure 6.1.

Fetal monitoring

Fetal monitoring should indicate any fetal compromise due to insufficient utero-placental circulation. Regular cardiotocographs (CTGs) to assess the fetal heart rate pattern should be undertaken as a reduction in fetal movements may indicate a degree of fetal hypoxia. The detection of growth restriction may necessitate corticosteroid administration to improve fetal lung maturity in anticipation of

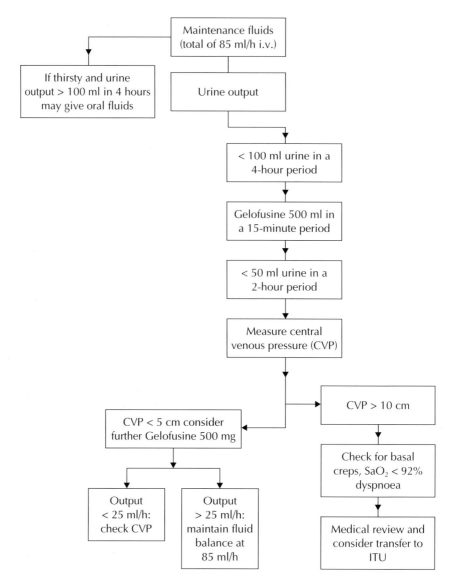

Figure 6.1   Example of a fluid management flow chart.

early delivery (Royal College of Obstetricians and Gynaecologists 1999). It may be necessary to organise either an *in utero* or neonatal transfer if the maternity unit is unable to cope with preterm neonates.

Treatment of hypertension

The objective of antihypertensive therapy in pre-eclampsia or eclampsia is to reduce the risk of cerebral haemorrhage, which may occur as the blood pressure becomes uncontrolled, thus lessening the risks of cerebral haemorrhage to the mother, and to maintain uteroplacental perfusion thus enabling continued fetal oxygenation. Antihypertensive therapy may be indicated with an elevated diastolic blood pressure of > 110 mmHg or an elevated systolic blood pressure of > 160 mmHg.

However, the use of medication to stabilise fluctuating blood pressure measurements remains a controversial process. Varying studies (Sibai 1996; Abalos et al. 2001) have indicated no clear successful benefits of using antihypertensive medication in the management of hypertension in pregnancy. First-line management tends to rely upon the use of centrally acting antihypertensive drugs such as methyldopa. Believed to be safe in pregnancy for both mother and fetus, doses can be increased to 3 g daily (British Medical Association (BMA) & Royal Pharmaceutical Society of Great Britain 2005), but drowsiness can occur with the increased doses.

If the woman's condition deteriorates or if stability is not obtained, hospitalisation needs to be maintained and second-line management may be considered to include the use of oral beta-blockers such as labetalol. Oral labetalol tablets may be increased up to a maximum dose of 2.4 g daily. Long-term usage is not advised due to the potential of fetal growth restriction and fetal bradycardia (Wells et al. 2002). The aim of hypertensive management should be to reduce the blood pressure to around 130–140/90–100 mmHg. A sharp reduction using medication can cause fetal heart rate abnormalities that will require management.

Treatment with intravenous antihypertensive medication should be considered if the blood pressure is not generally maintained below 160/100 mmHg or mean arterial pressure (MAP) at less than 125 mmHg. MAP can be defined as the average pressure in the arterial system during one complete cardiac cycle. The result will be closer to the diastolic recording because the diastolic (relaxed) state of the ventricle lasts twice as long as the systolic (contracted) state of the ventricle. It is generally perceived that MAP will reflect the degree of hypovolaemia associated with the disorder.

MAP is calculated as:

$$\frac{\text{Systolic BP} - \text{Diastolic BP}}{3} + \text{Diastolic BP}$$

For example, for a woman with a BP recording of 145/105 mmHg, the calculation would be:

145 – 105 (= 30) divided by 3 (= 10) + 105, which equals a MAP of 115

Evidence has found that the use of antihypertensive drugs in women with pre-eclampsia does not inhibit or change the natural pattern of events surrounding the disorder in women with mild pre-eclampsia. (Magee et al. 1999; Sibai 2003). However it should aim to prevent potential cerebrovascular and cardiovascular complications.

Hydralazine

Hydralazine tends to be the medication of choice for intravenous management of moderate to severe hypertension as it controls blood pressure in 95% of patients with pre-eclampsia (Fugate & Chow 2004). This is a vasodilator antihypertensive drug whose actions include increasing the cardiac output and heart rate, relaxing the smooth muscle and decreasing MAP. The side effects can include an abrupt and profound decrease in the blood pressure, and again caution needs to be taken in light of fetal wellbeing. The onset of the drug's action is within 15 minutes. It has its peak effect between 30 and 60 minutes and lasts between 4 and 6 hours. Volume expansion in the form of a plasma expander prior to hydralazine administration may be used to reduce the risk of poor placental perfusion (Cotton et al. 1985).

- Drug administration is 5–10 mg of hydralazine diluted with 10 ml of 0.9% normal saline (BMA & Royal Pharmaceutical Society of Great Britain 2005) intravenously as a bolus over a period of 1–2 minutes.
- The dose can be repeated at intervals of every 20 minutes until the diastolic blood pressure is between 90 and 100 mmHg or 30 mg of the drug has been administered. The diastolic blood pressure should not be allowed to fall below 90 mmHg as this may further reduce the blood flow to the placenta, kidneys and cerebrum.
- Caution needs to be taken as the side effects of hydralazine include tachycardia, palpitations and headaches. Blood pressure recordings should be obtained every 5 minutes whilst bolus doses are being administered.
- If the blood pressure or MAP stabilises with the administration of bolus dose(s), monitoring in the form of 15-minute BP recordings + MAP should continue.
- However, if there are difficulties maintaining a MAP below 125 mmHg, a maintenance infusion will need to be considered. Hydralazine is diluted with 0.9 normal saline to allow titration of the solution as 1 mg hydralazine per millilitre. Dosage may commence at 10 ml/h, and can be increased at increments until a satisfactory, responsive BP has been obtained. However, if the maximum dosage of 40 ml/h has been achieved or the maternal heart rate has increase to more than 120 beats/min, further intervention in the form of labetalol may be prudent.

Labetalol

Labetalol is often considered for second-line management in cases of uncontrolled blood pressure recordings (after hydralazine). A beta-adrenoceptor-blocking drug, labetolol works by reducing peripheral resistance by vasodilatation. However, caution needs to be considered as, following hydralazine administration and the resulting vasodilatation, labetalol may diminish the cardiac output resulting in a brisk reduction in blood pressure.

Labetolol has a prompt onset of action at 5 minutes, with a peak effect at 10 to 20 minutes. The duration of action is between 45 minutes and 6 hours.

- If labetalol is required, an intravenous bolus dose of 20 mg may be slowly administered.
- If stability is still not achieved, further intermittent doses at 10-minute intervals (40 mg at 10 minutes after the first dose, followed by 80 mg and then further incremental doses up to a total maximum dose of 300 mg) can be administered (Lewis 2001).
- Some units may utilise a continuous infusion of labetalol, which can be implemented at 1–2 mg/min.

Nifedipine

Nifedipine should be used with caution, orally in 1 mg doses. The response should be obtained within 30 minutes after administration. The aim of nifedipine is to reduce peripheral resistance and thus lower blood pressure. It should not be administered in combination with magnesium sulphate due to the risk of profound hypotension, muscle weakness and fetal distress (Waisman et al. 1988; Khurana & Graham 1999; BMA & Royal Pharmaceutical Society of Great Britain 2005).

A meta-analysis comparing hydralazine against other antihypertensive medications (Magee et al. 2003) questions the use of hydralazine as the drug of choice for controlling severe hypertension yet fails to provide adequate evidence to support the routine use of alternative medication such as labetalol.

Anticonvulsive therapy

The aim of the care and management of a woman with pre-eclampsia is to prevent the condition from deteriorating further into eclampsia. Seizures can be prevented with the expectant use of anticonvulsant therapy in the form of magnesium sulphate. Trials such as the MAGPIE trial (Magpie Trial Collaborative Group 2002) provide substantial evidence to establish that the use of magnesium sulphate can reduce the risk of women developing eclampsia and prevent recurrent seizures. Historically, diazepam and phenytoin have been used in the treatment or prevention of eclamptic seizures, nevertheless they are viewed as less effective (Sibai 1996).

The action of magnesium sulphate aims to decrease the irritability of the central nervous system, cause peripheral vasodilatation and increase uterine and renal blood flow (Eclampsia Trial Collaborative Group 1995). Of note, magnesium is contraindicated in clients with renal failure (magnesium is mainly excreted by the kidneys and therefore retained in renal failure potentially causing hypermagnesaemia), hence phenytoin may need to be used.

Magnesium sulphate regimes across the country may differ to a degree but should encompass the following:

- One bolus dose administered intravenously (4 g $MgSO_4$ and 12 ml dilutant such as 0.9% NaCl to equal 20 ml total volume for administration) over a period of 5–10 minutes. This equates to approximately 16 mmol of magnesium being administered (BMA & Royal Pharmaceutical Society of Great Britain 2005).
- Following the bolus dose, a maintenance dose of 1–2 g/h needs to be infused to maintain the serum magnesium levels within a therapeutic range of 2–4 mmol/L.
- Once magnesium sulphate administration has commenced, monitoring of the deep tendon reflexes, respiratory rate and oxygen saturation should occur. Some maternity units may choose to undertake blood sampling to assess serum magnesium levels at timed opportunities during therapy.
- Attention needs to be paid for the onset of any clinical signs of magnesium toxicity. Therapeutic magnesium levels lie between 2.0 and 4.0 mmol. With increasing magnesium levels up to 5 mmol, the client may complain of feeling warm, flushing, experiencing double vision or possessing slurred speech.

Tendon reflexes may be lost as magnesium concentrations exceed 5 mmol. Respiratory depression followed closely by respiratory arrest can occur with magnesium levels in excess of 6.0 mmol. Cardiac arrest will occur at levels above 12 mmol of magnesium.

- With the detection of any form of magnesium toxicity, the magnesium sulphate infusion should be immediately halted. Maternal (and fetal) monitoring should be instigated. Electrocardiographic recording should be commenced to detect cardiac arrhythmias. Duley et al. (2003) proposed that therapeutic levels of magnesium might affect the fetal heart rate variability; hence CTG recording of the fetal heart needs to be maintained through the labour to delivery.
- If a respiratory or cardiac arrest occurs, 1 g of calcium gluconate (10 ml of 10% solution) can be administered in the form of a slow intravenous bolus over a 3-minute period. The patient should be intubated, ventilated immediately and transferred to the intensive treatment unit.
- Magnesium sulphate should be continued for 24 hours following delivery or the last seizure.

Delivery will depend upon the condition of the mother and the fetus. A fine balance needs to be achieved so as to not compromise the fetus, yet ensuring the maternal condition does not deteriorate to the detriment of the maternal physiology, e.g. renal impairment following untreated oliguria. For a premature fetus, decisions may be made surrounding prolonging the pregnancy by a short period of time until fetal lung maturation has been encouraged by the administration of corticosteroids. Odendaal (2001) advocates that systemic corticosteroid administration has no benefit after 34 weeks of fetal gestation. However, O'Brien et al. (2000) have indicated that higher doses of dexamethasone (10 mg every 12 hours for 36 hours, as opposed to the regular 8 mg × 2 doses) may be of value in the presence of HELLP syndrome by improving platelet counts and liver function enzymes. Although not routinely practiced in the UK, such practice may be worthy of consideration if a woman's condition continues to deteriorate and may necessitate urgent delivery with a severely depleted platelet count.

Close monitoring post-delivery is needed to ensure that pathological changes due to the disorder revert to within normally expected ranges, such as effective diuresis, and that no further deterioration occurs. It has been recognised that within the postnatal phase, 30–40% of eclampsia cases develop (Douglas & Redman 1994; Chames et al. 2002) so vigilance is of the utmost importance. If blood pressure had been controlled in labour or for delivery, it may be prudent to continue antihypertensive therapy with medication such as oral labetalol (initially 200 mg daily but increased at intervals of 14 days up to 800 mg daily (BMA & Royal Pharmaceutical Society of Great Britain 2005).

Eclampsia

Eclampsia is the occurrence of convulsions during pregnancy or within 10 days of delivery in association with pre-eclampsia (Robson 2002) or convulsions in any woman who has, or who later presents with, hypertension in pregnancy

(Walker 2000). The convulsions are precipitated by cerebral ischaemia due to vasoconstricition and/or hypertensive encephalopathy. This is damage to the blood–brain barrier secondary to severe hypertension, which is associated with loss of cerebral autoregulation. There is pressure-driven extravasation of fluid resulting in cerebral oedema (Robson 2002). It is postulated that eclamptic convulsions in women with normal or mildly elevated blood pressure are likely to be due to cerebral ischaemia, while those in women with severe hypertension are more likely to be due to hypertensive encephalopathy (Robson 2002).

The incidence of eclampsia is approximately 1:2000 of all pregnancies (Douglas & Redman 1994; Katz et al. 2000). A study of all cases of eclampsia in the UK in 1992 ($n = 383$) found that nearly 1:50 (1.8%) women died and that 35% had at least one major complication. Preterm and antenatal eclampsia was associated with higher maternal complications and higher neonatal mortality (Douglas & Redman 1994).

Douglas and Redman's (1994) study found that 38% of seizures were antepartum, 18% were intrapartum and 44% occurred following delivery, with 12% of the postpartum cases occurring more than 48 hours after delivery and 2% more than 7 days after delivery. In contrast, a retrospective study of 53 pregnancies complicated by eclampsia in the USA (Katz et al. 2000) found that seizures occurred antepartum in 28 women (53%), intrapartum in 19 (36%) and postpartum in six (11%). The differences may be due to differences in the management of confirmed cases of pre-eclampsia, including timing of delivery, as removal of the placenta is the only recognised 'cure'.

The traditional view that pre-eclampsia progresses from a mild to a severe form and then on to eclampsia is questioned. In Katz et al.'s study, only 13% ($n = 7$) of women were considered to have severe pre-eclampsia before seizure, while seizure was the first sign of pre-eclampsia in 60% ($n = 32$). On the basis of this, and acknowledging that five women had no antenatal care and a further two had only one antenatal visit prior to seizure, Katz et al. (2000) suggest that rather than being a condition of worsening pre-eclampsia, eclampsia may be a cerebrovascular pathological condition. Similarly, Douglas and Redman (1994) found that in 43% of women, seizures occurred before both hypertension and proteinuria had been documented, while in 11% there was no recorded hypertension or proteinuria (although this included 13 women who had no antenatal care).

The recurrence rate of eclampsia in subsequent pregnancies is unknown, largely because the overall occurrence of the condition is so rare. However, APEC (2005b) suggest that one in 20 will develop pre-eclampsia in a subsequent pregnancy, with a higher risk factor for women who developed eclampsia relatively early in pregnancy.

Morbidity and mortality

Serious respiratory complications occur in up to 5% of women with eclampsia, coagulation problems in 10–15% and renal failure in 5–8% (Robson 2002). Renal failure is associated with haemorrhage and/or HELLP syndrome. Fetal morbidity relates mainly to preterm birth and growth restriction.

Although mortality and morbidity have fallen steadily over the last 30 years, hypertensive disorders remain a leading cause of direct maternal death (Lewis 2001, 2004). Exact cause of death can be difficult to determine as there may be multisystem failure (Robson 2002). Cerebral haemorrhage is the principal cause of death, but death may also result from cerebral infarction, cerebral oedema, pulmonary causes and renal or hepatic failure.

Care and management

Management of eclampsia is based upon the ability to manage the immediate fit and to avert further seizures. However, due to the uncertainty of the disorder, prediction is difficult as warning signs may not be portrayed prior to the onset of the seizure.

Immediate care of a woman with eclampsia should be based on basic ABC resuscitation guidelines (see Chapter 11) and suitable medication administered.

- Send for appropriate aid (Nursing and Midwifery Council 2004), resuscitation equipment and eclampsia medication. (Many units have implemented an 'eclampsia box' where appropriate medication is present and is easily portable to the room as required.)
- Remain with the woman.
- Maintain a patent *airway* and reduce the risk of aspiration. This may need to be achieved by removing the pillow, turning the woman's head to the left and clearing any mucus/vomit from the mouth and airway.
- *Breathing* needs to be assessed and post-seizure oxygen may be administered at 10 L/min to ensure adequate maternal (and fetal) oxygenation.
- Pulse oximetry may be appropriate to gain a visual value of maternal oxygenation. The oximetry probe will only offer clear recordings post seizure as good skin surface contact is required which may be difficult during the seizure.
- Prevent maternal injury – if the woman is in an area of danger, prompt moving of obstructions will be necessary thus preventing injury from other sources.
- *Circulation* – cardiac output needs to be observed and cardiopulmonary resuscitation commenced if the pulse rate is absent.
- If the woman has no venous access, cannulation needs to be urgently performed to enable bloods to be drawn and drugs to be administered.
- If the seizure occurs whilst the woman is pregnant, consideration needs to be paid to positioning post-seizure as aorta vena caval compression may occur. In such incidences, uterine displacement will need to be considered in the form of placing a wedge under the woman's right side of the back.

Seizure management

The control of convulsions was traditionally managed with either intravenous diazepam or phenytoin. However, the findings from recent scientific-based studies promote the fact that magnesium sulphate should be used for the prevention and treatment of seizures in women with severe pre-eclampsia or eclampsia (Eclampsia Trial Collaborative Group 1995) The Magpie trial findings (Magpie

Trial Collaborative Group 2002) proposed that the use of magnesium sulphate can reduce the incidence of eclampsia developing by half in women with pre-eclampsia. Nevertheless, the unwanted side effects from magnesium administration, such as nausea, vomiting, dizziness, hypotension or tachycardia (Magpie Trial Collaborative Group 2002), need to be explicitly explained to the woman prior to commencing therapy. This can allow true informed choice to be made and not simply to comply with the practitioners' wishes.

Therapy should be initiated with a seizure in the form of a bolus dose of magnesium sulphate 4 g given slowly over a 5–10-minute period. The action of magnesium sulphate is not clearly apparent. Belfort and Moise (1992) believe that the drug's action initiates vasodilatation and thus reduces the potential of cerebral ischaemia.

Prevention of further seizures

A continuing infusion of magnesium sulphate (1 g/h) is recommended by the Eclampsia Trial Collaborative Group (1995). Comparison against other anticonvulsant agents indicated that magnesium sulphate reduced the risk of recurrent seizures in excess of 50%, although within the confines of the study the results were not considered statistically significant.

Management of a seizure in a pregnant woman

If the woman is pregnant and experiences an eclamptic seizure, consideration needs to be paid to the following two points.

- *Assessment of fetal condition*. Evidence has been provided to substantiate the risks of maternal and fetal mortality and morbidity (Sibai 1996). Placental abruption has been recognised as occurring in almost one-quarter of eclamptic women. Clinical signs should be checked for, such as vaginal bleeding or fetal bradycardia. Post seizure a decision will be necessary regarding the need to deliver the fetus. The mode of delivery will depend upon fetal gestation, but should also consider maternal wishes.
- *Assessment of maternal condition*. HELLP syndrome and DIC are recognised conditions that may accompany the eclamptic disorder, thus blood sampling should be undertaken to confirm/refute the development or progress of either condition. Frequent maternal observations (every 15 minutes) should be undertaken with the use of magnesium sulphate to reduce the risk of magnesium toxicity occurring (see above). Urinary output should also be monitored hourly to ensure adequate renal function.

Postpartum management

It is recommended that the woman's lungs should be auscultated after the convulsion has ended to check for aspiration.

Close observation needs to be paid to the woman's condition, as 40% of eclamptic seizures have been noted to occur in the postnatal period (Douglas & Redman 1994). Magnesium sulphate should be continued for at least 24 hours post seizure as the theoretical risk of seizure decreases after 48 hours to 12% and then further by the end of a week to 2% (Royal College of Obstetricians and Gynaecologists 1999).

Skilful psychological care in the postnatal period is imperative as the experience may have been, or seemed to the partner to have been, traumatic. Explanations and justification may be required not only pertaining to maternal care but also to the neonate's condition.

HELLP syndrome

HELLP, an acronym for the complication of pregnancy which manifests itself as *h*aemolysis, *e*levated *l*iver enzymes and *l*ow *p*latelets, was introduced by Weinstein in 1982, although the condition was first described in three women with eclampsia in 1954 (Portis et al. 1997). HELLP syndrome is generally regarded as a variant of severe pre-eclampsia or eclampsia, which is associated with multisystemic dysfunction due to arterial vasospasm, endothelial damage and platelet aggregation (Nutt 1997). Maternal and fetal conditions can deteriorate rapidly and outcomes are generally poorer than for pre-eclampsia alone.

Sibai et al. (1986) comment upon the rate of occurrence (between 2 and 12%) and that maternal mortality has been estimated to be between 3.5 and 24%. Perinatal mortality ranges from 79 to 367 per 1000 live births (Portis et al. 1997). The wide variation in estimated mortality is due to the difficulties of diagnosis and differences of diagnostic criteria (Nutt 1997). Neonatal complications correlate with the severity of the maternal condition (Portis et al. 1997).

Physiopathology

Haemolysis

Haemolysis occurs as a result of vasospasm and endothelial damage. Platelets aggregate at the site of damage and fibrin deposits form. Fragmentation of red blood cells occurs as the cells are forced through the fibrin network at high pressure (Nutt 1997; Portis et al. 1997). However, the haemolysis is rarely sufficient to cause severe anaemia (Nelson-Piercy 2002).

Haemolysis is indicated by the presence of Burr cells (crenated and distorted red cells with spiny projections along the borders) and/or schistocytes (small, irregularly shaped red cell fragments), and a rise in bilirubin (> 1.2 mg/dl), SGOT (serum glutamic oxalo-acetic transaminase), SGPT (serum glutamic pyruvic transaminase) and lactate dehydrogenase (LDH). These are regarded as abnormal if they are more than 3 standard deviations (SD) above mean for the local laboratory (Sibai et al. 1993). Nutt (1997) suggests that there may also be a reduction in haematocrit.

Elevated liver enzymes

There is periportal or focal parenchymal necrosis, and hyaline deposits of fibrin-like material, multiple microthrombi and fibrin deposits in the sinusoids (Fraser & Caunt 1996). Obstruction of blood flow in the sinusoids causes liver distension, which leads to right upper quadrant pain. It is important to note that some women experience this as back pain. Liver enzymes are raised (Sibai et al. 1993), and hepatic failure and jaundice may occur, although rarely. In severe cases, spontaneous hepatic rupture may occur (Portis et al. 1997).

Low platelets

Low platelets appear to be due to increased peripheral vascular destruction in addition to increased platelet activation (Portis et al. 1997). Platelet levels are regarded as abnormal if less than $100 \times 10^9/L$, and severely abnormal if less than $50 \times 10^9/L$ (Sibai et al. 1993). Nutt (1997) suggests that unlike DIC, prothrombin time (PT), partial thromboplastin time and bleeding time usually remain normal.

Other pathophysiology

- Reduced renal blood flow and glomerular filtration
- Reduced cardiac output and increased vascular resistance
- Neurological involvement due to platelet and fibrin deposition, leading to headaches, cerebral oedema, seizures and stroke (Nutt 1997)

Predisposing factors and clinical features

Sibai et al. (1993) described 442 pregnancies complicated by HELLP syndrome. One in six women had pre-existing hypertension and a disproportionate number of women were white. Nutt (1997) suggests (although cites no evidence) that older, white multiparous women are most at risk.

Clinical features include the following (Sibai et al. 1993):

- Right upper quadrant or epigastric pain: 65%
- Nausea or vomiting: 36%
- Headache: 31%
- Visual changes: 10%
- Other: bleeding, jaundice, diarrhoea, weakness and fatigue

However, like pre-eclampsia, presentation may be very variable making initial diagnosis difficult. In some women the classic pre-eclamptic picture is absent (Portis et al. 1997). Sibai et al. (1993) found that 70% of all cases presented in pregnancy and 30% after delivery. From these statistics, 20% of women had neither hypertension nor proteinuria present before delivery.

Fraser and Caunt (1996) suggest that evidence of hepatic involvement should be sought in all women with severe pre-eclampsia through screening for hepatic enzymes, serum bilirubin, blood sugar, platelet count, coagulation studies and plasma protein levels (especially albumin).

Diagnostic testing

As the acronym suggests, HELLP relates to an altering blood picture: haemolysis (break down of red cells), elevated liver enzyme levels and a low platelet count.

To summarise, the laboratory criteria for confirming the presence of the syndrome are:

- A total bilirubin level of > 1.2 mg/dl and a lactate dehydrogenase level of > 600 U/L for the haemolysis aspect.
- Elevated liver function tests, for example a serum aspartate aminotransferase level of > 70 µg/L.
- A level of < 100×10^9/L may indicate a falling platelet count. Any further reductions in the level should be observed for.

Care and management

Prompt intervention is required with the detection of HELLP syndrome. Management is similar to that of severe pre-eclampsia with regard to stabilising the woman's condition and preparing for fetal delivery. Blood pressure and seizure control with appropriate fluid balance should be the primary goal of managing HELLP syndrome.

Attention needs to be paid to the potential differential diagnosis of acute fatty liver of pregnancy (AFLP) where the symptoms may be similar (pain, nausea and vomiting, reduced urine output) yet the blood results will indicate differing values depending upon the disorder. For example, it would be expected that in HELLP syndrome a normal PT would be present, as opposed to AFLP where the PT is increased. Jaundice would not be expected for HELLP syndrome yet could be present with AFLP (Witlin & Sibai 1999). It is crucial that a correct diagnosis is made to allow accurate and effective management of care to take place.

The presence of a subcapsular haematoma of the liver will need to be looked for. Clewell (1997) clarifies the signs of a haematoma as severe epigastric or right upper quadrant abdominal pain, or an unexplained hypotension. Such signs may indicate the potential of hepatic capsule rupture, thus emergency surgery will be necessary to prevent maternal mortality and morbidity.

Antepartum management

- Stabilise the maternal condition.
- Make a decision regarding fetal maturity and planned management. If > 34 weeks' gestation, delivery will generally be expedited. However, if fetal gestation is < 34 weeks, steroids to accelerate fetal lung maturity will need to be considered.
- Delivery of the fetus.

Postpartum management

Close monitoring needs to be continued to detect any further deviations of the maternal condition.

Complications of HELLP syndrome

Maternal complications may include:

- Progressive DIC: 21%
- Placental abruption: 16%
- Acute renal failure: 8%
- Acute pulmonary oedema
- Pleural effusions
- Cerebral oedema
- Subcapsular liver haematoma
- Liver rupture
- Acute respiratory distress syndrome

Severe cases of HELLP syndrome can have features of multiorgan failure (Sibai et al., cited by Fraser & Caunt 1996).

Neonatal complications include death due to placental infarction, placental abruption, intrauterine growth restriction, asphyxia and preterm birth. Thrombocytopenia and leukopenia occur in 25–30% (Portis et al. 1997).

Conclusion

There is an increased likelihood of pre-eclampsia developing in subsequent pregnancies, which may be as high as 75% if there is pre-existing hypertension. However, the risk of recurrence of HELLP syndrome is much lower at 3–5% (Nelson-Piercy 2002).

It is of utmost importance that midwives recognise, refer and record their actions in relation to the detection of any degree of hypertensive disorder in pregnancy. Once detected, the aim is to prevent any alteration or deterioration in the maternal condition that could cause maternal/fetal mortality and morbidity. By working in collaboration with the multidisciplinary team to ensure that evidence-based practice is implemented, and by using clear guidelines, policies and procedures, best possible care can be made available to the woman and reduce the risk of causing harm.

References

Abalos, E., Duley, L., Steyn, D. and Henderson-Smart, D. (2001) Antihypertensive drug therapy for mild to moderate hypertension during pregnancy. *Cochrane Database of Systematic Reviews*, Issue 2.

Action on Pre-eclampsia (APEC) (2005a) *About Pre-eclampsia*. Action on Pre-eclampsia, London (also available at http://www.apec.org.uk).

APEC (2005b) *Eclampsia*. Action on Pre-eclampsia, London (also available at http://www.apec.org.uk).

Belfort, M. and Moise, K. (1992) The effect of $MgSO_4$ on brain flow in pre-eclampsia: a randomised placebo-controlled study. *American Journal of Obstetrics and* Gynaecology, **167**: 661–6.

Bennett, P. (1994) Pre eclampsia II: the midwife and detection. *Modern Midwife*, **Oct**: 20–22.

Bennett, P. (1995) Pre eclampsia IV: the midwife's role after diagnosis. *Modern Midwife*, **Jan**: 25–6.

Bird, J. (1997) Intensive care problems in obstetric patients. *Care of the Critically Ill*, **13** (6): 241–4.

Briley, A., Chappell, L., Kelly, F., Shennan, A. and Poston, L. (2001) The vitamins in pre eclampsia study. *Midwives*, **4** (9): 288–91.

British Medical Association (BMA) and Royal Pharmaceutical Society of Great Britain (2005) *British National Formulary*, No. 49. BMA and Royal Pharmaceutical Society of Great Britain, London.

Brown, M., Buddle, M., Farrell, T., Davis, G. and Jones, M. (1998) Randomised trial of management of hypertensive pregnancies by Korotkoff phase IV or phase V. *Lancet*, **352** (9130): 777–81.

Chames, M.C., Livingstone, J.C., Ivester, T.S., Barton, J.R. and Sibai, B.M. (2002) Late postpartum eclampsia: a preventable disease? *American Journal of Obstetrics and Gynecology*, **186**: 1174–7.

Chernecky, C. and Berger, B. (2001) *Laboratory Tests and Diagnostic Procedures* (3rd edn). W.B. Saunders, Philadelphia.

Clewell, W. (1997) Hypertensive emergencies in pregnancy. In: M. Foley and T. Strong (Eds) *Obstetric Intensive Care: A practical manual*. W.B. Saunders, Philadelphia.

Cotton, D., Gonik, B. and Dorman, K. (1985) Cardiovascular alterations in severe pregnancy induced hypertension seen with intravenously given hydralazine bolus. *Surgery, Gynecology and Obstetrics*, **161**: 240–44.

Davies, L., Waugh, J. and Kilby, M. (2002) Assessing proteinuria in hypertensive pregnancy. *British Journal of Midwifery*, **10** (7): 441–5.

Dekker, G. and Sibai, B. (2001) Primary, secondary and tertiary prevention of pre-eclampsia. *Lancet*, **357**: 209–21.

Dekker, G. and Walker, J. (1997) Maternal assessment in pregnancy induced hypertensive disorders. In: J. Walker and N. Gant (Eds) *Hypertension in Pregnancy*. Chapman & Hall, Oxford.

Douglas, K. and Redman, C. (1994) Eclampsia in the UK. *British Medical Journal*, **309**: 1395–400.

Duley, L. (2003) Pre eclampsia and the hypertensive disorders of pregnancy. *British Medical Bulletin*, **67**: 161–76.

Duley, L., Gulmezoglu, A. and Henderson-Smart, D. (2003) Magnesium sulphate and other anticonvulsants for women with pre-eclampsia. *Cochrane Database of Systematic Reviews*, Issue 2.

Eclampsia Trial Collaborative Group (1995) Which anticonvulsant for women with eclampsia? Evidence from the collaborative eclampsia trial. *Lancet*, **345**: 1455.

Fraser, R. and Caunt, A. (1996) The HELLP syndrome. *Care of the Critically Ill*, **12** (6): 188–9.

Fugate, S. and Chow, G. (2004) Eclampsia. http://www.emedicine.com/med/topic633.htm

Hankey G., Eikelboom J., Khoon Ho W. and van Bockxmeer F. (2004) *Clinical usefulness of plasma homocysteine in vascular disease*. http://www.mja.com.au/public/issues/181_06_200904/han10269_fm.html

Higgins, H. and de Swiet, M. (2001) Blood pressure measurement and classification in pregnancy. *Lancet*, **357**: 131–5.

Katz, V., Farmer, R. and Kuller, J. (2000) Preeclampsia into eclampsia: toward a new paradigm. *American Journal of Obstetrics and Gynecology*, **182** (6): 1389–96.

Khurana, R. and Graham, D. (1999) Managing hypertensive disorders in pregnancy. *Womans Health Primary Care*, **2**: 559.

Larrabee, K. and Monga, M. (1997) Women with sickle cell trait are at increased risk for preeclampsia. *American Journal of Obstetrics and Gynecology*, **177** (2): 425–8.

Levine, R., Ewell, M., Hauth, J., Curet, L., Catalano, P. and Morris, C. (2000) Should the definition of preeclampsia include a rise in diastolic blood pressure >/= 15 mmHg to a level < 90 mmHg in association with proteinuria? *American Journal of Obstetrics and Gynecology*, **183**: 787–92.

Lewis, G. (2001) *Why Mothers Die 1997–1999: The Confidential Enquiries into Maternal Deaths in the United Kingdom.* Royal College of Obstetricians and Gynaecologists (RCOG) Press, London.

Lewis, G. (2004) *Why Mothers Die 2000–2002: Report on Confidential Enquiries into Maternal Deaths in the United Kingdom.* RCOG Press, London.

Lim, K., Friedman, S., Ecker, J., Kao, L. and Kilpatrick, S. (1998) The clinical utility of serum uric acid measurements in hypertensive disease of pregnancy. *American Journal of Obstetrics and Gynaecology*, **178**: 1067–71.

Magee, L., Cham, C., Waterman, E., Ohlsson, A. and von Dadelszen, P. (2003) Hydralazine for treatment of severe hypertension in pregnancy: meta analysis. *British Medical Journal*, **327**: 955.

Magee, L., Ornstein, M. and von Dadelszen, P. (1999) Management of hypertension in pregnancy. *British Medical Journal*, **318**: 1332–6.

Magpie Trial Collaborative Group (2002) Do women with pre eclampsia and their babies, benefit from magnesium sulphate? The Magpie trial: a randomised placebo-controlled trial. *Lancet*, **359**: 1877–90.

Mattar, F. and Sibai, B. (2000) Eclampsia: risk factors for maternal morbidity. *American Journal of Obstetrics and Gynecology*, **182** (2): 307–12.

McKay, K. (1999) Biochemical and blood tests in midwifery practice (1): Pre-eclampsia. *Practising Midwife*, **2** (8): 28–31.

Mosby (1986) *Mosby's Medical and Nursing Dictionary.* Mosby, St Louis.

National High Blood Pressure Education Program Working Group (1990) Report on high blood pressure in pregnancy. *American Journal of Obstetrics and Gynecology*, **163**: 1691–712.

Nelson-Piercy, C. (2002) *Handbook of Obstetric Medicine.* Martin Dunitz, London.

North, R., Taylor, R. and Schellenberg, J. (1999) Evaluation of a definition of pre-eclampsia. *British Journal of Obstetrics and Gynaecology*, **106** (8): 767–73.

Nursing and Midwifery Council (2004) *Midwives Rules and Standards.* Nursing and Midwifery Council (NMC), London.

Nutt, J. (1997) HELLP syndrome. *British Journal of Midwifery*, **5** (1): 8–11.

O'Brien, J.M., Milligan, D.A. and Barton, J.R. (2000) Impact of high-dose corticosteroid therapy for patients with HELLP syndrome. *American Journal of Obstetrics and Gynaecology*, **183** (4): 921–4.

Odendaal, H. (2001) Severe preeclampsia and eclampsia. In: B. Sibai (Ed.) *Hypertensive Disorders in Women.* W.B. Saunders, Philadelphia.

Portis, R., Jacobs, M., Skerman, J. and Skerman, E. (1997) HELLP syndrome (hemolysis, elevated liver enzymes, and low platelets) pathophysiology and anesthetic considerations. *Journal of the American Association of Nurse Anesthetists*, **65** (1): 37–47.

Redman, C. (1994) Pre-eclampsia: still a difficult disease. *Professional Care of Mother and Child*, **Jan/Feb**: 7–9.

Redman, C., Sacks, G. and Sargent, I. (1999) Preeclampsia: an excessive maternal inflammatory response. *American Journal of Obstetrics and Gynecology*, **180** (2): 499–506.

Roberts, J. and Cooper, D. (2001) Pathogenesis and genetics of pre-eclampsia. *Lancet*, **357**: 53–6.

Robson, S. (2002) Pre eclampsia and eclampsia. In: A. MacLean and J. Neilson (Eds) *Maternal Morbidity and Mortality.* RCOG Press, London.

Royal College of Obstetricians and Gynaecologists (1999) *Management of Eclampsia Clinical Guideline.* RCOG Press, London.

Rubin, P. (1996) Measuring diastolic blood pressure in pregnancy. *British Medical Journal,* **313** (7048): 4–5.

Saudan, P., Brown, M., Farrell, T. and Shaw, L. (1997) Improved methods of assessing proteinuria in hypertensive pregnancy. *British Journal of Obstetrics and Gynaecology,* **104** (10): 1159–64.

Seidel, H. (2002) *Mosby's Guide to Physical Examination.* Mosby, St Louis.

Shennan, A., Gupta, M., Halligan, A., Taylor, D. and de Swiet, M. (1996) Lack of reproducibility in pregnancy Korotkoff phase IV as measured by mercury sphygmomanometer. *Lancet,* **347**: 399–42.

Sibai, B. (1996) Treatment of hypertension in pregnant women. *New England Journal of Medicine,* **335**: 257.

Sibai, B. (2003) Diagnosis and management of gestational hypertension and preeclampsia. *Obstetrics and Gynecology,* **102**: 181–92.

Sibai, B., Lipshitz, J., Anderson, G., and Dilts, P. (1981) Reassessment of intravenous magnesium sulphate therapy in pre eclampsia–eclampsia. *Obstetrics and Gynaecology,* **57**: 199–202.

Sibai, B., Ramadan, M., Usta, I., Salama, M., Mercer, B. and Friedman, S. (1993) Maternal morbidity and mortality in 442 pregnancies with hemolysis, elevated liver enzymes, and low platelets (HELLP syndrome). *American Journal of Obstetrics and Gynecology,* **169**: 1000–1006.

Sibai, B., Taslimi, M., el-Nazer, A. et al. (1986) Maternal perinatal outcome associated with the syndrome of hemolysis, elevated liver enzymes and low platelets in severe pre eclampsia. *American Journal of Obstetrics and Gynecology,* **15** (5): 501–9.

Stamilio, D., Sehdev, H., Morgan, M., Propert, K. and Macones, G. (2000) Can antenatal clinical and biochemical markers predict the development of severe preeclampsia? *American Journal of Obstetrics and Gynecology,* **182**: 589–94.

Waisman, G., Mayorga, L., Camera, M., Vignolo, C. and Martinotti, A. (1988) Magnesium plus nifedipine: potential of hypotensive effect in preeclampsia. *American Journal of Obstetrics and Gynecology,* **159**: 308–309.

Walker, J. (2000) Pre eclampsia. *Lancet,* **356** (9237): 1260–65.

Warden, M. and Earle, B. (2005) Pre eclampsia (toxemia of pregnancy). www.emedicine.co/med/topic1905.htm

Wells, B., Dipiro, J., Schwinghammer, T. and Hamilton, C. (2002) *Pharmacotherapy Handbook.* Appleton & Lange, Connecticut.

Witlin, A. & Sibai, B. (1999) Diagnosis and management of women with hemolysis, elevated liver enzymes and low platelet count (HELLP) syndrome. *Hospital* Physician, **Feb**: 40–45, 49.

Further reading

Broughton Pipkin, F. (1995) Fortnightly review: the hypertensive disorders of pregnancy. *British Medical Journal,* **311**: 609–13.

Brown, M., Buddle, M., Farrell, T., Davis, G. and Jones, M. (1998) Randomised trial of management of hypertensive pregnancies by Korotkoff phase IV or phase V. *Lancet,* **352**: 777–81.

Brown, M., Reiter, L., Smith, B., Buddle, M., Morris, R. and Whitworth, J. (1994) Measuring blood pressure in pregnant women: a comparison of direct and indirect methods. *American Journal of Obstetrics and Gynecology,* **171**: 661–7.

Chesley, L. (1978) *Hypertensive disorders in pregnancy* Appleton Century Crofts, New York.

Egerman, R. and Sibai, B. (2001) Preconception counselling for women with a history of hypertensive disorders. In: B. Sabai (Ed.) *Hypertensive Disorders in Women*. W.B. Saunders, Philadelphia.

Green, L. and Fromen, R. (1996) Blood pressure measurement during pregnancy: auscultatory versus oscillatory methods. *Journal of Obstetric, Gynecology and Neonatal Nursing*, **25**: 155.

Nisell, H., Lintu, H., Lunell, N., Mollerstrom, G. and Pettersson, E. (1995) Blood pressure and renal function seven years after pregnancy complicated by hypertension. *British Journal of Obstetrics and Gynaecology*, **102**: 876–81.

O'Brien, E., Waeber, B., Parati, G., Staessen, J. and Myers, M. (2001) Blood pressure measuring devices: recommendations of the European Society of Hypertension. *British Medical Journal*, **322**: 531–6.

Raftery, E. and Ward, A. (1968) The indirect method of recording blood pressure. *Cardiovascular Research*, **2**: 210–18.

Royal College of Obstetricians and Gynaecologists (1999) *Antenatal Corticosteriods to Prevent Respiratory Distress Syndrome*. Guideline No. 7. RCOG, London.

Zuspan, F. (1999) Chronic hypertension. In: J. Queenan and J. Hobbins (Eds) *Protocols for High Risk Pregnancies* (3rd edn). Blackwell Science, Oxford.

7 Haemorrhagic Disorders and the Critically Ill Woman

Dianne Steele

This chapter concerns the midwife's role and responsibilities in the care and management of women where massive haemorrhage occurs. Antepartum and primary postpartum haemorrhage are addressed.

Massive obstetric haemorrhage ranks in the top three causes of maternal death in the United Kingdom, the number of deaths from haemorrhage being 8.5 per million maternities in the period 2000–2002 compared to 9.3 per million maternities in 1988–1990 (Lewis 2004). Although the statistical evidence demonstrates a reduction which may be attributed to better midwifery and obstetric care, a percentage of cases were associated with substandard care. Seventeen maternal deaths were reported, with seven deaths attributed to antepartum events (four placenta praevia and three placental abruption) and ten postpartum. Trends reported in the current Confidential Enquiry in into Maternal Deaths (CEMD) (Lewis 2004) that may be associated with haemorrhage in childbearing women are:

- Rise in mean maternal age
- Rise in the number of women becoming pregnant with complex medical disorders
- Rise in the number of multiple pregnancies due to assisted reproduction
- Rise in the number of caesarean sections leading to more cases of placenta praevia or accreta
- Maternal refusal of blood products

Assumed prior knowledge

- The physiological processes of separation and expulsion of the placenta, cord and fetal membranes
- Care and management during active and physiological third stage of labour

- Associated causes of ante- and postpartum haemorrhage
- Normal blood-clotting processes

Background

Definition

There appears to be no agreed definition for major ante- and postpartum haemorrhage with respect to quantity. However a range of 1000–2500 ml blood loss was reported by Mousa and Alfirevic (2003) and reflects the response within the United Kingdom. The working definition of antepartum haemorrhage (APH) is not disputed and is defined as 'bleeding from the genital tract at any time after the 24th week of pregnancy until the baby is born' (Tiran 2004, p. 13). Primary postpartum haemorrhage (PPH) is considered to be 'excessive bleeding from the genital tract from the birth of the baby and up to 24 hours following the birth' (Tiran 2004, p. 205). There is no consensus for a working definition where the term 'massive' or 'catastrophic' is used, nor the quantity of blood loss contributed to APH.

Incidence

Data on the incidence of antepartum and postpartum haemorrhage is difficult to determine since no national survey has been completed. A survey of maternity units in the United Kingdom by Mousa and Alfirevic (2003) missed the opportunity to establish national PPH rates. When considering risk management within local maternity units, incidence rates are helpful when considering best practice. Equally, publishing this data could be beneficial when comparing practices, particularly for high-risk cases.

Aetiology/pathophysiology

Normal changes in haemostasis

Healthy pregnant women can tolerate a blood loss of up to 1000 ml due to the physiological adaptations in pregnancy. These changes include an increase in plasma volume and red cell mass. Alterations in the haematological system and homeostasis are vital for the childbearing woman to tolerate normal blood loss at delivery. These adaptations also prevent excessive bleeding during and after placental separation. A blood loss of between 500 and 1000 ml is well tolerated by women, with minimal changes in blood pressure and heart rate (Duffy 1999).

During labour, haemoglobin levels rise due to haemoconcentration. This is partly due to an increase in erythropoiesis due a stress response, muscular action and dehydration. Clotting factors also increase during labour. This rise is attributed to the increase of thromboplastin in the placenta and decidua. The release of thromboplastin during placental separation activates coagulation via the extrinsic system. The concentration of clotting factors and a reduction in prothrombin time during placental separation assists in the clotting at the placental site. Correspondingly, the levels of fibringogen and plasminogen decrease due to the increase in their utilisation after the placenta has separated. Equally, clotting factors V and VIII increase and contribute to the clotting activity via the extrinsic system. Given the haematological changes during labour, Greer et al. (1991) recommend that all women with congenital coagulopathies should be managed in specialist units with access to haematological and haemophilia services.

Following labour and delivery, fibrinolytic activity reduces further. This reduction of activity allows the formation of small clots at the placental site and the deposit of fibrin forms a mesh over the placental site. Hathaway and Bonnar (1987) estimated about 5–10% of the total available fibrin is utilised at this site. The rise in fibrin degradation products (FDP) following delivery potentially gives rise to complications when haemostasis is not achieved. However, for the majority of childbearing women, the increase in FDPs is tolerated. The increase in FDPs can interfere with the formation of fibrin mesh at the placental site thus predisposing women to bleed from this site. The increased consumption of platelets by about 20% (Gerbasi 1990), due to clotting at the placental site, does not compromise the childbearing woman, given the physiological increase during pregnancy.

Generally the ability to hypercoagulate in the intrapartum phase enables the childbearing woman to cope with haemorrhage and an initial excessive blood loss around the time of delivery. The woman's ability to react to achieve haemostasis following the delivery of the placenta is only achieved because of the haemodynamic changes occurring during pregnancy and labour.

Predisposing/risk factors

When employing risk assessment strategies, an increasing number of women book and birth in consultant-led units where facilities are available to support them during a critical phase. Whilst midwives and obstetricians can anticipate predisposing factors, a number of women will present with a massive haemorrhage simply because they have never been tested.

Often it is the midwife who is best placed to recognise deviations and summon help in the early phase of profuse bleeding. The midwife's ability to initiate prompt treatment can prevent further manifestation of catastrophic haemorrhage (Stables & Rankin 2005).

The anticipation of haemorrhage can be identified through risk management processes and retrospective studies. Predisposing factors are reliant on the reporting of incidences, risk factors and associated complications. The reliance on mortality data is useful but 'near miss' cases are not widely reported. Recently the CEMDs reports in the United Kingdom (Lewis 2001, 2004) have included chapters on 'near miss' reporting.

When considering the causes and predisposing factors for haemorrhage these are confined to antepartum and primary postpartum haemorrhage.

Antepartum haemorrhage

The causes of APH are attributed to:

- Placenta praevia
- Placental abruption
- Other causes may be associated with extraplacental bleeding such as cervical erosions or polyps

Placenta praevia

Placenta praevia is where the placental location occurs in the lower uterine segment and/or borders the upper and lower uterine segment of the uterus. Placental location is graded according to its location within the uterus and is confirmed by ultrasound scan. Inevitably when uterine contractions commence, placental separation occurs and bleeding commences from the placental site. As the lower uterine segment is void of oblique muscles, the muscle is unable to contract and retract to seal the blood vessels and stem bleeding. The amount of blood loss is variable and unpredictable and therefore the risk of torrential haemorrhage is possible. Therefore, the reporting of placental location is noted on ultrasound scanning as part of the current antenatal screening provision. The possible causes are reported in Box 7.1.

Placental abruption

Placental abruption is where the placenta separates from the uterine wall before the birth of the baby and occurs before the onset of labour as well as during labour. Uterine bleeding may be revealed, concealed or mixed depending on the degree of placental detachment. The contributing causes are reported in Box 7.1.

Postpartum haemorrhage

The predisposing factors for PPH are related to:

- The failure of the myometrial muscles to contract and retract in order to arrest bleeding during and after placental separation
- Trauma to structures within the genital tract
- Coagulation disorders

Risks are noted in Box 7.1.

Placental location and separation

The sequence of placental separation has been studied using Doppler sonography and provides a better understanding of the mechanisms involved in the third stage of labour (Herman 2000). The location of the placenta is relevant to the time it takes for the placenta to separate. Lurie et al. (2003), using ultrasound, noted the

---

Box 7.1   Risk factors for antepartum and postpartum haemorrhage.

Antepartum haemorrhage	Postpartum haemorrhage	Contributing factors
Placenta praevia:	Previous history	Hypertensive disease
Multiparity	Previous retained	Use of tocolytic drugs
Multiple pregnancy	placenta	in preterm labour
Previous hysterotomy,	Current retained	Induced and
myomectomy, caesarean	placenta	augmented labours
section(s)	Large placental site	Clotting disorders
Bipartite placentae	Overdistension of	Instrumental delivery
Succenturiate placentae	uterus:	Disseminated
Enlarged placentae,	polyhydramnios, fetal	intravascular
associated with smoking	macrosomia	coagulation (DIC)
Increasing maternal age	Antepartum	Severe anaemia
	haemorrhage	Amniotic fluid
Placental abruption:	Prolonged labour	embolism
Maternal hypertension	Uterine fibroids	General anaesthesia
Trauma following external	Uterine infection	Mismanagement of
cephalic version	Inversion of uterus	third stage of labour
Trauma to the abdomen	Atony of uterine	Abdominal
Overdistension of uterus	muscles	pregnancy (rare)
with rupture of fetal	Genital tract trauma	
membranes	Chance	
Previous history		
Smoking		
Drug misuse		
(cocaine, crack)		
Chance		

---

third stage of labour was significantly longer if the placenta was located in the fundal area of the uterus. The location of the placenta may therefore assist in the recognition of third stage complications.

Uterine atony

Evidence suggests most cases of PPH are caused by uterine atony and associated with prolonged labour (Jouppila 1995). Haemorrhage is associated with manual removal of the placenta and the likelihood of occurrence is reduced with increasing gestational age (Dombrowski et al. 1995). Maternal soft-tissue injury is associated with the delivery of macrosomic babies (Lim et al. 2002), but equally their births may be complicated by difficult delivery of the shoulders, or instrumental and operative delivery. Coulter-Smith et al. (1996) noted a trend towards a greater chance of haemorrhage in parous women and previous caesarean section when studying the case notes following maternal deaths. Trauma linked with instrumental delivery has been disputed in two retrospective studies (Herabutya et al. 1988; Weerasekera 2002), the results revealing no significant difference in degree of soft-tissue trauma or PPH. Advanced maternal age, pre-eclampsia and obesity have also been cited as contributing factors to postpartum bleeding (Joippila 1995).

When summarising the predisposing factors, many women who experience a haemorrhage do so without any pre-existing cause, and occurrence purely by 'chance' still remains a phenomenon.

Clinical presentation

Hypovolaemic shock will present in an otherwise healthy childbearing woman when the intravascular circulating blood volume falls. A blood loss of up to 1 L is well tolerated. If fluids are not replaced or the cause of bleeding is not arrested the symptoms of hypovolaemic shock will intensify. A fall in blood pressure indicates a serious physiological event despite the body's attempt to compensate for blood loss from the cardiovascular system. The presenting symptoms include a weak tachycardic pulse diminishing in strength. The rise in the heart rate is related to the sudden surge of catecholamines produced by the adrenal glands. Catecholamines directly increase the heart rate and the vascular resistance of the blood vessels, thus attempting to increase the circulating blood volume to the vital organs. However, the uterus is not a vital organ and a pregnant woman may lose 1200–1500 ml of blood before changes in maternal vital signs indicate hypovolaemia, although the fetus will show signs of compromise (Advanced Life Support in Obstetrics 2000).

In order for the body to increase its falling circulatory volume, fluid moves from the interstitial spaces into the vascular space. Depending on the degree of blood loss and the movement of interstitial fluid, this often cannot be sustained for long before the woman becomes symptomatic.

A further attempt is made by the body to reinstate blood volume by ejecting stored red blood cells and plasma from the spleen and liver back into the circulatory system. Equally the body attempts to conserve water and sodium levels by increasing production of renin from the kidneys, which incites aldosterone production. In turn, aldosterone activity stimulates water retention and increases plasma volume, thereby increasing blood pressure.

The physiological events cause the capillaries and small blood vessels to constrict, forcing blood away from the skin back to the major organs. In childbearing women this is usually accompanied by alterations in pallor, restlessness and air hunger, all of which are symptoms of falling oxygen. These latter symptoms relate to the further deterioration in cell metabolism.

The quantity of blood seen may not reveal the true clinical picture, as unrevealed blood loss is unquantifiable. Therefore, the early signs of hypovolaemic shock are useful markers for the midwife to note in order to implement immediate action.

Care and management

The main goal is to restore the collapse within the circulatory system. Midwives are best placed to undertake venous cannulation in order to expedite commencement of prescribed crystalloid and colloid fluids.

The monitoring of vital signs has advanced with the advent of continuous electronic monitoring equipment which, if available, must be used. Criticism in failing to use equipment was a contributory factor for one maternal death:

> "Clinical detection of post-operative cyanosis may have been difficult as she had dark skin. She would clearly have benefited from pulse oximetry." (Department of Health 1996, p. 89)

The midwife requires knowledge of obstetric management in order to provide the necessary midwifery care. This includes the use of contemporary drugs (see below) noting the dosage, route and side effects. Equally, where medical treatment fails, surgical intervention is required. The midwife needs to be equipped with the necessary knowledge to anticipate procedures suggested by Tamizian and Arulkumaran (2002), such as aortic compression, embolisation techniques, uterine compression sutures and procedures such as uterine tamponade. The possibility of hysterectomy should be considered in severe cases. Midwifery support is vital not only for the woman and her family, but also in providing key support to obstetricians when faced with life-threatening events.

Guidance for the management for massive haemorrhage is available (Department of Health 1994; Lewis 2001, 2004) and all maternity units should have protocols in place to deal with such emergencies. Subsequent authors have disseminated good practice and templates for units to construct their own protocols (Macphail & Fitzgerald 2001). Midwives should be familiar with these protocols, and Hutchon and Martin (2002) propose that familiarity and rehearsal of protocols with designated staff would test the robustness of such protocols and may contribute to the reduction of near misses and maternal deaths.

The initial assessment of visible blood loss and the reference to the woman's physical response does not change the midwife's actions – whether bleeding is profuse, massive or catastrophic, the initiation of action must be unprompted.

If antepartum haemorrhage presents the midwife should:

- Call medical and additional midwifery assistance
- Assess and record maternal vital signs
- Assess and treat associated pain to reduce neurogenic shock
- Assess and record fetal wellbeing
- Palpate the abdomen noting any tenderness and consistency
- Gain intravenous access at two sites for drug administration and fluid replacement
- Obtain venous blood for coagulation screen, blood group and cross-match
- Prepare and assist the woman for ultrasound scan
- Catheterise the urinary bladder

Depending on the diagnosis and proposed management by the obstetric team, the midwife may need to consider preparing the woman for surgery under general anaesthesia to deliver the baby and placenta, and possibly further measures to control bleeding. The midwife should refer to hospital policy for preoperative care, ensuring antacids are given prior to surgery. Examination per vaginam should never be performed as this may increase bleeding in cases where the placenta is sited near the cervical os.

In cases of postpartum haemorrhage, prompt action could arrest bleeding and prevent further blood loss (Fig. 7.1). The actions of the midwife should be to:

- Call medical and additional midwifery assistance
- Assess uterine contractility
- Determine if the bleeding is uterine or due to trauma
- Administer oxytocic drugs (including Syntocinon 40 iu i.v. in 500 ml Hartmann's solution) if the cause is uterine
- Apply pressure and prepare for suturing if the cause is trauma
- Gain intravenous access for drug administration and fluid replacement
- Obtain venous blood for coagulation screen, blood group and cross-match

The midwife should anticipate probable blood screening such as:

- Full blood count with platelets and fibrin degradation products
- Prothrombin time
- Partial thromboplastin time and thrombin time and fibrinogen titre
- Blood group and rhesus factor for cross-matching of blood

Clotting studies will determine the best fluid replacement, which is prescribed by the anaesthetist in collaboration with the haematologist and obstetrician.

It is advocated in the early stages of management to secure intravenous access using 16 G cannulae in no less than two sites to enable maximum and quick delivery of crystalloid and colloid fluids. Where severe blood loss is anticipated, or has occurred, then the siting of the central venous pressure (CVP) line by an anaesthetist should be standard practice in order to monitor fluid balance.

The initial assessment by the midwife detailed in Fig. 7.1, enables prompt action, relay of information to medics and anticipation of appropriate treatment. It also enables the midwife to assess the condition of the woman, through assessment of measured blood loss and observing whether or not clotting of blood continues.

Summoning appropriate staff, such as the consultant obstetrician, anaesthetist and haematologist, is seen as good practice. In addition, notifying other workers such as theatre staff, porters and blood transfusion service prepares all for impending care. The assessment of the placenta and membranes will determine its degree of completeness, and the measure of blood loss by volume and weight will assist in the estimation of blood loss.

Drug management for postpartum haemorrhage

Myometrial contractility is vital for the successful delivery of the placenta and the arrest of subsequent haemorrhage, and in the majority of births this is successfully achieved. However, there is evidence that the use of ergotic drugs since their

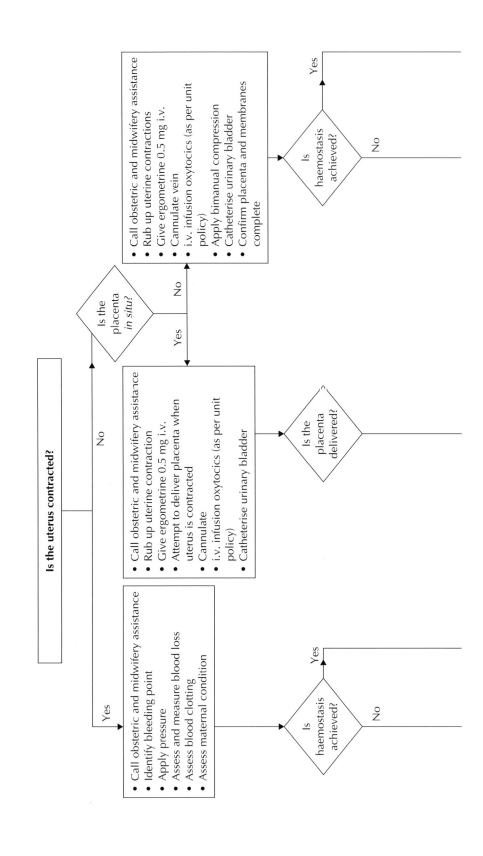

Is the uterus contracted?

Yes

- Call obstetric and midwifery assistance
- Identify bleeding point
- Apply pressure
- Assess and measure blood loss
- Assess blood clotting
- Assess maternal condition

Is haemostasis achieved?

Yes / No

No

Is the placenta *in situ?*

Yes / No

Yes:
- Call obstetric and midwifery assistance
- Rub up uterine contraction
- Give ergometrine 0.5 mg i.v.
- Attempt to deliver placenta when uterus is contracted
- Cannulate
- i.v. infusion oxytocics (as per unit policy)
- Catheterise urinary bladder

Is the placenta delivered?

No:
- Call obstetric and midwifery assistance
- Rub up uterine contractions
- Give ergometrine 0.5 mg i.v.
- Cannulate vein
- i.v. infusion oxytocics (as per unit policy)
- Apply bimanual compression
- Catheterise urinary bladder
- Confirm placenta and membranes complete

Is haemostasis achieved?

Yes / No

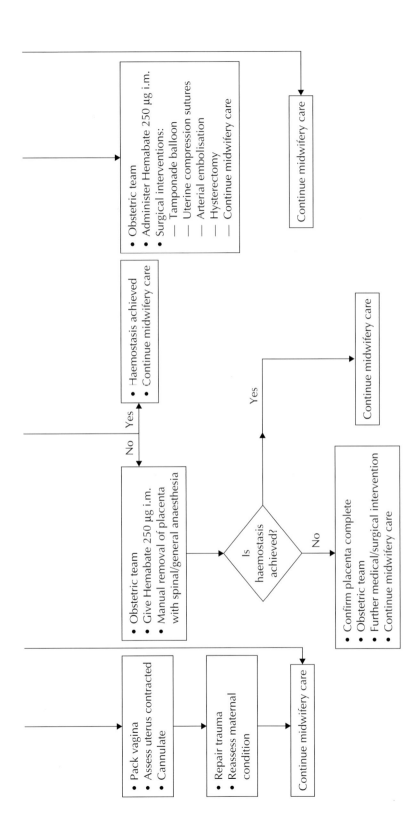

Figure 7.1 Midwifery management and primary postpartum haemorrhage.

introduction in the 1930s by Chassar Moir (Dunn 2002) has reduced morbidity and mortality rates amongst childbearing women. Equally, drug management is one contributing element in reducing maternal mortality in the United Kingdom (Lewis 2004). The use of oxytocin with or without ergometrine has been beneficial in reducing and arresting PPH. However, these drugs are not without side effects and there is increasing interest in the use of prostaglandins such as misoprostol in the management of the third stage. This section will examine the evidence as to which is the best pharmacological choice to reduce PPH.

A comparison study by Soriano et al. (1996) was conducted to determine the efficacy of intramuscular oxytocin 5 iu plus ergometrine 0.5 mg (Syntometrine) versus intravenous oxytocin (Syntocinon 10 iu) in preventing PPH. The findings confirmed the use of oxytocin is as effective as Syntometrine; however, the reported maternal side effects were less in the oxytocic group (7.2%) compared with the Syntometrine group (22.9%). The side effects included elevated blood pressure, nausea, vomiting, chest pain and excessive sweating. Similar findings have been reported by McDonald et al. (1993). A Cochrane review (McDonald et al. 2003), noted that the routine use of combined oxytocin and ergometrine in active management did statistically reduce the incidences of PPH when compared to oxytocin where blood loss was estimated below 1 L. Equally, where the blood loss was greater than 1 L, there was no difference between the groups when either using 5 or 10 iu oxytocin. Given the side effects of combined oxytocin and ergometrine, a review of current drug management in maternity units is worth consideration. Whilst several studies refer to the reduction of blood loss and similar reporting of side effects, Yuen et al. (1995) noted a small increase in the incidence of manual removal of placenta when Syntometrine was used, compared to Syntocinon. The use of intraumbilical diluted oxytocin or saline seems to have no benefit over the traditional intramuscular and intravenous routes and its use has been largely abandoned (Ozcan et al. 1996).

Another drug worth considering where ergometrine and oxytocin have been unresponsive in treating uterine atony is carboprost (Hemabate). This has proved useful in augmenting contractility of the myometrial muscles. It is administered by deep intramuscular injection in a dose of 250 µg at intervals of 15–90 minutes. Reported side effects include nausea, vomiting and hyperthermia. Carboprost seems to fare better compared with ergometrine and other oxytocic drugs as it produces less side effects pertaining to hypertension (British Medical Association (BMA) & Royal Pharmaceutical Society of Great Britain 2005).

There is a growing interest in the use of misoprostol, a synthetic prostaglandin analogue, for the management of the third stage of labour (BMA & Royal Pharmaceutical Society of Great Britain 2005). In one study, oral misoprostol, when compared with intramuscular oxytocin 10 iu in low risk women, was found to be as effective in reducing blood loss (Walley et al. 2000). The literature reports unwanted side effects of mistoprostol as shivering, pyrexia, nausea, vomiting and diarrhoea (Lumbiganon et al. 2002). When comparing the administration of mistoprostol intrarectally with conventional oxytocics, rectal mistoprostol was found to be significantly less effective than oxytocin plus ergometrine for the prevention of PPH (Caliskan et al. 2002). Equally when comparing rectal mistoprostol against intravenous oxytocin, rectal mistoprostol was no more effective than intravenous oxytocin in preventing postpartum bleeding (Gerstenfeld & Wing 2001).

How well misoprostol performs in massive or unresponsive haemorrhage has yet to be studied. Rectally, misoprostol appears to be effective treatment for PPH where oxytocin and ergometrine have been unresponsive (O'Brien et al. 1998). This concurs with findings from a Cochrane review by Mousa and Alfirevic (2003), that rectal misoprostol 800 µg given as a prime drug for the management of post-partum haemorrhage has had some success.

Determining the best choice of drug for the management of PPH requires further randomised controlled trials, particularly for massive or unresponsive haemorrhage. However, recruitment into such trials may be problematic as the number of subjects is likely to be small and therefore skews findings. It is noted that where a combination of drugs are used such as intramuscular syntometrine, oxtyocin intravenous infusion and rectal misoprostol, there is a reduction in the number of women who continue to bleed after interventions such as internal iliac artery ligation, uterine packing or hysterectomy (Mousa & Alfirevic 2003).

Fluid replacement

As hypovolaemic shock is a major cause of maternal mortality, the priority is to replace fluids rapidly. The replacement of blood products and haemodynamic monitoring is the same for any event where massive blood loss and resuscitation is required. These principles include that the management of fluid replacement is by the anaesthetist in collaboration with the haematologist and obstetrician. The management of massive obstetric haemorrhage includes the arrest of subsequent events such as disseminated intravascular coagulation (DIC) and further maternal collapse requiring resuscitation.

Where severe blood loss is anticipated or has occurred, then the siting of a CVP line by the anaesthetist should be standard practice in order to monitor fluid balance.

As long ago as 1994, the CEMD report (Department of Health 1994) recommended that all acute maternity units should have available continuous monitoring display for CVP, intra-arterial pressure, electrocardiogram, heart rate, blood gases and acid base status. Where monitoring equipment is available and its use is advocated, early use of continuous monitoring should commence.

In many cases, following the identification of the source of bleeding and prompt repair and/or use of oxytocic drugs, further bleeding will be arrested. In conjunction with fluid management and stabilisation of the maternal haemodynamic state, often no further treatment is required. In cases where maternal bleeding continues, further obstetric action is required and is outlined in Box 7.2.

The midwife's role will be to provide midwifery care to the woman and participate in obstetric care. In some maternity units where 'high risk' midwifery teams are established, protocols are established to enable midwives to function within frameworks and working practices that have been agreed by the multi-professional team.

Box 7.2   Management of massive postpartum haemorrhage.

Resuscitation (see Chapter 11)
Identify cause and augment obstetric treatment
Commence prostaglandin treatment
Consider compression techniques
Internal iliac artery ligation
Angiographic embolisation (if facilities available)
Hysterectomy

Compression techniques

Bimanual compression techniques are applied postpartum when uterine bleeding persists and the placenta is either partially adhered to the uterine wall or separated and the uterus is atonic. Where previous management – such as 'rubbing up' a contraction, giving an oxytocic drug and emptying the urinary bladder – has been unresponsive, the midwife must consider applying pressure techniques. Midwives should be familiar with external and internal bimanual compression methods and be able to apply these techniques in an emergency. Internal bimanual compression may be more effective than external compression but can only be attempted if the woman has effective anaesthesia. Before commencing bimanual compression the midwife must summon medical help (Nursing and Midwifery Council (NMC) 2004a) and ensure an intravenous infusion is sited.

In extreme cases where the placenta is partially separated, the midwife in the absence of a doctor may attempt to manually remove the placenta and also carry out a manual examination of the uterus (NMC 2004a). It is stressed that in the UK these actions should only occur if the woman's condition is life threatening (NMC 2004a).

External bimanual compression

The midwife should choose this method where the woman does not have adequate pain relief available. The aim of this technique is to apply pressure to the uterus and compress the blood vessels in an attempt to achieve haemostasis. The left hand is placed on the fundus and then moved behind the uterus. At the same time the right hand is positioned flat on the abdominal wall just below the umbilicus and both hands apply pressure. As pressure is applied the uterus is pulled upwards in order to straighten any kinked blood vessels to allow drainage.

The midwife should continue compression observing the condition of the woman and noting whether blood loss is diminishing.

Internal bimanual compression

This technique is usually adopted when the placenta has been delivered either spontaneously or after manual removal and when the uterus continues to bleed. However, this method should not be attempted without adequate anaesthesia.

The aim of this technique is to apply pressure between the uterus and the abdominal wall in order to compress uterine blood vessels. Using universal sterile precautions, the midwife places the right hand into the vagina, closing the hand to form a tight fist. The fist should be directed upwards to the anterior fornix. The left hand is initially placed flat on the abdominal wall near the fundus. The left hand should then firmly dip behind the uterus pulling it forward and towards the symphysis pubis. Both hands should attempt to meet and apply pressure on the uterine muscle in an effort to compress the blood vessels at the placental site. The midwife should continue to apply pressure until the uterus contracts or instructed otherwise by the medical team.

Abdominal aortic compression

Abdominal aortic compression can be used as a temporary emergency measure, for a short period to arrest bleeding while waiting for blood replacement or transfer to theatre. The midwife can adopt this technique under the guidance of a medical practitioner and, as with other emergency procedures, it should be rehearsed.

Due to the anatomy of the blood supply to the uterus and genital tract the occlusion of the aorta will obstruct the blood flow to the uterus. Compression of the aorta is achieved by forming a fist, which is pressed against the abdomen about 3 cm above the umbilicus. The pressure is directed backwards towards the vertebral column.

Musculoskeletal discomfort

When applying compression techniques the midwife should be aware of the possibility of developing or experiencing musculoskeletal discomfort as the techniques adopted may cause the worker to adopt a fixed working posture. Evidence of sustained and repetitive loading on the spine can lead to chronic muscle dysfunction (Adams & Dolan 2005). To avoid injury the midwife should adopt the best working posture in the circumstances for the emergency. Factors to be considered include:

- Avoid forward and side flexion and rotation of the spine
- Get close access to the woman to avoid forward flexion
- Consider the bed height and adjust for maximum personal comfort
- Adopt a stable base by selecting a step stance

Alternatively the bed height can be lowered to mid-thigh – the midwife places one knee on the bed and the other foot on the floor. This will keep the worker's spine straight but allows flexion at the hips. If musculoskeletal discomfort is experienced the worker's posture must be changed or another midwife recruited to undertake the compression technique.

Surgical management

After medical interventions have been implemented and where the arrest of bleeding has failed, surgical intervention is required. The surgical management discussed here includes tradition and less radical surgical options such as embolisation techniques, uterine compression sutures and uterine tamponade. They are all considered to be less hazardous to perform than initially opting for hysterectomy and they have the advantage of preserving the reproductive system. Traditional management includes surgical repair of the tissue and blood vessels including uterine packing and hysterectomy.

Surgical repair and its success is largely dependent on the ability to locate and isolate trauma and arrest bleeding. The successful use of haemostatic cervical sutures has been reported (Kafali et al. 2003). Suturing of the anterior and posterior lips of the cervix using chromic catgut was used in three women with intractable haemorrhage. The authors report the techniques as safe and easy to execute and it may be an alternative to hysterectomy, particularly where the preservation of the uterus is paramount. However, in many instances where haemorrhage is intractable, hysterectomy is the only option to prevent mortality.

Uterine packing

Uterine packing may be used when the uterus is partially contracted with the upper segment contracted but the lower segment continuing to bleed. This is more likely to arise when the cervix is bleeding or the placenta has been sited in the lower uterine segment. Uterine packing may be chosen prior to other surgical interventions and when oxytocic drugs have proved ineffective. Hsu et al. (2003) report on nine obstetric cases with reasonable outcomes and recommend uterine packing as an alternative to other surgical intervention and/or where the preservation of fertility is requested.

The midwife may be required to assist in the procedure and therefore should be conversant with the technique. The woman will require intravenous fluids and additional intravenous access. Adequate anaesthesia should be administered and the woman placed in the lithotomy position. The aim is to pack the uterus with sterile roll gauze which applies pressure to the uterine wall. The rolls can be tied together ensuring the pack is continuous, leaving no spaces. When packing, an assistant may be required to provide counterpressure on the fundus to ensure the pack fills the cavity. For uterine packing to be successful a degree of tension is required in the cervix otherwise the pack is likely to slip if the cervix is fully dilated. The midwife is required to care for the woman, monitoring vital signs, and looking for persistent or episodes of new bleeding vaginally.

Tamponade balloon

There has been reported success with the use of fluid-filled tamponade balloons in the management of PPH (Bakri et al. 2001). The balloon is inserted into the uterus and filled with sterile saline. The drainage holes at the tip of the balloon enable measurement of blood loss, an advantage when comparing blood loss where uterine packing is employed. The strength of the balloon is designed to exert an internal and external pressure of 300 mmHg. As the balloon inflates it exerts pressure on the uterine wall in an attempt to stem blood flow. The decision to use a tamponade balloon may be selected when previous attempts to achieve uterine pressure by packing the uterus have failed. The tamponade balloon has been reported to be successful in arresting bleeding in cases where placenta praevia is the initial cause of bleeding.

A small study ($n = 16$) by Condous et al. (2003) investigated whether the insertion of a Sengstaken–Blakemore stomach tube into the uterus would arrest catastrophic bleeding sufficiently to reduce the need for further major surgery. The technique was successful in 14 of the 16 women, and proved life saving for two women as it allowed time to correct consumption coagulopathy when balloon tamponade was not successful.

Although reports have been based on small numbers of cases, there is evidence to suggest this method is successful and reduces the need for further invasive procedures (Marcovici & Scoccia 1999). Particular success in achieving haemostasis has been reported in cases where bleeding originated from the lower uterine segment in association with placenta praevia and cervical ectopic pregnancy (Bakri et al. 2001). The period of time for insertion varies and if bleeding is not arrested then further surgical measures will be considered. If the tamponade balloon stems bleeding, the tamponade balloon is likely to remain *in situ* for 12–24 hours before deflation is considered. The midwife will need to continue observing and measuring blood loss and to monitor vital signs.

Uterine compression sutures

The use of B-Lynch uterine compression sutures is recommended where uterine atony persists. The aim is to exert pressure on the uterine muscles and thus control pelvic arterial pressure. The sutures are applied via a lower segment incision in the uterus; prior to applying sutures, bimanual compression is applied to assess whether this arrests bleeding. Using Vicryl or Dexon suture material, straight sutures are inserted the length of the uterus. Once *in situ* the sutures are pulled to compress the uterus. The sutures are tied off and haemostasis is noted before the abdomen is closed (Lynch et al. 1997). The literature reports favourably on its use and outcome (Lynch et al. 1997; Danso & Reginald 2002; Hayman et al. 2002; Smith & Baskett 2003). Authors report the technique as easy to apply, relatively safe and life saving. The preservation of the uterus is seen as an advantage. It is a technique that can be tried before proceeding to hysterectomy. There is one reported case where a combination of uterine compression sutures and tamponade balloon were used with a reported successful outcome (Danso & Reginald 2002). Consequentially, in the postpartum period, women appear to pass normal lochia and resume normal menstruation.

Arterial embolisation

Embolisation of the uterine arteries may be considered in the treatment of intractable PPH where vaginal packing and administration of uterotonic drugs have failed (Corr 2001). Embolisation entails the insertion of intravascular catheters into the internal iliac arteries under radiological guidance. Therefore, arterial embolisation can only be offered where suitable radiological skills and equipment are available. Ideally, embolisation is completed before surgery and where massive haemorrhage is anticipated, such as in cases of caesarean section for placenta accreta.

The aim is to halt blood flow temporarily by inflating balloons at the end of the catheters and to release them when haemostasis is achieved (Dubois et al. 1997).

Benefits include low complication rates (Vedantham et al. 1997), avoidance of surgical risks, fertility preservation and shorter hospitalisation. The evidence suggests maternal outcome is favourable although it is based on only a small number of case histories. Pelage et al. (1998) and Picone et al. (2003) both report successful fetal growth in subsequent pregnancies after embolisation. It appears the mode of delivery has no relevance to cases where intractable bleeding occurs (Tourne et al. 2003) and where embolisation was not effective hysterectomy was the only option to avoid mortality.

Hysterectomy

Removal of the uterus is considered to be the last resort and is only carried out in order to preserve life. The preservation of the ovaries in the younger woman is considered and a subtotal hysterectomy may be best practice. Given the nature of bleeding from the uterine site, a total hysterectomy rather than a subtotal one is the usual management. Where the decision is to proceed to hysterectomy, this is usually performed under general anaesthesia. The midwife should be familiar with postoperative recovery and management of the airway following instructions by the anaesthetist (see Chapter 11). The provision of adequate pain relief preferably by patient-controlled analgesia is considered best practice. The choice and dosage is the remit of the anaesthetist; however the midwife should act as an advocate to ensure women undergoing medical and surgical procedures during emergencies have adequate pain relief.

Complications

Childbearing women who have difficulty maintaining haemostasis are likely to develop DIC. This is a life-threatening condition resulting from an uncontrolled activation of the haemostatic process triggered by tissue damage, which could be maternal, fetal or placental in origin. As a result of massive tissue damage the intrinsic and extrinsic clotting pathways are activated. The midwife requires knowledge of the normal blood-clotting mechanism to appreciate coagulation disturbances associated with DIC (Marieb 2002).

Once the trigger mechanism has activated the coagulation system, both fibrin and thrombin circulate freely within the plasma. The excessive quantity of circulating thrombin causes fibrinogen to produce fibrin. Due to the overproduction of circulating fibrin, microvascular thrombosis occurs, leading to peripheral ischaemia and organ damage. With the excessive quantities of fibrin deposits throughout the circulatory system, platelets become trapped, and this is followed by thrombocytopenia. Excessive quantities of plasmin, which is required to assist in the activation of FDPs to disperse fibrin once blood vessels are sealed, is released. The interference between FDP production and overproduction of fibrin further impairs haemostasis and leads to haemorrhage.

Thus the quantities of circulating thrombin and plasmin means the childbearing woman who develops DIC will suffer from both thrombosis and haemorrhage. The clotting mechanism is overwhelmed and is no longer able to compensate due to the excessive consumption of fibrinogen, platelets, coagulation factors and fibrinolytic enzymes. The utilisation of the latter will eventually lead to the catastrophic demise of the woman once platelet and clotting factors are depleted, leading to shock, further bleeding and occlusion of blood vessels due to multiple microemboli.

The midwife needs to appreciate the sudden onset of DIC and is probably best placed to notice the signs and symptoms of DIC. Although it is not the remit of the midwife to diagnose DIC, it is important the obstetric team is alerted. The midwife may note changes in blood clotting following delivery when handling the expelled blood from the uterus. A woman with fulminating DIC usually bleeds from other sites such as venepunctures, wounds and mucous membranes. Petechiae may develop in the skin and bleeding will persist from the uterine cavity.

To arrest DIC, the source of tissue injury must be identified and corrected using available medical and surgical interventions. Haematological studies will confirm coagulation failure and inform appropriate fluid replacement. Coagulation screening should include:

- Whole blood film including platelet count
- Fibrin degradation products
- Prothrombin time (normal 10–14 seconds)
- Thrombin time (normal 10–15 seconds)
- Partial thromboplastin time (normal 35–45 seconds)
- Fibrinogen levels (normal 2.5–4 g/L)

It is the remit of the senior obstetrician, anaesthetist, haematologist and midwife to instigate the rehearsed policy for catastrophic haemorrhage. The midwife's role remains primarily with caring for the woman, delivering midwifery care, and responding to and working with the multiprofessional team. Midwives should familiarise themselves with their unit policy concerning the care and management of women receiving blood products.

Further information on hypovolaemic shock and DIC can be found in Chapter 8, and on principles of fluid management in Chapter 9.

Midwifery care

The midwife's role is to ensure the best care for women when they become acutely ill. In some instances where women require prolonged respiratory support, admission to a high dependency unit or intensive care unit is usual practice. The principles of midwifery care are outlined below.

- Undertake or assist in intravenous cannulation using two large-bore cannulae, and the ongoing care of intravenous lines and fluids.
- Record vital signs using continuous electronic monitoring equipment to assess adequacy of circulating volume, oxygenation and effects of any interventions.
- Catheterise the urinary bladder.

- Monitor fluid balance to determine signs of dehydration and/or fluid overload, including hourly urine output, wound drainage, wound sites, vaginal loss, vomit and perspiration.
- Care of wounds and wound drains – assessment of fluid loss, wound healing and signs of infection.
- Assess vaginal loss noting the difference between lochia and significant blood loss.
- Recognise pain and provide adequate pain relief noting its effectiveness.
- Assess and record levels of consciousness by measuring motor and verbal responses and eye opening using a designated assessment tool such as the Glasgow Coma Scale (Teasdale & Jennett 1974).
- Maintain body alignment to gain an optimal position in order to maintain respiration, nutrition, hydration, posture, skin integrity and elimination.
- Assist with or provide personal hygiene for women when unable to self-care.
- Minimise infection through the use of aseptic techniques and handwashing before and after undertaking procedures.
- Provide and maintain privacy and dignity as far as possible during obstetric emergencies in accordance with the *Code of Professional Conduct* (NMC 2004b) and *Midwives Rules and Standards* (NMC 2004a).
- Record accurately events detailing the midwifery care provided in accordance with the *Midwives Rules and Standards* (NMC 2004a).

References

Adams, M. and Dolan, P. (2005) Biomechanics of low back pain. In: J. Smith (Ed.) *The Guide to Handling People* (5th edn). BackCare, National Back Pain Association, Royal College of Nursing, London.

Advanced Life Support in Obstetrics (ALSO) (2000) *Advanced Life Support in Obstetrics Provider Manual* (4th edn). American Academy of Family Physicians, Kansas City.

Bakri, Y., Amri, A. and Jabbar, F. (2001) Tamponade-balloon for obstetrical bleeding. *International Journal of Gynecology and Obstetrics*, **74** (2): 139–42.

British Medical Association (BMA) and Royal Pharmaceutical Society of Great Britain (2005) *British National Formulary*, No. 49, March. BMA and Royal Pharmaceutical Society of Great Britain, London.

Caliskan, E., Meydanli, M., Dilbaz, B. et al. (2002) Is rectal misoprostol really effective in the treatment of third stage of labor? A randomized controlled trial. *American Journal of Obstetrics and Gynecology*, **187** (4): 1038–45.

Condous, G., Arulkumaran, S. and Symonds, I. (2003) The "Tamponade Test" in the management of massive postpartum hemorrhage. *Obstetrics and Gynecology*, **101** (4): 767–72.

Corr, P. (2001) Arterial embolization for haemorrhage in the obstetric patient. *Best Practice and Research Clinical Obstetrics and Gynaecology*, **15** (4): 557–61.

Coulter-Smith, S., Holohan, M. and Darling, M. (1996) Previous caesarean section: a risk factor for major obstetric haemorrhage? *Journal of Obstetrics and Gynaecology*, **16** (5): 349–52.

Danso, D. and Reginald, P. (2002) Combined B-Lynch suture with intrauterine balloon catheter triumphs over massive postpartum haemorrhage. *British Journal of Obstetrics and Gynaecology*, **109** (8): 963.

Department of Health (1994) *Report on Confidential Enquiries into Maternal Deaths in the United Kingdom 1988–1990*. Her Majesty's Stationery Office (HMSO), London.

Department of Health (1996) *Report on Confidential Enquiries into Maternal Deaths in the United Kingdom 1991–1993*. HMSO, London.

Dombrowski, M., Bottoms, S., Saleh, A. et al. (1995) Third stage of labor: analysis of duration and clinical practice. *American Journal of Obstetrics and Gynecology*, **172** (4): 1279–84.

Dubois, J., Garel, L., Grignon, A. et al. (1997) Placenta percreta: balloon occlusion and embolization of the internal iliac arteries to reduce intraoperative blood losses. *American Journal of Obstetrics and Gynecology*, **176**: 723–6.

Duffy, T. (1999) Hematologic aspects of pregnancy. In: G. Burrows and T. Duffy (Eds) *Medical Complications during Pregnancy* (5th edn). W.B. Saunders, London.

Dunn, P. (2002) John Chassar Moir (1900–1977) and the discovery of ergomentrine. *Archives of Diseases in Childhood, Fetal and Neonatal Edition*, **87**: F152–F154.

Gerbasi, F. (1990) Changes in hemostasis during delivery and the immediate postpartum period. *American Journal of Obstetrics and Gynecology*, **162**: 1158.

Gerstenfeld, T. and Wing, D. (2001) Rectal misoprostal versus intravenous oxytocin for the prevention of postpartum hemorrhage after vaginal delivery. *American Journal of Obstetrics and Gynecology*, **185** (4): 878–82.

Greer, A., Lowe, G. and Walker, J. (1991) Haemorrhagic problems in obstetrics and gynaecology in patients with congenital coagulopathies. *British Journal of Obstetrics and Gynaecology*, **98** (9): 909–18.

Hathaway, W. and Bonnar, J. (1987) *Hemostatic Disorders of the Pregnant Woman and Newborn Infant*. Elsevier, Edinburgh.

Hayman, R., Arulkumaran, S. and Steer, P. (2002) Uterine compression sutures: surgical management of postpartum haemorrhage. *Obstetrics and Gynaecology*, **99** (3): 502–6.

Herabutya, Y., Prasertsawat, P. and Boorangsimant, P. (1988) Keilland's forceps or ventouse – a comparison. *British Journal of Obstetrics and Gynaecology*, **95** (5): 483–7.

Herman, A. (2000) Complicated third stage of labor: time to switch on the scanner. *Ultrasound in Obstetrics and Gynecology*, **15** (2): 89–95.

Hsu, S., Rodgers, B. and Lele, A. (2003) Use of packing in obstetric haemorrhage of uterine origin. *Journal of Reproductive Medicine*, **48** (2): 69–71.

Hutchon, S. and Martin, W. (2002) Intrapartum and postpartum bleeding. *Current Obstetrics and Gynaecology*, **12** (5): 250–5.

Jouppila, P. (1995) Postpartum haemorrhage. *Current Opinion in Obstetrics and Gynecology*, **7** (6): 446–50.

Kafali, H., Demir, N., Soylemez, F. et al. (2003) Hemostatic cervical suturing techniques for management of uncontrolled postpartum haemorrhage originating from the cervical canal. *European Journal of Obstetrics and Gynaecology and Reproductive Biology*, **110** (1): 35–8.

Lewis, G. (2001) *Why Mothers Die 1997–1999: The Confidential Enquiries into Maternal Deaths in the United Kingdom*. Royal College of Obstetricians and Gynaecologists (RCOG) Press, London.

Lewis, G. (2004) *Why Mothers Die 2000–2002: Report on Confidential Enquiries into Maternal Deaths in the United Kingdom*. RCOG Press, London.

Lim, J., Tan, B., Jammal, A. et al. (2002) Delivery of macrosomic babies: management and outcomes of 330 cases. *Journal of Obstetrics and Gynaecology*, **22** (4): 370–4.

Lumbiganon, P., Villar, J. and Piaggio, G. (2002) Side effects of oral misoprostol during the first 24 hours after administration in the third stage of labour. *British Journal of Obstetrics and Gynaecology*, **109** (11): 1222–6.

Lurie, S., Gomel, A. and Sadan, O. (2003) The duration of the third stage of labor is subject to the location of placental implantation. *Gynecology and Obstetric Investigation*, **56** (1): 14–16.

Lynch, C., Coker, A., Lawal, A. et al. (1997) The B-Lynch surgical technique for the control of massive postpartum haemorrhage: an alternative to hysterectomy. *British Journal of Obstetrics and Gynaecology*, **104** (3): 372–5.

Macphail, S. and Fitzgerald, J. (2001) Massive post-partum haemorrhage. *Current Obstetrics and Gynaecology*, **11** (2): 108–14.

Marcovici, I. and Scoccia, B. (1999) Postpartum hemorrhage and intrauterine balloon tamponade: a report of three cases. *Journal of Reproductive Medicine*, **44** (2): 122–6.

Marieb, E. (2002) *Human Anatomy and Physiology* (7th edn). Benjamin/Cummings Publishers, London.

McDonald, S., Prendiville, W. and Blair, E. (1993) Randomised controlled trial of oxytocin alone versus oxytocin and ergometrine in active management of the third stage of labour. *British Medical Journal*, **307** (6913): 1167–71.

McDonald, S., Prendiville, W. and Elbourne, D. (2003) Prophylactic syntometrine versus oxytocin for delivery of the placenta. *Cochrane Library*, Issue 2. Update Software, Oxford.

Mousa, H.A. and Alfirevic, Z. (2003) Treatment for primary postpartum haemorrhage. *Cochrane Database of Systematic Reviews*, Issue 1.

Nursing and Midwifery Council (2004a) *Midwives Rules and Standards*. Nursing and Midwifery Council (NMC), London.

Nursing and Midwifery Council (2004b) *The NMC Code of Professional Conduct: Standards for conduct, performance and ethics*. NMC, London.

O'Brien, P., El-Rafaey, H., Gordon, A. et al. (1998) Rectally administered misoprostol for the treatment of postpartum haemorrhage unresponsive to oxytocin and ergometrine: a descriptive study. *Obstetrics and Gynecology*, **92** (2): 212–14.

Ozcan, T., Sahin, G. and Senoz, S. (1996) The effect of intraumbilical oxytocin on the third stage of labour. *Australian and New Zealand Journal of Obstetrics and Gynaecology*, **36** (1): 9–11.

Pelage, J., Le Dref, O. and Mateo, J. (1998) Life-threatening primary postpartum hemorrhage: treatment with emergency selective arterial embolization. *Radiology*, **208** (2): 359–62.

Picone, O., Salmon, L. and Ville, Y. (2003) Fetal growth and Doppler assessment in patients with a history of bilateral internal iliac artery embolization. *Journal of Maternal-Fetal and Neonatal Medicine*, **13** (5): 305–308.

Smith, K. and Baskett, T. (2003) Uterine compression sutures as an alternative to hysterectomy for severe postpartum haemorrhage. *Journal of Obstetrics and Gynaecology (Canada)*, **25** (3): 197–200.

Soriano, D., Dulitzki, M. and Schiff, E. (1996) A prospective cohort study of oxytocin plus ergometrine compared with oxytocin alone for prevention of postpartum haemorrhage. *British Journal of Obstetrics and Gynaecology*, **103** (11): 1068–73.

Stables, D. and Rankin, J. (2005) *Physiology in Childbearing with Anatomy and Related Biosciences* (2nd edn). Bailliere Tindall, London.

Tamizian, O. and Arulkumaran, S. (2002) The surgical management of post-partum haemorrhage. *Best Practice and Research Clinical Obstetrics and Gynaecology*, **16** (1): 81–98.

Teasdale, G. and Jennett, B. (1974) Assessment of coma and impaired consciousnesses. *Lancet*, **ii**: 81–4.

Tourne, G., Collet, F. and Seffert, P. (2003) Place of embolization of the uterine arteries in the management of post-partum haemorrhage: a study of 12 cases. *European Journal of Obstetrics and Gynecology and Reproductive Biology*, **110** (1): 29–34

Tiran, D. (2004) *Bailliere's Midwives Dictionary* (10th edn). Bailliere Tindall, London.

Vedantham, S., Goodwin, S. and Lucas, B. (1997) Uterine artery embolization: an underused method of controlling pelvic hemorrhage. *American Journal of Obstetrics and Gynecology*, **176** (4): 938–48.

Walley, R., Wilson, J. and Crane, J. (2000) A double-blind placebo controlled randomised trial of misoprostol and oxytocin in the management of the third stage of labour. *British Journal of Obstetrics and Gynaecology*, **107** (9): 1111–15.

Weerasekera, D. (2002) A randomised prospective trial of the obstetric forceps versus vacuum extraction using defined criteria. *Journal of Obstetrics and Gynecology*, **22** (4): 344–5.

Yuen, P., Chan, N., Yim, S. et al. (1995) A randomised double blind comparison of Syntometrine and Syntocinon in the management of the third stage of labour. *British Journal of Obstetrics and Gynaecology*, **102** (5): 377–80.

8 Shock and the Critically Ill Woman

*Terry Ferns**

The diagnosis and subsequent management of shock may provoke anxiety for some midwives. Prompt recognition and intervention is required in an attempt to prevent maternal mortality and morbidity.

Although each form of shock has a particular pathophysiology and presentation, there is considerable overlap in the management of shock from whatever cause, which midwives need to appreciate. This chapter will explore the various types of shock and discuss the management required to maintain maternal homeostasis.

Assumed prior knowledge

- Physiology of the adult cardiovascular and renal systems
- Physiological adaptations of the cardiovascular and renal systems in the normal pregnancy

Introduction

Globally, shock has been defined as acute circulatory failure with inadequate or inappropriately distributed tissue perfusion resulting in generalised hypoxia (Hinds 1999). The net effect of the shocked state is that tissue cells are deprived of oxygen, leading to a resultant increase in anaerobic metabolism to produce adenosine triphosphate, a subsequent byproduct creation of lactic acid, a metabolic acidosis and, finally, cell swelling, necrosis, end organ failure and death.

---

* With thanks to Allison Letford of Queen Elizabeth Hospital, Woolwich, for midwifery input.

Each form of shock has a specific pathophysiology and presentation although there is considerable overlap. This chapter will examine the physiological changes that occur during pregnancy, the components of a comprehensive assessment of the pregnant shocked patient and the presentation and management of the resulting state of shock.

Shock can be classified by the cause:

- *Cardiogenic shock* can result from pump (heart) failure following an acute myocardial infarction or embolism.
- *Hypovolaemic shock* can be caused by loss of circulating volume. These losses may be exogenous (e.g. haemorrhage or burns) or endogenous (through leaks in the microcirculation or into body cavities as occurs in intestinal obstruction). Hypovolaemic shock is associated with severe obstetric haemorrhage, antepartum or postpartum haemorrhage, ruptured ectopic pregnancy, genital tract trauma or following coagulopathy.
- *Distributive shock* is caused by abnormalities of the peripheral circulation. Examples include anaphylaxis, sepsis and neurogenic shock. Anaphylaxis is a consequence of an antigen/antibody response, sepsis is due to an overwhelming infection and neurogenic shock is associated with uterine inversion, regional anaesthesia and the aspiration of gastric contents (Hinds 1999; Beringer & Patteril 2004).

The three phases of shock: an overview

Shock is a progressive syndrome but it can be divided into three phases:

- Stage 1: compensated (non-progressive)
- Stage 2: uncompensated (progressive)
- Stage 3: irreversible (irreversible)

Stage 1

Following an insult such as trauma that results in a loss of circulating volume and a subsequent fall in blood pressure, baroreceptor stimulation results in systemic vasoconstriction of the arterioles, kidneys and other abdominal viscera and an increase in the release of adrenaline and noradrenaline by the adrenal medulla. Vasoconstriction maintains preload by increasing systemic vascular resistance, which maintains an adequate venous return. This results in the patient presenting with minimal signs and symptoms such as subtle changes in colour and skin temperature, minimal increases in heart rate and increased stroke volume. Vital signs may only alter slightly and the patient may complain of nausea and be mildly agitated and restless. The rennin–angiotension pathway and the release of antidiuretic hormone stimulates the kidney to retain water and sodium resulting in a reduced urine output and the client possibly complaining of a dry mouth or thirst. If cells experience hypoxia they will liberate vasodilators that increase regional blood supply, which might lower systemic vascular resistance leading to a drop in blood pressure. The lowered perfusion state and subsequent lactic acid formation stimulates an increased respiratory rate and sympathetic stimulation may manifest as dilated pupils and sweating.

Compensatory mechanisms can take from 30 seconds to 48 hours to work providing the level of shock does not worsen to stage 2.

Stage 2

As the shocked state progresses, the patient will experience cardiac depression as a compromised blood pressure and excessive tachycardia leads to poor coronary artery perfusion leading to myocardial ischaemia, a weakened myocardium and reduced cardiac output. A consequence of poor myocardial function is the release of myocardial depression factor, further compromising cardiac function. Manifestations may include ST depression or T-wave inversion and cardiac arrhythmias. As mean blood pressure falls the vasomotor centre in the medulla oblongata begins to lose control of tone leading to generalised vasodilatation and further reductions in preload/afterload and cardiac output.

As stage 2 shock progresses, hypoxia leads to an increase in blood capillary permeability leading to inappropriate fluid shift and further blood volume loss; this in turn leads to a falling cardiac output and intensified hypoxia. Fluid shift may lead to a ventilation/perfusion mismatch and the sluggish cardiac output encourages platelet aggregation, pooling of blood peripherally and the release of acid metabolites. The release of catacholamines, the production of lactic acid and the loss of cell wall permeability contribute to acidosis. The patient will display symptoms ranging from reduced neurological function and tachypnoea, to peripheral oedema. Medical intervention is required to reverse the above changes otherwise the patient will deteriorate to stage 3 shock.

Stage 3

During stage 3 there is a rapid deterioration in cardiovascular function that cannot be reversed by medical intervention. The heart is unable to pump effectively, cell perfusion reaches critical levels and cell death is inevitable.

General considerations in the assessment of shock

Each form of shock has a specific pathway that can be further complicated during pregnancy, and differing management strategies will need to be considered. However, general principles can be applied in the first instance to each form of shock.

The principle of assessment of a woman presenting with potential or established shock is to apply a comprehensive, systematic approach with an emphasis on attention to detail. The woman should be approached with a high index of suspicion and the practitioner should remain vigilant throughout the assessment. *Midwives should approach the pregnant woman with the viewpoint that she is shocked*

(and the fetus distressed) until formal assessment proves otherwise. A confident practitioner will eliminate the signs and symptoms of the shocked state by using a
systematic approach employed to conduct a comprehensive assessment. Hudak
et al. (1998) recommends that the assessment should comprise:

- Inspection
- Palpation
- Auscultation
- Percussion

The following will set the tone for completing a professional assessment:

- Always wash your hands and put on gloves (and aprons) prior to conducting
  the assessment.
- Introduce yourself and explain what you want to do and gain consent.
- Optimise the environment (pump up the bed to a comfortable height, turn on
  the light, etc.).
- Position the pregnant woman in the most appropriate position for assessment.
- Have any equipment clean and available for use.
- Always maintain the client's privacy and dignity.

The above statements can all be independently justified as, for example, failure
to wash one's hands prior to personal contact may lead to a healthy woman developing a shocked state in the future due to nosocomial infection. Subsequently,
although the four classic vital signs and pain assessment are extremely important,
secondary symptoms (neurological function, colour, urine output, perfusion) are
increasingly relevant. The experienced practitioner will use these as a basis of
assessment in conjunction with vital signs applying a holistic approach. In essence,
vital sign recording confirms what you can see and feel.

It is crucial to assess the shocked pregnant woman with a clear understanding
of the physiological changes that occur as a consequence of pregnancy, which may
underpin management. Assessing the pregnant woman by applying the same
set of physiological values that apply to non-pregnancy or early pregnancy will
result in inaccurate diagnosis and a poor outcome. Jiva (2000) comments on the
potential difficulties experienced when diagnosing a shocked pregnant woman
due to the potential physiological adaptations – such as the presence of oedema,
an increased heart rate, mid-systolic murmur and shifted apical pulses – which
are all expected findings in pregnancy. The normal cardiovascular changes in
pregnancy can complicate the evaluation of intravascular volumes, blood loss
and extent of the shocked state.

Due to pregnancy-related physiological changes, there may appear to be a
much closer relationship between the pregnant woman and the early stages of
shock as opposed to a non-pregnant woman's baseline observations and the
diagnosis of a shocked state. Although one could suggest that the increased blood
volume that occurs during pregnancy might mean that the pregnant woman is
better prepared to withstand haemorrhage, those with anaemia, prolonged labour,
dehydration, or with a reduced blood volume and contracted intravascular space
associated with, for example, pre-eclampsia may not tolerate quite small blood
loss, especially if this loss is rapid (Baskett 2004).

Approximately 10% of pregnant woman at term manifest signs of shock when placed supine. Sharma (2003) notes how pregnant women have a greater tendency for pooling venous blood, and subsequently when moving from a lying to a sitting position may experience dizziness, pallor, tachycardia, sweating, nausea or hypotension. Nelson-Piercy (2002) identifies that towards term, turning from the lateral to the supine position may result in a 25% reduction in cardiac output that is associated with a reduction in uterine blood flow, which can compromise the fetus. Sharma (2003) also notes how pain and anxiety during the birthing experience can make diagnosis difficult. Edwards (1998) elaborates on this issue, emphasising that a pregnant woman in shock may present with warm, dry skin rather than cool, clammy skin, due to circulating progesterone, which causes vasodilatation and a decrease in systemic vascular resistance. Inherent delays associated with diagnosis and treatment decisions and the potential for misdiagnosis are likely to contribute to increased maternal morbidity and mortality and fetal loss, emphasising the importance of vigilance in our care.

Midwives care for a client group whose presentation may mask clinical deterioration and who have a narrower scope for deterioration to become life threatening. The dilemma is separating the dizzy, pregnant woman experiencing 'normal' pain experienced during pregnancy to the truly shocked patient. Assessment should be based on clinical presentation and knowledge of how current presentation differs from previous baseline observations. Attention should be paid to trends and to viewing the patient holistically, not simply focusing on one abnormal vital sign. One must always consider that the mother maintains homeostasis at the expense of the fetus.

Clinical competence, vigilance and expertise are the key. This is particularly important in the management of the shocked client as recognition and intensive treatment of shock is an indisputable priority (Ratcliffe 1999). Ratcliffe (1999) elaborates on this issue, suggesting that the following factors will contribute to successful management of shocked pregnant woman:

- The knowledge that certain clinical conditions may lead to the acute onset of shock
- The development of a rapid process to evaluate the degree of shock
- The institution of effective management in the care of a shocked client

Subsequently, Ratcliffe suggests that midwives should continue to assess the following:

- Airway
- Breathing
- Circulation (Resuscitation Council UK 2001, 2005a)

ABC is a globally recognised gold standard for assessment. The Intensive Care Society (2002) issued guidelines for the introduction of outreach services where they note that clients at risk of deterioration can be identified by:

- The exhibition of abnormal physical signs
- Their condition and history
- Intuition that the patient is not 'quite right' (patterns observed from previous experience)

However, midwives can only assess women for signs of deterioration if they have the assessment skills, time, motivation, comprehension of their role and the role of other practitioners within the team, and an understanding of the consequences of what they are seeing.

What do we want to know when being confronted with a potentially shocked pregnant woman? Ask the woman how she feels. This will complete a major component of the assessment: airway. Simply put, an unconscious patient will not respond, demonstrating an inability to maintain one's airway. However, if the woman responds, she can tell you other important information. A confused woman may answer inappropriately or a woman may suggest they are in pain. Further, you are also conducting a respiratory assessment because, if the woman has to pause for breath to speak, this is also giving you information.

The *primary assessment* should include:

- Respiratory rate, depth and pattern
- Blood pressure (systolic/diastolic, mean) and pulse pressure
- Heart rate, rhythm and amplitude
- Temperature (peripheral or central)

The *secondary assessment* should also include:

- Level of consciousness, orientation and evidence of pain.
- Colour, perfusion and peripheral warmth.
- Urine output and quality. Renal function is sensitive to perfusion and urinary output during pregnancy is the best non-invasive indicator of circulatory volume. An output of less than 30 ml/h indicates decreased circulatory volume to the uterus (Gilbert & Harmon 2003).

To assess a woman comprehensively you must lay your hands on them and look under the covers. This is why we emphasise maintaining the client's dignity. You cannot conduct a comprehensive assessment by standing at the end of the bed. The circulation component of the assessment includes pulse, blood pressure, how warm the woman feels, evidence of blood loss and urine output.

It is vital that good communication is maintained between anaesthetists, obstetricians, midwives, neonatologists and other specialists, such as haematologists and intensivists, both during emergency situations and in preparation for anticipated problems. The overall aim is to ensure that appropriate care and management are delivered without delay (Robson & Holdcroft 2000).

Assessment summary

To summarise, the information to be gathered from (or about) the pregnant woman in a shocked condition should include:

- The patient's neurological state: can they maintain their airway, are they conscious and are they lucid?
- Are they warm or cold? What about their urine output?
- Is the patient in pain? What does a comprehensive pain assessment tell me?

- What are the patient's vital signs, respiratory rate, pulse, blood pressure and temperature?
- Is there evidence of blood loss?
- Fetal evaluation.

Principles of shock reversal

- Treat the cause
- Oxygen therapy
- Cardiac output restoration by fluid resuscitation/inotrope therapy
- Restore perfusion and offer supportive therapy
- Ensure adequate pain relief

Signs of improvement

- Stabilising pulse (rate of 90/min or less)
- Increased blood pressure (systolic 100 mmHg or more)
- Improving mental status (less confusion or anxiety)
- Increasing urine output

Hypovolaemic shock

Hypovolaemic shock refers to a medical or surgical condition in which rapid fluid loss results in multiple organ failure due to inadequate perfusion (Kolecki & Menckhoff 2005). It is a clinical state in which tissue perfusion is rendered relatively inadequate by loss of blood or plasma after injury to the vascular tree. Hypovolaemic shock should also stimulate consideration of the differential diagnosis of fluid deprivation (severe dehydration, excessive vomiting and diarrhoea) and conditions causing inappropriate fluid shift such as pre-eclampsia, sepsis or anaphylaxis.

Physiological pathway of hypovolaemic shock

Hypovolaemia leads to a decreased circulatory volume reducing venous return. Subsequent adaptive mechanisms lead to an increased heart and respiratory rate but the reduced preload and tachycardia leads to a decreased stroke volume and cardiac output. As cardiac output falls, the adrenal glands release catecholamines causing arterioles and venules in the skin, lungs, gastrointestinal tract, liver and kidney to constrict, thus diverting available blood flow to the brain and heart. This leads to reduced systemic cell perfusion, oxygenation and impaired cellular metabolism leading to anaerobic metabolism, lactic acid formation, loss of cell integrity and, if not corrected, cell death.

Causes of hypovolaemic shock in pregnancy

Obstetric haemorrhage (from placenta praevia or placental abruption) is cited as the major contributory factor in hypovolaemic shock (Bird 1997; Kolecki & Menckhoff 2005). Seventeen maternal deaths in the 2000–2002 Confidential Enquiry into Maternal Deaths (CEMD) report (Lewis 2004) were caused by ante-partum or postpartum haemorrhage. A ruptured ectopic pregnancy can also cause a significant blood loss, which in turn can result in a shocked state.

Clinical features

Ratcliffe (1999) and Baskett (1991) identify the clinical signs of hypovolaemia as restlessness, anxiety, confusion, coma, tachypnoea and air hunger, skin changes, sweating, cold peripheries, peripheral oedema, dry mouth and thirst, tachy-cardia, hypotension, oliguria, anuria and low volume pulses peripherally, and at a more advanced stage, centrally. Peripheries are cool with at least a 2°C gap between core and peripheral temperatures, capillary refill is slow (greater than 2 seconds after 5 seconds' pressure) and often pallor or peripheral cyanosis is present. The woman may be irritable with a reduced conscious level or may pre-sent unconscious. Reduced tissue perfusion leads to cellular hypoxia, anaerobic glycolysis, lactic acid production, metabolic acidosis and elevated lactate (Hinds 1999). Due to altered physiology, the assessment of the shocked pregnant woman is complicated as, for example, peripheral oedema is frequently present during normal pregnancy. The importance of the woman's mental state is paramount as altered levels of consciousness and lucidity may manifest before the later stage changes of altered vital signs. Clinical presentation is the most important factor and the consequences of allowing the shocked state to progress emphasises the need for midwives to remain with their clients to offer clinical and psychological care. Women should not be left alone.

Estimating blood loss

Estimating blood loss from the haemorrhaging pregnant woman is difficult. Almost 40% of maternal blood volume may be lost prior to the signs of maternal shock becoming apparent (Sharma & Mink 2004). Up to 3000 ml of blood may remain concealed in the uterus, while a small blood loss of 100 ml may not cause maternal symptoms but may jeopardise the fetus (Robson & Holdcroft 2000). Visual assessments include estimates of stained bedding and linen protectors or amount of blood pooling on the floor. It is not easy to assess the blood loss from the genital tract unless it is overt. The measured blood loss plus an estimate of the concealed blood loss should be considered and a prediction of the continuing risk and extent of blood loss should be made in order not to delay treatment. Swabs should be weighed (1 g = 1 ml). Any blood clots represent blood cells without plasma and their measured volume can be doubled to estimate actual loss.

Direct measurements of haemoglobin concentration and haematocrit levels can be made after blood transfusion through laboratory studies. Suction volume can be calculated subtracting estimations for amniotic fluid volume. Vaginal inspection or uterus palpation for intrauterine collections can offer further information (Holdcroft and Thomas 2000; Robson & Holdcroft 2000; Gilbert & Harmon 2003).

Care and management

Clinical principles of management include:

- Comprehensive assessment and monitoring
- Goal-related therapy
- Fluid replacement and correction of lost coagulation factors
- Diagnosis and treatment of the bleeding cause (medical or surgical therapy)

Time is precious particularly during the development of hypovolaemic shock. Virtually all causes of acute gynaecological/obstetric bleeding that cause hypovolaemia require surgical intervention (Kolecki & Menckhoff 2005). In all cases of circulatory insufficiency, the objective is to restore oxygen delivery to the tissues while correcting the underlying cause (Hinds 1999). As assessment is made following ABC, goal-related therapy should be initiated in the same order of priority. First, maintain the patient's airway and administer high flow inspired oxygen (15 L/min) through a facemask with a reservoir bag. Consider raising the woman's legs to increase blood perfusion to vital organs until fluid replacement can be achieved (Gilbert & Harmon 2003).

The woman will require aggressive fluid resuscitation. At least two large-bore intravenous cannulae must be inserted. The choice of peripheral or central cannulation depends on the experience of the anaesthetist. Peripheral access to a central line is preferred, unless experienced staff and facilities for treating complications of inserting internal jugular or subclavian lines are readily available (Holdcroft & Thomas 2000).

Blood samples for cross-match, clotting studies and full blood count (FBC), including platelets, should be sent urgently to the haematologist at the time of cannulation. Fluid-warming devices and pressure infusors should be used, initially to give 2 L of crystalloid and colloid while awaiting the arrival of blood (Holdcroft & Thomas 2000). Depending on time constraints, blood for transfusion may be cross-matched or group-specific. In dire emergencies, O-negative blood, which may be available for immediate use on the labour ward, can be administered. A more rapid rate of infusion is required in the management of shock resulting from bleeding.

The consequences of not replacing lost fluid are an increased period in the shocked state and the subsequent development of, for example, maternal renal failure due to hypotension. Overly aggressive fluid resuscitation can also predispose the patient to postshock complications such as acute respiratory distress syndrome. Midwives need to consider possible complications of massive fluid resuscitation such as immunological disturbances, citrate toxicity, acid base disturbances, hyperkalaemia, hypothermia and jaundice.

Throughout fluid resuscitation, a left lateral tilt of the pelvis is essential if the baby has not been delivered. Supine hypertension occurs when the mother remains in the flat position. The side lying position is recommended, but if the mother must be supine, the uterus should be tilted away from the inferior vena cava by using a wedge under the hip (Hudak et al. 1998).

Monitoring in the form of electrocardiogram (ECG), pulse oximetry and continuous arterial line pressure wave monitoring will almost certainly be required. A urinary catheter should be placed to allow the patient's urine output to be assessed and to facilitate a comprehensive fluid input/output chart to be maintained alongside the fluids being introduced. Empirical oxygen may also be required.

The health care team is dependent upon the quality of the personnel who make up the team. Staff with poor assessment skills and a poor understanding of the consequences of their patient's presentation will hinder a successful outcome.

The clinical signs and symptoms of blood loss and hypovolaemia in the pregnant woman at term are shown in Table 8.1.

Table 8.1   Clinical signs and symptoms of blood loss and hypovolaemia in the pregnant woman term (adapted from Fcrouz 1999).

Mild bleeding Class 1	Moderate bleeding Class 2	Severe bleeding Class 3	Massive bleeding Class 4
15% of blood volume (up to 1000 ml)	20–25% (up to 1600 ml)	30–35% of blood volume (up to 2400 ml)	40% of blood volume (over 2400 ml)
Mild/absent tachycardia	Tachycardia (heart rate 110–130/min)	Marked tachycardia (heart rate 120–160/min)	Marked tachycardia
Normal blood pressure and respiration, no change in pulse pressure	Decreased pulse pressure Moderate tachypnoea Positive capillary blanching test Decreasing pulse pressure	Hypotension Tachypnoea (respirations > 30/min) Pronounced changes in pulse pressure	Systolic blood pressure < 80 mmHg Peripheral pulses absent Excessive changes in pulse pressure
Negative tilt test	Positive tilt test	Cold, clammy, palid skin, colour changes	Mental status changed/disorientated/ confused
Normal urine output	Urine output < 1 ml/kg/h)	Oliguria	Oliguria or anuria
No change in baseline vital signs	Moderate compensation of vital signs	Marked changes in vital signs	Life-threatening changes in vital signs

Organisational issues

Clinical assessment must be supported with organisational management and resource allocation. The CEMD report (Lewis 2004) provides key recommendations surrounding the management of women at known risk of haemorrhage and therefore the potential risk of developing hypovolaemic shock:

- Every unit should have a protocol for the management of haemorrhage and this should be reviewed and rehearsed on a regular basis. It should also be included in life support training. All members of staff, including those in the blood bank, must know exactly what to do to ensure that large quantities of cross-matched blood can be delivered without delay.
- The speed with which obstetric haemorrhage can become life threatening emphasises the need for women at known high risk of haemorrhage to be delivered in a hospital with a blood bank on site and appropriate laboratory facilities, including haematological advice and therapy.
- Placenta praevia, particularly in women with previous uterine scars, may be associated with uncontrollable uterine haemorrhage at delivery or caesarean section and a hysterectomy may be necessary. A very experienced operator is essential and a consultant must be readily available.
- On-call consultant obstetricians must consider all available interventions to stop haemorrhage, such as radical surgery or embolisation of uterine arteries, involving surgical or radiological colleagues as required.
- It is essential that both obstetricians and anaesthetists be involved, at an early stage, in planning the elective management of very high risk cases.
- If haemorrhage occurs, experienced consultant obstetric and anaesthetic staff must attend.

The effects of obstetric haemorrhage may be further exacerbated by the development of thrombocytopenia, coagulopathy or sepsis (Sharma 2003). Coagulation defects such as disseminated intravascular coagulation (DIC) have the potential to cause further complications such as tissue damage to the major organs.

Disseminated intravascular coagulation

Baglin (1996) describes DIC as an unregulated thrombin explosion causing the release of free thrombin into the circulation. This extensive microvascular thrombosis can produce tissue ischaemia, organ damage and finally result in mortality. Haemorrhage appears to be the commonest presentation and is caused by the generation of free plasmin and the depletion of coagulation factors and platelets in fluid loss.

Diagnosis

Any degree of abnormal bleeding or clotting in a sick childbearing woman should alert doctors and midwives to the possibility of the development of DIC. The diagnosis of DIC is made with laboratory tests, providing positive evidence as to the presence of the syndrome.

Treatment

Treatment of the underlying cause is essential for treating DIC. The condition will not resolve until the trigger mechanism is removed, and mortality from DIC is often the result of the underlying disease. Patients may be treated with blood components to replace depleted coagulation factors, platelets and natural inhibitors of thrombin and plasmin in an attempt to reduce bleeding while the underlying problem is corrected.

Cardiogenic shock

Cardiogenic shock is characterised by a decreased pumping ability of the heart causing a shock-like state with inadequate perfusion of the tissues (Hostetler 2004). Cardiac complications in pregnancy tend to fall into two categories: complications due to clients presenting pregnant with pre-existing disease and those who become compromised during pregnancy.

Causes in pregnancy

Despite the increased workload of the heart during gestation and labour, the healthy woman has no impairment of cardiac reserve. In contrast, for the gravida with heart disease and low cardiac reserve, the increase in the work of the heart may cause ventricular failure and pulmonary oedema (Ciliberto & Marx 1998). Nelson-Piercy (2002) notes that the ability to tolerate pregnancy is related to the following:

- Presence of cyanosis (arterial oxygen saturation 80%)
- Presence of pulmonary hypertension
- Haemodynamic significance of any lesion
- Functional class (New York Heart Association (NYHA) classification)

Predictors of cardiac events in pregnant woman with heart disease can also include the following (Nelson-Piercy 2002):

- History of transient ischaemic attacks or arrhythmias
- History of heart failure
- Left heart obstruction
- Myocardial dysfunction

If cardiac reserve is limited, increased cardiac work may precipitate cardiac failure (Woodrow 2000). Poor cardiac function that cannot tolerate excessive stress will fail when confronted with the increased preload and increased left atrial pressure induced by pregnancy and the patient may develop pulmonary oedema and right heart failure.

During the intrapartum phase, cardiac function is elevated due to increased intravascular volume and in the immediate postpartum period there is a risk for fluid volume overload in the pregnant woman presenting with cardiac disease (Gilbert & Harmon 2003). Duffy (2002) notes that pregnant women with pre-existing cardiovascular disease may decompensate during pregnancy because of these physiological demands. This is especially true for women with stenotic valvular lesions.

Women presenting with cardiogenic shock will manifest complicated, interrelated, systemic symptoms requiring high quality medical and midwifery management/care. Mitral valve disease is the most frequently seen valve defect in pregnant women (Gilbert & Harmon 2003), and if either parent has a congenital heart defect the fetus has an increased risk for also developing such a defect (Gilbert & Harmon 2003).

The causes of cardiac disease in pregnancy can be summarised as follows (Gilbert & Harmon 2003):

- Rheumatic fever
- Valve deformities
- Congenital heart disease
- Developmental abnormalities
- Congestive cardiac myopathies
- Cardiac dysrhythmias

Peripartum cardiomyopathy can develop in previously fit women in the last month of pregnancy or up to 5 months' postpartum (Bird 1997). Dilatation and poor function of the left ventricle are characteristic and the prognosis depends on the speed of resolution, although mortality rates are high at 50–60%. Risk factors for the development of the condition include age, multiparity, twin pregnancy, African descent, long-term tocolytic therapy and cocaine abuse (Gilbert & Harmon 2003).

Classification

Cardiogenic shock can be divided into two broad categories:

- *Coronary.* The cause of the shock is intrinsic to the heart itself. The most frequently cited cause in this category is acute myocardial infarction secondary to atherosclerotic disease. Other causes include severe heart failure due to coronary disease, valve defects, arrhythmias, endocarditis, ventricular septal defects or cardiomyopathies. Coronary heart disease is uncommon in women of reproductive age but myocardial infarction may occur because of the excessive haemodynamic stress of pregnancy (Gilbert & Harmon 2003).
- *Non-coronary.* The cause of the cardiogenic shock is extrinsic to the heart. Examples include hypovolaemia, trauma, drug overdose, respiratory acidosis, pulmonary embolism, cardiac tamponade, tension pneumothorax, or swelling or inflammation around the heart impeding the heart's ability to pump.

The NYHA identifies maternal risk subgroups, which may be found in mid-wifery clientele groups although the incidence is rare. The resulting mortality for each complication has been reported (Gilbert & Harmon 2003):

- *Group 1*, with a mortality rate of less than 1%, includes atrial septal defects and pulmonary/tricuspid disease.
- *Group 2* (two groups), with a mortality rate of between 5 and 15%, includes disorders such as previous myocardial infarction, coarction of the aorta without valve involvement or the presence of an artificial valve.
- *Group 3*, with a mortality rate of 25–50%, includes disorders such as pulmonary hypertension, coarction of the aorta with valvular involvement or Marfan's syndrome with aortic involvement.

The CEMD report (Lewis 2004) identified 44 deaths due to cardiac disease in pregnancy and care was found to be substandard in 40% of these cases. Learning points surrounding the variants in cardiac diseases are clearly identified in the report, and indicate the need for the development of protocols for the management of pregnant women with cardiac diseases who can become extremely ill for non-obstetric reasons.

Physiological pathway of cardiogenic shock

A clear understanding of the pathophysiology related to this condition is vital if midwifery staff are to be involved in care as effective members of the multidisciplinary team. Postmortem studies by Harnarayan et al. (1970) found that cardiogenic shock manifested with the loss of 40% of the left ventricular myocardium.

Taking the presentation of myocardial infarction for example, necrosed myocardium that does not contract has two major implications. For myocardium damage predominantly on the left side of the heart, first, the cardiac output falls and second, stroke volume and ejection fraction is reduced. The reduction in volume ejected by the left side of the heart leads to hypotension and increased pooling of blood in the ventricles, eventually elevating ventricular filling pressures.

As myocardial oxygen demands are affected by heart rate, contractility and wall tension, stretching of the cardiac chamber due to increased ventricular filling pressure will reduce heart wall compliance, raise oxygen requirements and lead to an already strained tachycardic heart to fail. Further, in an attempt to maintain vital organ perfusion, the body responds by vasoconstricting and increasing systemic vascular resistance, increasing afterload and making the heart work even harder to eject blood out of the ventricles.

Clients experience a 'double whammy' of compromised cardiac function and respiratory distress as the elevated ventricular filling pressures eventually result in the manifestation of pulmonary oedema.

With right ventricular damage the right ventricle is unable to pump blood through the pulmonary circulation to the left side of the heart. In simple terms, as the left side of the heart can only eject what enters it (Starling's law) cardiac output falls, tissue perfusion is reduced and cardiogenic shock manifests. Subsequently the inability of the heart to pump effectively manifests as the classic symptoms of shock identified earlier.

Presentation

The woman presenting with cardiogenic shock will suffer from a range of symptoms that vary in severity but may include:

- Hypotension, tachycardia, a rapid and thready pulse, arrhythmias, decreased stroke volume, cardiac index, cardiac contractility, ejection fraction and hence cardiac output, reduced tissue perfusion, increased systemic vascular resistance, vasoconstriction, decreased peripheral pulses and cool extremities, and the presence of systemic emboli.
- Increased respiratory rate, increased work of breathing, pulmonary congestion/oedema, cyanosis, acidosis, decreased PaO_2 decreased SvO_2, deteriorating chest radiograph, hyperlactataemia and tissue hypoxia.
- Reduced renal perfusion leading to salt and water retention and circulating volume redistribution culminating in acute renal failure.
- Altered mental status, pain, fear and anxiety.
- Postpartum patients may have a localised abscess, resistant organisms or pelvic thrombophlebitis and persistent fever.
- Fetal distress.

Care and management

Treatment of the cause and optimalisation of the woman's current health status is a fundamental goal of critical care. Women will need to be cared for in facilities offering advanced monitoring and therapies. Treatment will be guided by information taken from patient assessment, monitoring equipment and diagnostic evidence. Particularly relevant to the management of cardiogenic shock is the ability of the facility to treat the cause of the shocked state. If the cause requires cardiac surgery, for example, facilities lacking this service must aim for early stabilisation and transfer. An elemental principle of critical care is that it is the response to therapy, not patient presentation, that is important. Is the therapy working? How do you know? The multidisciplinary team must have clear goals in relation to care. Specific therapy goals in relation to cardiogenic shock include (Nimmo 1993; Holmes & Walley 2003):

- Stimulation of myocardial function
- Improvement of pre/afterload
- Maintenance of valvular function and structure
- Improvement of coronary artery perfusion and the increase of oxygen supply to the myocardium
- Improvement of oxygen delivery ($SvO_2 > 60\%$)

From a cardiovascular perspective, dilemmas may occur in the choice of fluids, inotropes, diuretics, beta-blockers or vasodilators in relation to the cause of the cardiogenic shock. However, supporting the heart is vital regardless of the therapy – systemic perfusion must be optimised together with support for the pumping mechanism of the heart itself. Evidence of improved cardiovascular perfusion would come from a haemodynamically stable, pain-free, warm and well-perfused woman producing a reasonable urine output.

From a respiratory perspective, midwives should be vigilant for the development of respiratory failure and pulmonary oedema. Cardiogenic shock can result in major increases in respiratory muscle oxygenation requirements; it has been demonstrated through experimentation that respiratory arrest due to diaphragmatic exhaustion is frequently the cause of death as opposed to cardiac dysfunction (Nimmo 1993).

From a neurological perspective, pain relief is vital as a woman in pain may be uncompliant and will have increased myocardial oxygen requirements. Further changes or deterioration in a woman's mental status may, however, indicate a shocked state, which will require urgent management.

From a renal perspective, a reduced renal output is a further indication of a shocked state. A drop in cardiac output of 10–20% can have a direct effect on the glomerular filtration rate by up to 20% (Darovic 1995). If untreated, this reduction in secreted urine can result in the retention of damaging metabolic waste products and potentially acute renal failure.

Immunosupression has been recommended for women with peripartum cardiomyopathy and myocarditis diagnosed by biopsy (Gilbert & Harmon 2003).

Post-event care may revolve around counselling due to the potential dangers of future pregnancies with compromised cardiovascular function.

Neurogenic shock

Causes

Neurogenic shock is caused by the interruption of autonomic sympathetic control from central nervous system injury or oedema (Woodrow 2000). Causes include any disruption to the systemic nervous system such as trauma, spinal anaesthesia, drugs, stress, pain or central nervous system dysfunction (Urden et al. 2002). Neurogenic shock is an infrequent occurrence in pregnancy (Urden et al. 2002) and will only be dealt with briefly here.

Physiology

A disruption of the sympathetic nervous system leads to a loss of sympathetic tone, venous and arterial vasodilatation, decreased venous return, decreased stroke volume and a fall in cardiac output. As this large increase in blood vessel capacity is not matched by increased volume, perfusion falls and bradycardia from excessive and uncontrolled vagal tone further reduces blood pressure (Woodrow

2000). The loss of vasomotor tone also impairs thermoregulation, with the woman becoming dependent on the environment for temperature regulation (Urden et al. 2002). This leads to impaired tissue perfusion, cell oxygenation, impaired cellular metabolism and cell death.

Presentation

The woman presenting with neurogenic shock will manifest profound hypotension, bradycardia and loss of temperature control (Hudak et al. 1998).

Care and management

Management will depend on the type of injury experienced by the patient. Traumatic injuries may require transfer to specialised units. Management is generally the same as for other forms of shock considered in this chapter. The failure of autonomic response makes inotropes ineffective but fluid resuscitation may compensate for the increased blood vessel capacity (Woodrow 2000).

Anaphylactic shock

Lieberman (2002) defines anaphylaxis as 'a systemic, immediate hypersensitivity event produced by the union of antigen and IgE affixed to basophil and mast cells.' Following manifestation of the condition, the host may experience a wide range of symptoms from anxiety and restlessness to respiratory depression and cardiac arrest (Jones 2000). Severe anaphylaxis represents a life-threatening experience and, therefore, midwifery staff require in-depth knowledge and a clear understanding of the presentation and management of the condition in order to maximise the opportunity for the safe recovery of mother and child.

Box 8.1 shows the common causes of anaphylaxis.

Pathophysiology

When an antigen is first introduced to the body it stimulates the production of immunoglobulin IgE. This attaches to mast and basophil cells (Carroll 1994). Once the body has manufactured IgE and it is attached to the surface of mast and basophil cells, the body now has a primary immune response. Initial exposure to the antigen is referred to as sensitisation (Henderson 1998) and, as Carroll (1994) notes, mast and basophil cells combined with IgE on their surface are like bombs waiting to explode and deposit their cell contents into the circulatory system.

During the primary response, a memory is laid down for further encounters with the same antigen. When the body encounters the antigen again, the IgE recognises it and an allergic reaction takes place.

> **Box 8.1   Common causes of anaphylaxis (Fisher 1986; Wyatt 1996; Docherty & Hall 2002).**
>
> Drugs
> Penicillin and cephalosporin antibiotics are the most commonly reported medical agents
> Aspirin and non-steroidal anti-inflammatory drugs
> Anaesthetics
> Opiates
> Muscle relaxants
> Intravenous radiocontrast media can cause an anaphylactoid reaction that is clinically identical to true anaphylaxis
> Plasma expanders
> Blood products
> Latex
> Food allergies (e.g. nuts, fish, eggs, dairy products)
> Insect stings

Mast cells and basophils are found primarily in the lungs, small intestine, skin and connective tissue (mast cells, interstitial, basophils, intravascular) (Henderson 1998; Jones 2000). As the mast and basophil cells are activated, they degranulate. Degranulation occurs when the surface of the cells ruptures, allowing substances found inside to leak out (Dreskin & Palmer 2005). Inside the cells are found histamine in an ionic complex with heparin. When degranulation occurs, this complex is released and the histamine and heparin separate. Histamine mediates its effects by acting on histamine 1 (H1) and histamine 2 (H2) receptors resulting in smooth muscle contraction, increased vascular permeability, increased gastric acid secretion, systemic vasodilatation and cardiovascular stimulation (Dreskin & Palmer 2005). The anticoagulant activity of heparin and the vasodilating and smooth muscle properties of histamine are easily identified in persons presenting with severe anaphylaxis through a characteristic flushing of the skin and systemic vasodilatation leading to circulatory collapse. Box 8.2 summarises the additional substances released following mast and basophil degranulation.

Clinical features

Potentially fatal reactions result in severe upper airway obstruction due to angioedema leading to asphyxiation, and/or lower airway obstruction, wheezing and chest tightness caused by bronchospasm (Wyatt 1996). The cardiovascular system may manifest tachycardia, arrhythmias and reduced cardiac contractility (Henderson 1998; Edwards 2001). Profound hypotension may also be present, caused by selective systemic vasodilatation/vasoconstriction and inappropriate fluid shift from the intravascular to the extravascular space due to mediator effects on capillary permeability (Edwards 2001). Significant upper and lower respiratory

---

Box 8.2   Additional substances released following mast and basophil degranulation (Dreskin & Palmer 2005; Krause 2005).

Slow reactive substances of anaphylaxis (SRS-A)
Eosonophil chemotactic factor of anaphylaxis (ECF-A)
Prostaglandins
Leukotrines
Platelet-activating factor
Tumour necrosis factor
Serotonin
Mast cell kininogenase
Basophil kallikrein
Tryptase

---

obstruction represents the cause of death in 70% of cases, and cardiac arrhythmia and dysfunction is present in 24% of cases (Krause 2005).

General presentation depends on the severity of the reaction. Patients may present as anxious and restless with a sense of impending doom particularly if they have experienced these symptoms before. Severe air hunger, hoarseness, dyspnoea, stridor, altered levels of consciousness, rhinitis and conjunctivitis may manifest. Urticaria (hives) may develop as red, raised lesions that may have central blanching. Intense pruritus occurs with these lesions, which may be prominent on the lips, palms, soles and genitalia. Abdominal pain, nausea, vomiting and diarrhoea may also be present (Henderson 1998; Edwards 2001; Resuscitation Council UK 2005a).

Care and management

The Resuscitation Council UK (2005b) provides clear guidance on the management of anaphylaxis:

- The use of adrenaline, which should be administered intramuscularly to all patients with clinical signs of shock, airway swelling or definite breathing difficulty.
- The consideration of other medication such as antihistamines and hydrocortisone in an aim to reduce symptoms.

A flowchart on management is available on http://www.resus.org.uk/pages/anafig1.pdf.

Why is adrenaline important?

As an alpha-receptor agonist, adrenaline reverses peripheral vasodilatation and decreases oedema. Its beta-receptor activity dilates the airways and increases the force of myocardial contraction. Adrenaline also attaches to and stimulates the adrenergic receptors on the mast cells. This allows the buildup of cyclic adenosine monophosphate (cAMP) that in turn stabilises the mast cells, thus reducing the release of cell contents (Jones 2000).

Intramuscular adrenaline is generally regarded as safe (except in coronary heart disease) whilst intravascular adrenaline is considered hazardous as therapy can be complicated by reactions or response to the drug (Resuscitation Council UK 2005b).

Recommended doses of adrenaline

Adrenaline should be administered intramuscularly to all patients with clinical signs of shock, airway swelling or definite breathing difficulty. Manifestations such as inspiratory stridor, wheeze, cyanosis, pronounced tachycardia and decreased capillary refilling time indicate a severe reaction. A dose of 0.5 ml adrenaline 1:1000 solution (500 μg) should be administered intramuscularly and repeated after 5 minutes in the absence of clinical improvement or if deterioration occurs after the initial treatment, particularly if consciousness becomes or remains impaired as a result of hypotension (Docherty & Hall 2002; Resuscitation Council UK 2005b). In some cases several doses of adrenaline may be needed.

Antihistamines

Antihistamines act by combining with histamine receptors (H1, H2) and competitively inhibiting them. An antihistamine such as chlorpheniramine should be administered either intramuscularly or slowly if given intravenously in order to avoid drug-induced hypotension (Jevon 2000). The recommended dose is 10–20 mg (Resuscitation Council UK 2005b).

Hydrocortisone

Hydrocortisone works by inhibiting virtually every step of the inflammatory pathway. Steroids inhibit SRS-A (slow acting substance of anaphylaxis), bradykinins and prostaglandins, and increase cAMP production (Palmer & Dreskin 2004). Hydrocortisone should be given by intramuscular injection or slowly intravenously to avoid inducing further hypotension (Resuscitation Council UK 2005b). The current recommended dose for adults is 100–500 mg (Docherty & Hall 2002; Resuscitation Council UK 2005b).

Other drugs

Salbutamol, ipratropium and aminophylline may all improve respiratory function, while aminophylline also increases cAMP production (Jones 2000). Fifty percent of intravascular volume can be lost within 10 minutes of anaphylaxis presenting. Therefore, if there appears to be little clinical improvement, further supportive measures of fluid, inotropes and antiarrhythmic drugs should be considered (Lieberman 2002) in an attempt to stabilise failing systems.

Principles of management

The key to the successful management of severe anaphylaxis revolves around appropriate staff education. Early identification, comprehensive assessment and prompt treatment are the goals of care. Midwifery staff encountering severe anaphylaxis should summon expert assistance, remove the likely allergen and administer high flow 100% oxygen (Docherty & Hall 2002). Above all, staff should ensure that they are familiar with current best practice guidelines for managing anaphylaxis published by bodies such as the Resuscitation Council UK.

When faced with severe anaphylaxis the following acronym (adapted from Ferns & Chojnacka 2003) may help:

- **E**: *e*xpertise in management and *e*arly treatment is of paramount importance.
- **A**: *a*ssess following airway, breathing, circulation (ABC). Ensure intravenous *a*ccess and initiate goal-related therapy.
- **R**: *r*emove the likely allergen.
- **L**: consider *l*ong-term (24-hour post event) monitoring.
- **Y**: as a qualified professional midwife it is *y*our responsibility to ensure women presenting with anaphylaxis receive high quality care. Take personal responsibility.

Post-event care

About 40% of patients have a further episode of anaphylaxis within 24 hours (Carroll 1994). Treatment and support/monitoring should continue and staff should approach with a high index of suspicion, with staff vigilant and careful to identify further manifestations of anaphylaxis early. Clients should be cared for by appropriately educated staff in areas with access to suitable monitoring/resuscitation equipment. Prevention of the condition will rely heavily on avoidance of harmful agents and midwives should offer health promotion advice. Referral to specialist allergy clinics and organisations such as the Anaphylaxis Campaign may help (Docherty & Hall 2002). Women experiencing severe reactions should consider carrying self-administrative adrenaline syringes (Jones 2000).

Midwifery teams should hold debriefing sessions to discuss particular incidents in order to review performance to ensure future high quality care is ensured. Severe episodes of anaphylaxis can be traumatic for staff and the opportunity to share the experience with colleagues through reflection may be both personally helpful and a positive team-building experience. It is particularly important that staff understand their professional responsibilities when such situations occur.

Septic shock

The definition of sepsis is complicated by a number of variables and the severity of the insult. Systemic inflammatory response syndrome (SIRS) is the hypermetabolic state that follows a severe insult and is defined as the presence of two or more of the following (American College of Chest Physicians and Society of Critical Care Medicine Consensus Conference 1992):

- Temperature > 38 or < 36°C
- Heart rate > 90 beats/min
- Tachypnoea respiratory rate > 20 breaths/min
- $Paco_2$ < 4.25 kPa
- Raised white cell count

The term sepsis refers to SIRS plus evidence of documented infection. Severe sepsis can be defined as sepsis associated with acute organ dysfunction, and results from a generalised inflammatory and procoagulant host response to infection (Bone 1997). Septic shock refers to sepsis induced hypotension (systolic blood pressure < 90 mmHg or a reduction of > 40 mmHg from baseline) despite adequate fluid resuscitation (Evans & Smithies 1999). Altered physiology of pregnancy must be considered when applying these variables and the fact that frequently an infective source cannot be identified (Evans & Smithies 1999). Data related to the incidence of severe sepsis are complicated due to the condition's frequent association with other insults such as acute respiratory distress syndrome or severe trauma.

In the USA, mortality rates for severe sepsis range from 30 to 50% (Linde-Zwirble et al. 1999), and Angus et al. (2001) estimates that there are now an estimated 751 000 cases (three per 1000 people) of sepsis or septic shock in the United States each year, responsible for as many deaths each year as acute myocardial infarction (215 000 or 9.3% of all deaths). Severe sepsis is the leading cause of severe illness and death in medical and surgical patients in intensive care (Bone 1997). A prevalence rate of severe sepsis in adult intensive care units has been cited at 27.1%, which equates to an estimated 23 000 cases annually (Padkin et al. 2003); ultimate hospital mortality for admissions who met the criteria for severe sepsis within the first 24 hours of admission to ICUs in England, Wales and Northern Ireland was 45% (Padkin et al. 2001).

Severe sepsis is a significant midwifery challenge and prevention of the development of the condition is always the best course of action. Numerous factors predispose the pregnant client to developing the condition. Initial insults such as trauma or the need for positive pressure ventilation are important but other factors to be considered include poor infection control policies, staffing levels, length of hospital stay, invasive equipment or monitoring equipment utilised (urinary catheters, central venous pressure lines), resident populations of micro-organisms, inappropriate antibiotic therapy, poor nutritional status, contaminated supplies/equipment or the need for immunosuppression. The lung is the most common site of infection followed by the abdomen and urinary tract (Wheeler & Bernard 1999).

Generally, severe sepsis or septic shock is associated with a severe, overwhelming systemic infection. It is a vasogenic form of shock, grouped with neurogenic and anaphylactic shock and develops secondary to the body being invaded by a foreign body. Sepsis is caused by a wide variety of organisms:

- Endogenous: *Staphylococcus aureus, Haemophilus influenza, Escherichia coli* and *Streptococcus pneumoniae*
- Exogenous: *Klebsiella, Pseudomonas, Proteus, Serratia* and *Actinobacillus*

Gram-positive organisms are responsible for two-thirds of infections but other organisms implicated include Gram-negative bacteria, viruses, yeasts and fungi, and in 20–30% of cases there are multiple causative organisms increasing the difficulty in treatment.

Causes of severe sepsis in pregnancy

Sharma (2003) identified the commonest causes of severe sepsis in pregnant women as septic abortion, chorioamniotic and postpartum infections, pyelonephritis and respiratory tract infections. Prolonged rupture of membranes, retained products of conception and instrumentation of the genitourinary tract are other significant risk factors. If maternal infections occur, they usually develop during the post-partum period as endometriosis is more prevalent after a caesarean delivery (Robinson et al. 2000).

The CEMD report (Lewis 2004) indicates that 13 maternal deaths occurred at varying stages of pregnancy due to genital tract sepsis with the most common pathogen being identified as beta-haemolytic *Streptococcus*. Some degree of sub-optimal care was considered to have occurred in 80% of these cases. Recommendations include encouraging all maternity units to have a policy surrounding the use of antibiotics in cases of sepsis to prevent any further deterioration in the maternal condition.

Pathophysiology

There is still a great deal of argument and debate surrounding the pathway of severe sepsis. Evidence appears to centre on endotoxins, exotoxins and host mediators (Sharma & Mink 2004). Endotoxins are lipoproteins contained within Gram-negative organisms and not contained but released by Gram-positive organisms. Exotoxins are products of microorganisms that are harmful to the host, and host mediators include cytokines such as tumour necrosis factor, interleukin 1, 6 and 8, and myocardial depression factor.

The effects of systemic infection involve inappropriate fluid shift and profound vasodilatation compromising tissue perfusion and producing widespread systemic symptoms as part of the inflammatory response. The net result is impaired tissue oxygenation, hypoxia, acidosis, hypotension and hypovolaemia. At cell level reduced oxygenation and perfusion leads to falling adenosine triphosphate (ATP) levels and loss of cell membrane integrity. Despite the body compensating by increasing cardiac output, this rise fails to meet metabolic demands or to compensate for the decreased ventricular preload, leading to end organ subperfusion and failure. As underperfused organs lose integrity, further secondary insults such as acute tubular necrosis, translocation of bacteria through the alimentary tract and coagulopathy disorders manifest.

Clinical features

Clinical symptoms depend on the stage of illness but may include confusion/ drowsiness, pyrexia or hypothermia, tachycardia, tachypnoea, hypotension with a decreased systemic vascular resistance, increased cell permeability and inappropriate fluid shift, relative plus real hypovolaemia, myocardial depression, microcirculatory dysfunction, acidosis, oliguria, thrombocytopenia, rigors and end organ dysfunction with acute renal, liver, heart or respiratory failure. Midwifery care must centre on a comprehensive assessment of vital signs, consciousness levels, evidence of pain, poor perfusion and poor urine output.

Care and management

Conventional therapy follows the golden rule of treating the cause of the severe sepsis and initiating early goal-directed therapy. Supportive therapy will be unsuccessful without the appropriate use of antibiotics or surgery to remove the focus of the sepsis. However, antibiotic therapy is very complicated as inappropriate use can free further microorganisms or increase immunity. Treatment revolves around optimising cardiac output, PaO_2 and arterial pH. Fluids and inotropes are titrated to maximise tissue oxygenation and to correct hypovolaemia. Women require comprehensive assessment and monitoring in an appropriate facility and the diagnosis and treatment of the cause of the insult cannot be overemphasised. Comprehensive samples including mid-stream urine, high vaginal swabs and blood cultures to locate the site of infection should be requested, and microbiologist support is essential. Further support to prevent complications such as respiratory, heart or renal failure is the current staple treatment of this syndrome together with nutritional support.

However, treatment remains frequently ineffectual as the high mortality figures suggest. Recently, Bellomo and Uchino (2003) have questioned the fundamental aim of therapy in severe sepsis, which drives up cardiac output. They suggest that this may simply lead to an extra surge in cytotoxic plasma to several vital organs, which can increase rather than decrease organ injury. Recent studies suggest that activated protein C, low dose steroids and titrating blood glucose levels to below 6.1 mmol/L can all improve outcomes in sepsis but their effects in the presence of pregnancy remain controversial (Bernard et al. 2001; Annane et al. 2002; Van Den Berghe 2002).

Midwifery care should revolve around early detection of the early symptoms of severe sepsis to ensure prompt therapy is introduced and steps to maintain the comfort of the individual, such as the administration of antipyretic agents, should be considered. Strict infection control policies should be adhered to and as with all forms of severe shock, early fetal delivery and the fundamental philosophy that maternal wellbeing will encourage fetal wellbeing is the priority.

References

American College of Chest Physicians and Society of Critical Care Medicine Consensus Conference (1992) Definitions of sepsis and organ failure and guidelines for the use of innovative therapies in sepsis. *Critical Care Medicine*, **20**: 864–74.
Angus, D., Linde-Zwirble W., Lindicker J., Clermont G., Carcillo, J. and Pinsky, M. (2001) Epidemology of severe sepsis in the United States, analysis of the incidence, outcome and costs of care. *Critical Care Medicine*, **29** (7): 1303–10.
Annane, D., Sebille, V. and Charpentier, C. (2002) Effects of treatment with low doses of hydrocortisone and fludrocortisone in patients with septic shock. *Journal of the American Medical Association*, **288** (7): 862–71.
Baglin, T. (1996) Disseminated intravascular coagulation: diagnosis and treatment. *British Medical Journal*, **312**: 683–6.
Baskett, T. (2004) *Essential Management of Obstetric Emergencies* (2nd edn). Clinical Press, UK.
Bellomo, R. and Uchino, S. (2003) Cardiovascular monitoring tools; use and misuse. *Current Opinion in Critical Care*, **9**: 225–9.
Beringer, R. and Patteril, M. (2004) Puerperal uterine inversion and shock. *British Journal of Anaesthesia*, **92** (3): 439–41.
Bernard, G., Vincent, J. and Laterre, P. (2001) Efficacy and safety of recombinant human activated protein C for sepsis. *New England Journal of Medicine*, **344** (10): 759–62.
Bird, J. (1997) Intensive care problems in obstetric patients. *Care of the Critically Ill*, **13** (6): 241–4.
Bone, R.C. (1997) Managing sepsis; what treatments can we use today? *Journal of Critical Illness*, **12** (1): 15–24.
Carroll, P. (1994) Speed. The essential response to anaphylaxis. *Registered Nurse*, **57** (6): 26.
Ciliberto, C. and Marx, G. (1998) Physiolological changes associated with pregnancy. *Update in Anaesthesia*, Issue 9: Article 2. http://www.nda.ox.ac.uk/wfsa/html/u09/u09_003.htm
Darovic, G. (1995) Haemodynamic monitoring. In: *Invasive and Non-invasive Clinical Application* (2nd edn). W.B. Saunders, London.
Docherty, B. and Hall, S. (2002) Anaphylaxis in adults. *Professional Nurse*, **18** (2): 73–4.
Dreskin, S. and Palmer, G. (2005) Anaphylaxis. http://www.emedicine.com/med/topic128.htm
Duffy, P. (2002) Nonobstetric surgery during pregnancy and obstetric trauma (unpublished). *Anaesthesia Core Program.*
Edwards, S. (1998) Haemodynamic monitoring of the pregnant woman in intensive care. *Nursing in Critical Care*, **3** (3): 112–16.
Edwards, S. (2001) Shock: types, classifications and explorations of their physiological effects. *Emergency Nurse*, **9** (2): 29–38.
Evans, T. and Smithies, M. (1999) Clinical review ABC of intensive care organ dysfunction. *British Medical Journal*, **318**: 1606–9.
Ferns, T. and Chojnacka, I. (2003) The causes of anaphylaxis and its management in adults. *British Journal of Nursing*, **12** (17): 1006–12.
Ferouz, F. (1999) Peripartum haemorrhage and maternal resuscitation. In: M.C. Norris (Ed.) *Obstetric Anaesthesia*. Lippincott, Williams & Wilkins, Philadelphia.
Fisher, M. (1986) Clinical observations of the pathophysiology and treatment of anaphylactic cardiovascular collapse. *Anaesthesia and Intensive Care*, **14**: 17–21.
Gilbert, E. and Harmon, J. (2003) *Manual of High Risk Pregnancy and Delivery* (3rd edn). Mosby, St Louis.
Harnarayan, C., Bennett, M., Pentecost, B. and Brewer, D. (1970) Quantitative study of infarcted myocardium in cardiogenic shock. *British Heart Journal*, **32**: 728–32.

Henderson, N. (1998) Anaphylaxis. *Nursing Standard*, **12** (47): 49–53.

Hinds, C. (1999) Circulatory support. *British Medical Journal*, **318**: 1749–52.

Holdcroft, A. and Thomas, T. (2000) *Principles and Practice of Obstetric Anaesthesia and Analgesia*. Blackwell Science, Oxford.

Holmes, C. and Walley, K. (2003) The evaluation and management of shock. *Clinics in Chest Medicine*, **24**: 775–89.

Hostetler, M. (2004) Shock, cardiogenic. http://emedicine.com/EMERG/topic530.htm

Hudak, C., Gallo, B. and Morton, P. (1998) *Critical Care Nursing: a holistic approach* (7th edn). Lippincott, Philadelphia.

Intensive Care Society (2002) *Guidelines for the Introduction of Outreach Services*. Intensive Care Society, London.

Jevon, P. (2000) Anaphylaxis: emergency management. *Nursing Times*, **96** (14): 39–40.

Jiva, T. (2000) Critical care of pregnant women. Part 1: pulmonary oedema, ARDS, thromboembolism. *Journal of Critical Illness*, **15** (6): 316–24.

Jones, G. (2000) Anaphylactic shock. *Emergency Nurse*, **9** (10): 29–35.

Kolecki, P. and Menckhoff, C. (2005) Hypovolemic shock. http://www.emedicine.com/EMERG/topic532.htm

Krause, R. (2005) Anaphylaxis. http://www.emedicine.com/EMERG/topic25.htm

Lewis, G. (2004) *Why Mothers Die 2000–2002: Report on Confidential Enquiries into Maternal Deaths in the United Kingdom*. Royal College of Obstetricians and Gynaecologists (RCOG), London.

Lieberman, P (2002) Anaphylaxis. http://www.chestnet.org/downloads/education/online/Vol14_07_12.pdf

Linde-Zwirble, W., Angus D., Carcillo, J., Lindicker, J., Clermont, G. and Pinsky, M. (1999) *Critical Care Medicine*, **27** (Suppl. 1): 33A.

Nelson-Piercy, C. (2002) *Handbook of Obstetric Medicine* (2nd edn). Martin Dunitz, London.

Nimmo, G. (1993) Cardiogenic shock, pathophysiology and a therapeutic strategy. *British Journal of Intensive Care*, **Aug**: 294–6.

Padkin, A., Goldfrad, C., Brady, A., Young, D., Black, N. and Rowan, K. (2003) Epidemiology of severe sepsis occurring in the first 24 hours in intensive care units in England, Wales and Northern Ireland. *Critical Care Medicine*, **31**: 2332–8.

Padkin, A., Goldfrad, C., Young, J. and Rowan, K. (2001) The prevalence of severe sepsis in the first 24 hours in the ICU, in England, Wales and Northern Ireland. *Intensive Care Medicine*, **27**: S485.

Palmer, G.W. and Dreskin, S.C. (2004) Anaphylaxis. *eMedicine Website*. http://www.emedicine.com/med/topic128.htm (last updated 30/10/2004)

Ratcliffe, J. (1999) Focus on: Paediatric intensive care recognition and management of shock. *Current Anaesthesia and Critical Care*, **10**: 241–5.

Resuscitation Council UK (2001) *Advanced Life Support Course Provider Manual* (4th edn). Resuscitation Council UK (RCUK), London.

Resuscitation Council UK (2005a) *Advanced Life Support Guidelines*. RCUK, London. (Also available at http://www.resus.org.uk/pages/als.pdf)

Resuscitation Council UK (2005b) *The Emergency Medical Treatment of Anaphylactic Reactions for First Medical Responders and for Community Nurses*. RCUK, London.

Robinson, J., Svigos, J. and Vigneswaran, R. (2000) Prelabour rupture of membranes. In: D. James, P. Steer, C. Weiner and B. Gonik (Eds) *High Risk Pregnancy: Management options*. W.B. Saunders, London.

Robson, V. and Holdcroft, A. (2000) Focus on obstetric emergencies. *Current Anaesthesia and Critical Care*, **11**: 80–85.

Sharma, S. (2003) Shock and pregnancy. http://www.emedicine.com/med/topic3285.htm

Sharma, S. and Mink, S. (2004) Septic shock. http://www.emedicine.com/med/topic2101.htm

Urden, L., Stacy, K. and Lough, M. (2002) *Thelans Critical Care Nursing Diagnosis and Management* (4th edn). Mosby, St Louis.

Van Den Berghe, G. (2002) Beyond diabetes: saving lives with insulin in the ICU. *International Journal of Obesity and Related Metabolic Disorders*, **26** (Suppl. 3): 3–8.

Wheeler, A. and Bernard, G. (1999) Treating patients with severe sepsis. *New England Journal of Medicine*, **340** (3): 207–14.

Woodrow, P. (2000) *Intensive Care Nursing: A framework for practice.* Routledge, London.

Wyatt, R. (1996) Anaphylaxis. http://www.postgradmed.com/issues/1996/08_96/wyatt.htm

9 Fluid Balance and Management and the Critically Ill Woman

*Nick Rowe**

Midwives are often required to administer fluid replacement therapy in different situations such as shock and pre-eclampsia. Therefore, an understanding of the need for appropriate fluid replacement and the actual intended action of the fluid is crucial. Inappropriate fluid replacement could have the potential to compromise the woman's condition and lead to a clinical deterioration which would need further intensive management. This chapter will explain the physiology of fluid replacement and discuss the benefits and possible detrimental effects each fluid could cause.

Assumed prior knowledge

- Physiology of the cardiovascular and renal systems
- Physiological changes in the cardiovascular and renal system during pregnancy

Introduction

To maintain a state of physiological wellbeing, regular quantities of water, electrolytes and energy are required. A disproportionate or reduced fluid intake or loss can lead to serious physiological adjustments, significant morbidity and even mortality. A normal fluid balance should enable the body to maintain homeostasis. This chapter explores normal fluid balance and details of the fluids required to maintain this equilibrium.

* Thanks go to Dr Elizabeth Roberts of Queen Mary's Hospital Sidcup and Dr Pauline Vine of Princess Royal University Hospital Farnborough for their kind help and guidance through a controversial topic.

The process of normal fluid balance

The cardiovascular system is vital in its role for the distribution and absorption of gases, nutrients and metabolites, throughout the body. The normal passage of circulatory fluids is shown in Fig. 9.1. The passage between the arterial and venous systems is regulated by tube-like endothelial capillaries. The transfer of gases, nutrients and metabolites takes place at a cellular level. Oxygen, for example, carried by erythrocytes (red blood cells) is transported through the capillary wall to interact with tissue cells (Fig. 9.2). The medium through which

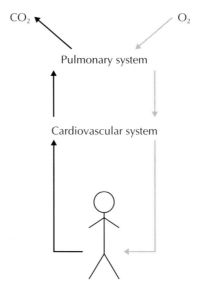

Figure 9.1   Normal passage of circulatory fluids.

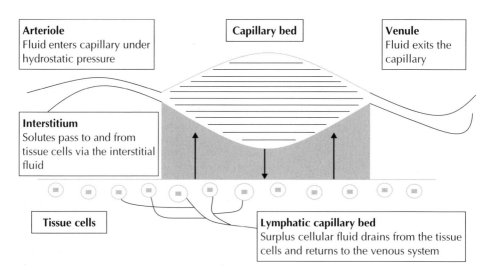

Figure 9.2   Transfer of fluids between the tissues and the arterial and venous systems.

the cells pass is the interstitium. The interstitium is a fibrous tissue and binds the capillary with the surrounding tissues. The fluid present in the interstitium allows the passage of solutes to and from the tissue cells, thus allowing the supply of gases, nutrients and hormones and the return of unused or waste products.

The fluid volume contained in the body is referred to as the total body water. This is divided between three compartments, with 25% in the vascular space, 8% in the interstitial space and 67% within the intracellular compartment. In a 70 kg male, the total body water is approximately 60% of the total body weight (around 42 L). In females, due to increased fat levels, this figure may be reduced to 50% (around 35 L).

Surplus tissue fluid is collected by the lymphatic system at the lymphatic capillary bed. Regulated by lymph nodes, the fluid is returned to the venous system, with the upper right body quadrant draining via the right lymphatic duct and the remainder via the thoracic duct.

The passage of fluid between the intracellular fluid (ICF) space and the extracellular fluid (ECF) space, which includes both plasma and interstitial fluid, is governed by osmosis. As both ICF and ECF are isotonic, an osmotic equilibrium exists at the cell membrane. ICF has potassium as its principle cat ion and is sensitive to changes in ECF sodium concentrations. A raise in serum or ECF sodium levels will cause water to pass from the ICF to the ECF. The reverse is also seen when ECF sodium concentrations are reduced. Albumin and a higher proportion of water with its dissolved oxygen are forced from the arterial end of the capillary by hydrostatic pressure, into the interstitium. The concentration of albumin remaining in the plasma is increased due to the water displacement, so increasing the colloid oncotic pressure. At the venous end of the capillary, the reduced blood pressure and raised oncotic pressure draw water containing carbon dioxide and metabolites back into the vasculature for transfer to the lungs, etc.

The extracellular space is regulated by both its tonicity and volume. Tonicity is governed by osmoreceptors in the brain, which serve to stimulate or suppress thirst, and to regulate water output. The smooth muscle that surrounds blood vessels controls either constriction (sympathetic nerve stimulation) or dilatation (parasympathetic nerve stimulation). An equal stimulus from both sympathetic and parasympathetic systems produces normal vascular tone. Reduced systemic arterial pressure in the renal system can lead to sodium and water retention in the kidney. Water retention itself can result in hyponatraemia (a sodium level of < 135 mmol/L) and, as previously mentioned, can result in a migration of water from the ECF to the ICF. Whilst this would impact upon the volume of the ECF, the total sodium level would not decrease in ratio to the fluid distribution, as electrolytes are unable to pass across the cell membrane. Other impacting factors relating to the ECF space are fluid intake (either oral or infusion therapy) and evaporation due to irregular thermoregulation and gastrointestinal conditions such as vomiting and diarrhoea. An imbalance of circulating fluid as either hypo- or hypervolaemia, will also impact on the normal process of fluid balance. This natural fluid balance may also be greatly disrupted by normal physiological changes in pregnancy related to conditions such as severe hypertensive disorders of pregnancy and postpartum haemorrhage.

Effective fluid balance in critically ill women

An effective fluid balance in any situation has but one aim; to maintain a normal balance that takes into account both the previous events and the current condition of the patient, and pre-empts foreseeable occurrences. Haemodynamics seen during pregnancy, whilst differing greatly from the baseline values, maintain a function that serves the needs of both mother and baby. In classifying a woman as being 'critically ill', we are therefore looking to have observed signs and symptoms that differ greatly from those we might normally expect to see, and can determine them to be an actual or imminent threat.

The physiology of fluid administration will show an initial expansion of the intravascular compartment. The subsequent passage across the capillary structure decrees the extent and duration of effect of the infusion. This differentiates between crystalloid and colloid solutions. Conditions that combine a decreased blood flow and oxygen transfer to the tissues that result in cellular hypoxia and potential organ dysfunction are represented as shock, which is explained at a greater depth in Chapter 8.

The most common pregnancy-related condition that affects fluid balance is pre-eclampsia. In respect of fluid management, the extremes that commonly guide treatment regimes are, on the one hand, pulmonary oedema versus renal failure on the other. Pearson (1992) argues that the woman with severe pre-eclampsia is at high risk of pulmonary oedema and as such should be fluid restricted with early diuretic therapy. Indeed, with women with a central venous pressure (CVP) of ≥ 4 mmHg, additional crystalloid infusion can raise the CVP to ≥ 10 mmHg, thus precipitating pulmonary oedema relating to the free passage of crystalloids between the intra- and extravascular spaces (Robson 1999).

However, the treatment of pre-eclamptic hypertension with hydralazine without a preload fluid dose can cause hypotension, fetal distress and oliguria (Magee et al. 2003). Reduced systemic arterial pressure in the renal system can lead to sodium and water retention in the kidney. This will cause a concentration of the urine output, seen as a darkening in colour and a thickened consistency; however this does not necessarily indicate renal failure, which affects approximately 1.5% of women in severe pre-eclampsia. Dehydration that manifests as thirst, however, indicates a depletion of 1 L or more and should be managed. Oral fluid intake will rarely result in toxicity and can be passed through the body; women can therefore be encouraged to drink at regular intervals. As such, maintenance fluids can be given as crystalloid fluids. In women with a urine output of < 100 ml/4 h, CVP can be measured. Readings of < 4 mmHg can be treated with 400 ml of 5% albumin. Careful challenges of colloid fluids, which remain in the intravascular space due to their higher molecular weight, will maintain colloid oncotic pressure – as opposed to crystalloids that are associated with a postpartum fall.

Pre-eclampsia can be considered to be a condition that illustrates a degree of distributive/vasogenic shock. Despite a relatively normal cardiac function and blood volume, the irregular distribution of blood can result in poor oxygenation of the tissues. Other shock-related disorders that can affect the distribution of body fluids are:

- *Septic shock.* As a result of the cardiac output and vasodilatation being depressed, a physiological attempt is made to direct the blood flow to critical organs at the expense of the pulmonary and renal systems. This results in an increased permeability of the capillaries, allowing water and large proteins such as albumin to migrate to the interstitium resulting in loss of proteins, hypovolaemia and interstitial oedema.
- *Anaphylactic shock.* The release of histamine, serotonin and other chemical mediators following the stimulation of the antibody–antigen complex, activates the cells of the immune system (such as mast cells and basophils) which causes vasodilatation and capillary permeability. This allows fluids to migrate from the intervascular compartment to the interstitium. The result is a fall in blood pressure and hypovolaemia resulting in tissue hypoxia.
- *Hypovolaemic shock.* This occurs when fluid leaves the cardiovascular space either to an internal space (as seen in distributive shock, burns or internal haemorrhage) or to external loss.

Fluid management

When considering the management of fluids in the critically ill woman, it is imperative not to lose sight of the fundamentals of fluid balance. The fluid volume contained in the body (total body water) is divided between three compartments, with 25% in the vascular space, 8% in the interstitial space and 67% within the intracellular compartment.

The composition of ECF and ICF is shown in Table 9.1.

Table 9.1   Composition of extracellular and intracellular fluids.

Intracellular fluid (28 L)		Extracellular fluid (14 L)	
Sodium	14 mmol/L	Sodium	150 mmol/L
Potassium	150 mmol/L	Potassium	4 mmol/L
Bicarbonate	10 mmol/L	Bicarbonate	27 mmol/L
Protein	74 mmol/L	Protein	Plasma = 16 mmol/L
			ISF = 2 mmol/L

ISF, interstitial fluid.

By looking at routine throughput of fluids and the metabolism of electrolytes (Table 9.2), a maintenance baseline of daily requirements can be identified. Intravenous fluids are distributed in differing ways between the intracellular, interstitial and plasma compartments (Table 9.3) and so the choice of fluid type is of vital importance.

Table 9.2   Example of daily input versus output.

Input H$_2$O 2500 ml/day	Output H$_2$O 2500 ml/day
Fluids 1400 ml	Urine 1500 ml
Food 750 ml	Skin 500 ml
Metabolism 350 ml	Lungs 400 ml
	Faeces 100 ml
	Sodium 50–90 mmol
	Potassium 50–90 mmol

Table 9.3   Distribution of fluid between the intracellular, interstitial and plasma compartments.

	Intracellular	Interstitial	Plasma
Isotonic saline	0%	80%	20%
Water (dextrose solution)	67%	25%	8%
Colloids	0%	0%	100%

From Table 9.3 we can see that a normal saline solution, whilst good for the maintenance of water and electrolyte homeostasis, will only be able to compensate for a blood volume loss of up to 20%. A colloid however, with a high molecular weight of > 10 000 Da, will stay entirely in the intravascular space. A combination therapy will therefore allow the crystalloid to provide tissue hydration, whilst a colloid infusion will hydrate the vasculature. It is important to note that simply infusing fluids will not correct electrolyte or component imbalance. Regular laboratory testing will show deficiencies or accumulations that result from the woman's condition and their response to fluid therapy. For example, during massive fluid resuscitation, full blood count tests will ensure that the woman's blood components are not simply diluted to an anaemic degree, simply for the sake of restoring volume. Any fluid infused must be able to perform its required function; that is, the distribution and absorption of gases, nutrients and metabolites throughout the body.

Principles of fluid management

Accurate fluid balance recording

This should include all oral/intravenous and otherwise introduced fluids. Balanced against these should be all excreted fluids such as urine output, vomit/diarrhoea and haemorrhage. It is best if all factors that relate to a patient's fluid balance are recorded on a single 24-hour sheet. In the critical care scenario, this should ideally be a component of their daily care record, which combines observations with treatment regimes, along with an area for staff to document their own comments. In this way, we reduce the possibility of events either being passed over or taken out of context. This should be implemented for any patient whose condition gives rise for concern.

Maintenance fluids

If a patient is able to safely drink fluids, they should be encouraged to do so. Any dehydration that manifests as thirst indicates a depletion of > 1 L. A background infusion of crystalloid fluid such as Hartmann's solution or 0.9% sodium chloride at 90 ml/h will offset the normal excretion of water by the body. In cases of vomiting or fasting, not only does the patient lose fluid but she is also prevented from any normal maintenance. During fasting a woman can lose 420 ml water in 4 hours, rising to 1260 ml in 12 hours. Sodium and potassium loss under the same conditions are equal at 12 mmol at 4 hours, rising to 35 mmol at 12 hours. In addition, stress may also induce the release of antidiuretic hormone (ADH), aldosterone and cortisol. This can then lead to water and sodium retention with the loss of potassium. Thus, if fluid balances are compromised for more than 24 hours, the potassium levels of the patient should be considered.

Possible invasive central venous monitoring

In cases of proven oliguria (< 0.5 ml/kg/h) or undue haemorrhage, the insertion of central venous monitoring should be considered. A low CVP, often indicative of left atrial filling pressures, could be indicative of a hypovolaemic state. However, when the reading rises above 6 cmH$_2$O, the filling pressures are often underestimated and there is an increased risk of pulmonary oedema. A raised CVP in isolation of supporting tests proves little in regard to fluid status but may be a precursor to fluid overload or myocardial dysfunction. As such, the insertion of a pulmonary artery catheter can be considered. In underloaded patients, the CVP will fall off soon after volume loading, despite a temporary rise being seen.

   The risks of insertion should, however, be taken into account. Coagulopathy may cause bleeding and be impossible to control. Poor oxygenation or lung disease may further deteriorate with accidental lung damage. The potential for sepsis is also increased with the introduction of invasive catheters. Unless there is expertise available in both the insertion and management of catheters, and the interpretation of results, central vein cannulation should not be attempted. In cases of severe refractory hypertension where drugs such as nitroglycerine or nitroprusside are used, invasive monitoring in an intensive care unit is required. A set protocol should be available for the implementation of invasive monitoring.

Selective colloid expansion

In cases of confirmed low blood pressures or low CVP readings, fluid challenges of 200–300 ml boluses of colloid can be administered. Colloid and plasma substitutes contain high molecular weight molecules (> 10 000 Da), together with electrolytes. The size of the molecules prevents passage through normal capillary membranes and, as a result, they remain in the intravascular space. The efficiency of colloids in volume replacement is, however, reduced in cases where damage to the capillary membrane has occurred (Vincent 2000). In pre-eclampsia, the combination of controlled vasodilatation (i.e. using hydralazine) with limited colloid loading can improve cardiac function whilst reducing vascular resistance. Whilst fluid overload is definitely to be avoided in light of the potential for the development of pulmonary oedema, limited fluid challenges prior to vasodilatation are imperative to prevent a sudden hypotensive crisis. In order to optimise intravascular volume, additional volume can be added and/or agents to cause vasoconstriction of the vessels can be used.

Any fluid administration should be managed with a specific end point in mind. To that end, fluids must be flexibly titrated with constant reference to the principle aims of administration and to the emerging physiological effects observed through measurements taken from the woman. Indiscriminate loading of fluids has in the past been the cause of fluid overload and ineffectual treatment and, hence, a move to severely restrict fluid therapy for fear of adverse outcome. Adult respiratory distress syndrome resulting from pulmonary oedema is second only to cerebral haemorrhage as the immediate cause of death in women with pregnancy-induced hypertensive disorders (Lewis, 2004).

Types of fluid

Accurate fluid selection must be made based on the expected function of the fluid, for example to replace electrolytes or to replenish volume. Fluids to be used consist of three categories: crystalloids, colloids and blood products.

Crystalloids

A large number of the crystalloid fluids are isotonic, which means that an equal solute concentration exists inside and outside the cell, encouraging the cell to stay the same size. Fluids found within this category include:

- Normal saline (0.9% sodium chloride in water): 154 mmol/L sodium and 154 mmol/L chloride.
- Ringer's lactate: 147 mmol/L sodium, 156 mmol/L chloride, 4 mmol/L potassium and 2.2 mmol/L calcium.
- Hartmann's solution: 131 mmol/L sodium, 111 mmol/L chloride, 5 mmol/L potassium, 2 mmol/L calcium and 29 mmol/L bicarbonate (lactate).
- Glucose 4%/NaCl 0.18%: 30 mmol/L sodium, 30 mmo/L potassium and 40 g/L glucose (164 kcal/L).
- Glucose 5%: 50 g/L glucose (205 kcal/L).

One significantly different fluid in this category is glucose 10% (100 g/L glucose (410 kcal/L)) which is considered *hypertonic*. Here, the solution on one side of the cell membrane has a solute concentration greater than on the opposite side. Care should therefore be taken with glucose (dextrose) solutions as the glucose is metabolised, leaving water. This quickly balances through the ECF and ICF spaces and can cause hyponatraemia and cellular oedema.

Normal saline can cause hypernatraemia and hyperchloraemic acidosis if given in excess (Gutteridge 2004).

Synthetic colloids

Synthetic colloids are used solely to expand the plasma volume as they have no oxygen capacity or clotting functions. They may be divided into three groups.

Hydroxyethyl starch (HES)

HES solutions are derived from a modified vegetable starch dissolved in 0.9% normal saline. This is similar to the glycogen found in liver and muscle, resulting in a reduced potential for immunological reactions. The different ratios of hydroxyethyl groups to glucose molecules within the starch will dictate how long the HES is maintained in the circulatory system. Available as 6% and 10% solutions, the former will expand the plasma volume by 500 ml with a 500 ml infusion, whereas the 10% solution acts similarly to 20% albumin in that 500 ml will cause an expansion of 750 ml volume. The difference in types available reflects the 'degree of substitution' of the hydroxyethyl groups to glucose molecules and their subsequent duration, with HES remaining up to four times longer in the system.

The molecular weight also covers a wide range (10–2000 kDa) compared to albumin (69 kDa). The amount of leakage through the capillaries is therefore much reduced, thus allowing HES solutions to remain longer in the vascular compartment. HES is eliminated via the kidney with molecules > 70 kDa being broken down by serum amylase. Again, the higher amount of HES groups present, the longer it takes for degradation to occur and hence there is a longer duration of effect.

Gelatins

This group of colloids derive from bovine proteins made soluble in 0.9% normal saline. Whilst molecular size varies, it tends to be approximately 30 kDa. Due to this relatively small size, gelatin molecules are not readily retained in the vasculature, leaking both into the interstitium and through the renal capillary system into the urine. As such, gelatines do not maintain their expansion properties for more than 3 hours. They are therefore useful for short-term expansion (e.g. to counteract the hypotension caused by spinal anaesthesia) but require long-term infusion for conditions such as sepsis. This sustained treatment may lead to a sodium buildup in women who have renal or hepatic impairment.

Dextrans

Dextrans are naturally occurring glucose polymers made by leucosoic bacteria. Simpler in structure than the hydroxyethyl groups, the molecular size is varied, so regulating its duration within the vasculature. Dissolved in 0.9% normal saline or 5% dextrose, dextrans are available in two molecular weights. Dextran 40 (low molecular weight) expands the blood by 150% of the infused volume in a similar manner to 10% HES, but will only remain active for 6–8 hours. The higher molecular weight dextran 70 expands the blood by only 100% of the infused volume, but has approximately 18 hours effective duration. A recognised chemical effect of dextran is the increased plasma viscosity seen during infusion. Whilst this definitely interferes with blood clotting functions, it is used occasionally during surgery to reduce the incidence of deep vein thrombosis. There is also an acknowledged incidence of anaphylaxis with the higher molecular weight dextrans.

Blood and blood products

In cases of significant haemorrhage, whole blood is an ideal choice due to it having the capacity to carry oxygen and the presence of clotting factors. Fresh blood is preferable to stored blood as, in time, stored blood breaks down, decreasing the concentrations of platelets and clotting factors. As a result of this breakdown, a rise in potassium, ammonium and cell debris is to be seen.

A cross-match and typing between the recipient and donor unit must be undertaken prior to transfusion. An initial infusion rate of 4 ml/kg/h should be used, unless a severe deficit is present, in which case the blood should be given as rapidly as possible. In cases where renal/cardiac disease or an acknowledged fluid overload is present, the infusion rate should be slowed to 1 ml/kg/h. One unit of packed red cells can be expected to raise the haematocrit level by approximately 3%. Targets for infusion should be set to reach a required haematocrit level without exceeding it. Except in extreme emergency, blood should be infused through both an infusion-warming device and a blood filtration system. The blood should not exceed 42°C and any units should be infused within a 4-hour period to prevent bacterial buildup. The woman should be carefully monitored for signs of transfusion reaction and/or fluid overload. If fresh frozen plasma is required, to correct coagulation deficiencies, it should be pre-thawed at room temperature or using a controlled method over 30 minutes.

Albumin

Albumin is naturally found in the body evenly divided with one-third found in the skin, one-third in the vasculature and one-third in the body tissues. Approximately 5% of the blood albumin transfers through the capillary per hour to the tissues (transcapillary escape rate). This acts as a buffer to the blood's oncotic pressure, so regulating its ability to attract water. The resulting effect is an even hydration of blood and tissues.

Albumin can be considered for use for the following conditions: hypoalbuminaemia, resuscitation in acute hypovolaemia and hypovolaemia occurring after the acute phase of critical illness. Available as 4.5% or 20%, the albumin is dissolved in saline and acts by drawing water from the interstitium back into the vasculature. Of the two concentrations, 100 ml of the 20% solution has the equivalent effect of 300 ml of the 4.5% solution, expanding to three times its volume in infusion. The molecular size of albumin is 69 kDa. This plays an important role in women suffering from oedema or sodium elimination conditions, as albumin levels affect the colloid oncotic pressure and thus the transfer of water to and from the interstitium with its dissolved gasses and metabolites. In cases of capillary leakage, the amount of colloid and water in the interstitium increases the distance between the capillary and the cells, thus causing reduced oxygen transfer between the two structures and resulting in hypoxia. In cases where the oedema is caused by sepsis, it is vital to address the cause in order to prevent the return of fluids from the interstitium and the subsequent restoration of normal gas exchange becoming a temporary state (Allison & Lobo 2000).

Diuretic usage

As denoted by the phrase 'fluid balance', there is a necessary correlation between administered or present fluids and those eliminated from the body. Concerns regarding fluid overload, and resulting pulmonary oedema, and pre-renal oliguria often result in the use of diuretic drugs to increase urine formation and output. The use of loop diuretics such as frusemide (furosemide) can promote diuresis by reducing the intravascular water and increasing the colloid oncotic pressure. This encourages water to be drawn from the interstitial space, back into the vasculature. In oliguria, it is important that the patient is fluid loaded (and still oliguric) prior to the administration of diuretics. Sodium reabsorbtion is inhibited in the loop of Henle in the medulla, enhancing the renal tubular oxygen balance, and diuresis often occurs despite renal impairment. Mechanically, this can help flush the renal tubules of any necrotic debris.

In cases of pulmonary oedema that result in adult respiratory distress syndrome, fluid restriction and diuretic administration are an advocated course of action. However, for critically ill pregnant women who become potentially oliguric, it is important that the cause (such as hypovolaemia) is treated or excluded prior to the use of diuretic drugs.

Summary

- Normal values in physiological measurements must be established as appropriate to the woman's condition.
- A normal balance should be sought, that takes into account both the previous events and the current condition of the woman, and pre-empts foreseeable occurrences.
- Fluids and treatments should be carefully administered with clearly defined end objectives. These should be determined by a multispeciality approach and laid out in policy.
- Fluids have individual properties and are not simply crystalloid or colloid. Choose with an aim in mind.
- Constant reassessment of the woman's condition must be undertaken to avoid potential harm.
- Expert help should be sought prior to implementing any stage of treatment.

References

Allison, S. and Lobo, D. (2000) Albumin administration should not be avoided. *Critical Care*, **4** (3): 147–50.

Gutteridge, G. (2004) Crystalloids, colloids, blood, blood products and blood substitutes. *Anaesthesia and Intensive Care Medicine*, **5** (2): 42–7.

Lewis, G. (2004) *Why Mothers Die 2000–2002: Report on Confidential Enquiries into Maternal Deaths in the United Kingdom*. Royal College of Obstetricians and Gynaecologists (RCOG), London.

Magee, L., Cham, C., Waterman, E., Ohlsson, A. and von Dadelszen, P. (2003) Hydralazine for treatment of severe hypertension in pregnancy: meta analysis. *British Medical Journal*, **327** (7421): 955.

Pearson, J. (1992) Fluid balance in severe pre-eclampsia. *British Journal of Hospital Medicine*, **48** (1): 47–51.

Robson, S. (1999) Fluid restriction policies in preeclampsia are obsolete. *International Journal of Obstetric Anaesthesia*, **8** (1): 49–55.

Vincent, J. (2000) Issues in contemporary fluid management. *Critical Care*, **4** (Suppl. 2): S1–S2.

10 Specialist Monitoring Technology and Skills for the Critically Ill Woman

Nick Rowe and Mandy Stevenson*

Caring for women whose condition is at risk of deteriorating often requires midwives to use their clinical skills in conjunction with medical technology. Knowledge and understanding of specialist monitoring technology and equipment will assist midwives in providing care for critically ill women as well as enabling them to recognise if the situation starts to deteriorate.

This chapter will explain the principles and practice surrounding the following methods of invasive and non-invasive monitoring which may be appropriate when caring for critically ill women in childbearing:

- Oxygen saturation
- Electrocardiogram (ECG)
- Non-invasive blood pressure
- Venous cannulation
- Arterial cannulation
- Central venous cannulation
- Pulmonary artery wedge pressure

Assumed prior knowledge

- Physiology of the cardiovascular and respiratory systems
- Physiological changes of the cardiovascular and respiratory systems in pregnancy

---

* With grateful thanks to Barbara Warncken for her valuable input on ECG interpretation.

Introduction

During any phase of critical illness, a range of diagnostic and therapeutic procedures will be required. It is therefore vital that baseline observations are known and viewed in the context of the medical setting. This takes into account all dimensions of physiology and wellbeing, not only those that are directly related to the condition being investigated. Once we have established what might be deemed as 'normal' for an individual, we are able to detect any deviation from the baseline figures.

The primary tool used in monitoring is direct observation. All members of staff within a department possess diagnostic skills to some degree. In dealing with people on a day-to-day basis, we have a natural acumen to detect when something is 'not right' with somebody. Someone who has fallen or who is having difficulty breathing is often noticed by non-medical people who react by getting help. With training and experience, we refine this diagnostic process so that we might pinpoint the cause of the trouble and facilitate prompt action to be taken. Whilst the application of specialist skills and technology can help us to reach diagnoses, it is vital that we do not disregard the skill of direct observation once we apply the available equipment. Despite the technology involved, we still must have knowledge of both patient and machine in order to detect any changes from the 'norm'. All too often in the investigation of incidents, patients attached to monitors have been found to have nobody watching them. The assumption is that simply because a piece of equipment has an alarm fitted, the woman 'should be alright'; this can often lead to complacency on the part of the carer, especially when a unit is busy or understaffed. In light of this, all staff should be equipped with the skills to use those items of equipment commonly used in their department. It must be acknowledged, however, that human error does occur, and in light of this, no culture should make a member of staff feel that it would look ill upon them to seek help or advice when they find themselves in an unknown situation. After all, when the monitor alarm sounds, it is performing exactly that function – drawing attention to something and summoning assistance.

Oxygen saturation: pulse oximetry

Pulse oximetry was introduced in 1976 as a non-invasive method of monitoring the arterial oxygen saturation (SpO_2) of blood. Originally measuring through the ear lobe, the eight wavelength Hewlett Packard ear oximeter eliminated both the need to draw regular blood samples and the expense of pathology analysis. In the early 1980s, technology advanced to enable the units to become more affordable, smaller in size and easier to use.

Technology

- Light-emitting diodes (LEDs) emit light at two wavelengths (visible red, 660 nm, and infrared, 940 nm). These flash every 30 seconds and are picked up by a photodetector on the opposite side of the clip or probe. A pause in the sequence, during which both LEDs are off, allows ambient light levels to be taken into account. Reflective measurement technology is available for measurement on more proximal anatomy as it uses a single-sided contact.

- The light is transmitted through the pulsatile tissue bed. Only the pulsatile flow is registered, with the non-pulsatile flow that results from venous and capillary flow and the absorption of light by the tissues being ignored. This results from the pulsatile tissues having a non-constant light absorption, whereas the absorption of the non-pulsatile flow is constant.
- The two (or more) light sources are absorbed at different levels dependent upon the oxygenation levels of the haemoglobin present in the arterial blood. One molecule of haemoglobin can carry up to four oxygen molecules. This would register as 100% saturated.
- The average percentage saturation (taken from the total molecules sampled) is processed by the microprocessor every 5–20 seconds and thus gives a saturation reading, expressed as a digital percentage figure.
- The heart rate is measured by averaging the number of emitted LED signals between successive pulsatile signals and an average taken in the same manner as the Sao_2 reading.

Use: performing pulse oximetry

Pulse oximetry can accurately determine SaO_2 in a range of 70–100% (± 2%). Below 70%, readings are extrapolated as the data for calibration were obtained from human volunteers and it was viewed as being unethical to test below this level. Once readings drop below 90%, the shape of the oxyhaemoglobin curve causes saturations to fall rapidly. Due to the time taken by the unit to average its readings, however, it will not measure acute desaturation. Women should have their oxygen therapy aimed at a maintenance level of > 95% to ensure effective oxygen perfusion of the tissues. Pulse oximetry will also provide a pulse rate. However, it has no function in the measurement of carbon dioxide and is therefore unable to provide information relating to ventilation (Fearnley 1995); breathing may stop prior to desaturation occurring.

- Units should be plugged into the mains when possible and have battery back-up.
- Each unit should perform a self-test when turned on. Ensure your unit is functioning correctly. Settings and alarm parameters should be checked. Never turn off an alarm simply because it is making a noise. Look to establish the cause.
- Probes or ear pieces should be fitted according to manufacturers' instructions. Normally, finger probes will measure 'top to bottom' through the finger tip. Ensure the area is clean and preferably free of nail varnish. If false nails are present, use an ear probe or rotate the finger probe 90° to measure 'side to side'. Do not cause pressure damage or reading impairment by applying force. Do not tape probes to extremities unless they are specifically designed for the purpose. If monitoring is intended to be long term, move the probe on a

regular basis to prevent pressure damage or burns, which have previously been reported.

- Ensure the unit displays a waveform in addition to providing a saturation figure. Without this, the figure cannot be trusted. Measurements have been observed from inanimate objects such as drip stands and bedside lockers in the past, when someone has 'parked' the probe for a moment whilst doing something else!
- Record the readings immediately. If possible, ensure that a printout accompanies the record sheet to verify any measurements taken.
- As in the use of all monitors, if there is a suspected discrepancy between the patient's clinical condition and those figures displayed by the unit, then you should trust clinical judgement rather than technology.

Complications

In any situation, check the woman first!

If no reading is obtained, check the unit is properly connected and that the probe is correctly positioned. Most units will show that no signal is being detected in the event of set-up problems.

Low readings can be caused by a variety of factors. Peripheral vasoconstriction can reduce pulsatile blood flow and so produce an inadequate signal. Venous congestion, high airway pressures and forced pressures such as the Valsalva manoeuvre during childbirth might cause venous pulsation, which can have a similar effect. Shivering will also cause signal interruption. Women with methaemoglobin presence will not show accurate readings, with the Sao_2 showing approximately 85%. High ambient light levels and the presence of false nails or nail varnish can also cause a falsely low reading (Pedersen et al. 2004).

False high readings can be obtained when haemoglobin is combined with carbon monoxide (CoHb or carboxyhaemoglobin). This is picked up as being 90% oxygenated haemoglobin and 10% desaturated haemoglobin, and as such, any readings are overestimated.

Electrocardiograms

An electrocardiogram (ECG) is a graph of the electrical activity of the heart. It is therefore a two-dimensional picture of something that occurs in three dimensions. In order to show a clearer picture of electrical activity, views are taken from a variety of places or leads. The same activity will therefore give a different picture from different leads. Electrical activity of the heart is recorded on the graph as movement away from the isoelectric line. An upward movement from the isoelectric line is called a positive deflection. A downward movement from the isoelectric line is known as a negative deflection.

As the ECG is attached to the body by electrodes, it will record any electrical activity inside (and sometimes outside) the body. All body muscles move by electrical impulses and activity; as a consequence if the woman makes any movement or shivers there will be resultant non-cardiac muscle movement. This will be recorded on the ECG as a jagged line and is known as an artefact. An artefact is anything appearing on the ECG trace that is not cardiac in origin.

Related cardiac physiology

To enable a practitioner to appreciate the relevance of ECG recording, an understanding of the related cardiac physiology is required. A brief overview of such physiology follows.

The cardiac cycle is divided into three main phases (Tortora & Derrickson 2005):

- Ventricular diastole (relaxation)
- Ventricular filling
- Ventricular systole (contraction)

For ease of reference the left side of the heart will be explained:

- *Ventricular diastole (relaxation).* This follows ventricular systole (contraction). The ventricles relax, resulting in pressure within the left ventricle falling below that of the aorta and thus the aortic valve closes and all valves within the heart are now closed (Tortora & Derrickson 2005). Simultaneously, blood is passively flowing into the left atrium via the pulmonary system. As the pressure and volume within the left atrium increases, the mitral valve opens and the second phase of the cardiac cycle begins.
- *Ventricular filling.* Ventricular filling has three phases (Tortora & Derrickson 2005). The first is referred to as rapid ventricular filling and involves passive filling of the left ventricle from the left atrium. The second stage of ventricular filling is known as diastasis and refers to slow ventricular filling. At the end of diastasis, the pressures in the left atrium and ventricle are now equal. The third stage of ventricular filling is due to the contraction of the atrium, with blood being forced into the left ventricle.
- *Ventricular systole (contraction).* As the left ventricle starts to contract, the mitral valve closes. The left ventricle is now a closed chamber. The muscles within the left ventricle begin to contract with an increasing resultant pressure. Once the pressure in the left ventricle is greater than that of the aorta, the aortic valve opens and blood is ejected out (known as the stroke volume). As pressure in the left ventricle falls with the expulsion of the blood, the aortic valve closes and the cardiac cycle begins again.

Electrical conduction system

The electrical conduction system consists of the sinoatrial (SA) node, the internodal pathways, the atrioventrical (AV) node, the bundle of His, the right bundle branch and the left bundle branch and its anterior and posterior divisions and the Purkinje fibres. All are necessary to initiate and continue rhythmic contraction of the heart.

Notable physiological adaptations in pregnancy

Pregnancy is characterised as a hyperdynamic (high flow), low resistance state. This occurs through an adaptive response in blood volume, cardiac structure, cardiac output, vascular resistance and heart rate. Other than blood volume changes, cardiac structural changes may occur that may affect the recording and interpretation of subsequent ECG recordings.

- The heart is displaced to the left and upwards and rotates anteriorly.
- There are no characteristic ECG changes (except left axis deviation may be seen).
- Left axis deviation may occur because of mechanical displacement.
- Cardiac volume increases slightly because of increased circulating volume and hypertrophy.

Cardiac ausculatory changes include the following (Thelan et al. 1998):

- Physiological S1 (first heart sound) split
- S3 (third heart sound) development is considered normal
- Systolic murmurs develop in 90% of all pregnant women
- Diastolic murmurs develop in 20% of all pregnant women
- Murmurs are physiological in nature and disappear after delivery

Use: performing an ECG

The basic three-lead ECG consists of three electrodes on bipolar leads, placed on the right shoulder (red), left shoulder (yellow) and the left lateral chest wall (black/green), in line with the apex of the heart. These detect impulses between a sensing point and a reference point, so triangulating across the heart using paths labelled as I, II and III. Used in routine cardiac monitoring, the three-lead ECG is standard on many defibrillators. Higher levels of information can be obtained by adding further unipolar leads to create a 12-lead ECG. This is more appropriate for the screening of high risk patients, and in reaching diagnoses in those with suspected or proven cardiac anomalies. All clinical staff should be comfortable in recognising the components of sinus rhythm (Lee 2000). Further to this, staff should be able to detect increases or decreases in normal heart rate, together with common rhythms that require emergency treatment. All hospital staff should have formal training in hospital basic life support, with clinical staff trained to immediate life support level. In addition, advanced life support (ALS) providers must be available to respond to any emergency situation.

How to undertake a 12-lead ECG

- Place the 10 electrodes onto the patient. While each of the six chest electrodes record one lead each, the three limb electrodes record six different views of cardiac electrical activity.
- Limb electrodes are colour coded to aid correct placement: right arm is red, left arm is yellow and left leg is green. When recording a 12-lead ECG the fourth limb electrode (black) is placed on the right leg.

- Lead I represents electrical activity from the right arm to the left arm.
- Lead II represents electrical activity from the right arm to the left leg. The bundle of His follows the main vector of electrical activity in the heart: the SA node to the AV node and down the bundle of His. This lead is the standard lead for understanding the principles of ECGs.
- Lead III represents electrical activity from the left arm to the left leg.
- The picture of electrical activity in the heart remains constant at any point in the limb (Woodrow 1998). An electrode placed on the right wrist will show the same waveform as one placed on the right elbow or shoulder.
- Leads AVR, AVL and AVF are known as unipolar leads. They read electrical impulses from one electrode, with the ECG machine calculating the effect of the other limb leads to give an average reading between the points of the triangle formed by the bipolar leads.

Components of a normal ECG

The ECG complex is made up of a sequence of electrical events occurring within the heart. As the atria depolarise, the P-wave is created, and because impulses spread from muscle fibre to muscle fibre, rather than through specialized conduction tissue, conduction is relatively slow in relation to the muscle mass of the atria. This makes a normal P-wave appear broad in relation to its height. A normal P-wave lasts 0.08 seconds (2 small squares wide on the ECG) (Marieb 2003).

The AV node filters and holds the atrial impulse to allow significant ventricular filling time prior to contraction. This is represented as a straight line (isoelectric line) on the ECG and is measured on the ECG by the distance from the start of the P-wave to the start of the R-wave, called the PR interval. The PR interval will normally last between 0.12 and 0.2 seconds (3–5 small squares) (Aehlert 2002).

The Q-wave, a negative deflection, is not always seen on ECGs; however its absence does not usually indicate a problem. A normal Q-wave (less than 1 small square wide) is caused by electrical activity moving across the muscle fibres of the septum (depolarisation).

The direction of the impulse travelling along the bundle of His is similar to that of lead II so the deflection is strongly positive; however, towards the end, the Purkinje fibres allow conduction to spread rapidly throughout the ventricular mass causing a final negative deflection of the RS line below the isoelectric line. The S-wave completes the electrical impulses through the muscle (Woodrow 1998). A normal QRS width lasts 0.12 seconds (within 3 small squares) (Aehlert 2002).

This illustrates the speed of ventricular impulses and allows coordinated contraction of the large ventricular muscle mass, ensuring an effective stroke volume (felt by the pulse). After the S-wave the ECG should return to the isoelectric line.

Repolarisation is represented by the T-wave; a normal T-wave should be positive and separated from the S-wave by a return to the isoelectric line. A normal T-wave lasts 0.16 seconds (4 small squares) (Marieb 1995). If the ST segment appears raised or depressed from the isoelectric line there is a problem with depolarisation, commonly due to infarction, ischaemia or abnormal potassium (or other electrolyte) levels.

Basic rhythm recognition

To analyse accurately cardiac activity, a 12-lead ECG is required. A rhythm strip shows only one view of the heart, which is dependent on the electrode positioning and, as such, myocardial stress or damage can be missed.

ECG tracings are standardised. Most ECG machines are set to pass paper through at 25 mm/s. As graph paper is standardised, one small square represents 0.04 seconds (1 mm of paper), one large square represents 0.2 seconds (5 mm of paper) and five large squares represent 1 second (25 mm of paper) (Schamroth 1990). Once the 12-lead ECG is obtained it is necessary to review each lead individually, examining each waveform to ensure any changes/abnormalities are recognised.

The application of a systematic framework will assist the health care professional in interpreting the ECG recording (Resuscitation Council UK 2005).

Is there any electrical activity?

If no electrical activity is identified, obviously the woman requires checking to ensure that there is no acute change in her condition; the gain control, ECG leads and electrical connections must be checked to ensure position and connection. A completely straight line usually demonstrates that a monitoring lead has become disconnected, because atrial and ventricular asystole usually coexist and this line is not usually completely straight as it becomes distorted by baseline drift, electrical interference, respiratory movement or resuscitation attempts. However, atrial activity (P-waves) may continue for a limited time after the onset of ventricular asystole. This P-wave asystole may respond to pacing.

If electrical activity is present, the activity should be examined for any recognisable complexes. If there are no recognisable complexes then the likely diagnosis is ventricular fibrillation – either coarse or fine, dependent on the amplitude of the complexes. If electrical activity is present and there are recognisable complexes then the following five questions should be applied in turn.

What is the ventricular rate?

The fastest approach to determine ventricular rate is to count the number of large (5 mm) squares between two consecutive QRS complexes and divide this number into 300; e.g. if there are four large squares between adjacent QRS complexes the rate is 300/4 = 75 per minute (Antunes et al. 1994).

Two alternative approaches are:

- To count the number of QRS complexes in a defined number of seconds and calculate the rate per minute. This approach can be useful if the rhythm is irregular; e.g. if 15 QRS complexes occur in 50 large squares (10 seconds) the rate is 15 × 6 = 90 per minute.
- Count the number of small (1 mm) squares between two consecutive QRS complexes and divide this number into 1500; e.g. if there are 15 small squares between adjacent QRS complexes the rate is 1500/15 = 100 per minute.

Is the rhythm regular or irregular?

This requires careful comparison of an adequate length of rhythm strip, as the faster the heart rate the beat-to-beat variation of irregular rhythms become less pronounced. Careful comparison of the R-R intervals of adjacent beats at different places in the recording will allow the detection of an irregular rhythm. Another option is to mark on a piece of paper two adjacent identical points in the cardiac cycle (e.g. the tips of the R-waves) and this paper can then moved along to another section of the rhythm strip. If the QRS rhythm is irregular, is it totally irregular with no recognisable pattern of R-R interval or is there a cyclical variation in the R-R intervals? A basic regular rhythm can become irregular by the occurrence of extra systoles (ectopic beats). Extra systoles can arise from any part within the heart and the position from which they arise will determine their morphology.

Is the QRS complex width normal or prolonged?

The normal upper limit for the QRS interval is 0.12 seconds (3 small squares). If the QRS width is less than this the rhythm originates from above the bifurcation of the bundle of His and may be from the sinoatrial node, atria or any part of the atrioventricular junction but not from the ventricular myocardium. If the QRS duration is 0.12 seconds or more the rhythm may be arising in the ventricular myocardium or may be a supraventricular rhythm with an aberrant conduction (Resuscitation Council UK 2005).

Is atrial activity present?

Having defined the rhythm in terms of rate, regularity and QRS width, a rhythm strip should then be examined carefully for atrial activity (Resuscitation Council UK (2005). The P-wave rate and regularity are determined in the same way as for the QRS complexes and any difference between the two identified. The shape of the P-wave may help to determine the rhythm. If atrial depolarisation originates in the sinoatrial node the P-wave will be upright in leads II and AVF. If the atria are being activated retrospectively (junctional or ventricular in origin), the P-waves will usually be inverted in these leads because atrial depolarisation takes place in the opposite direction to normal.

How is atrial activity related to ventricular activity?

If the time interval between each P-wave and the nearest QRS complex is constant, it is very likely that the atrial and ventricular depolarisation is linked. Inspection of the relationship between the P and QRS complexes should be made and if necessary the timings of the P-waves should be plotted separately and compared with the timings of the QRS complexes. Any recognisable patterns between the two should be identified, as well as the occurrence of any missed or dropped beats and PR intervals that vary in a repeated trend.

Complications

In any situation, check the woman first!

In matters of cardiac emergency, assumption is truly the mother of all errors. It cannot be presumed that simply because a member of staff is employed in critical care, they are necessarily competent to deal effectively with an emergency, or to detect important changes in cardiac state. To this end, all staff should maintain their knowledge and skills. Common errors stem from poor lead placement, which gives a distorted image of the actual cardiac conductivity, and a lack of knowledge on the part of staff who are monitoring the woman. The ECG will give no information in regard to cardiac output or efficiency. As with all clinical situations, if there is any doubt, seek help immediately.

Non-invasive blood pressure monitoring

In order to enable the function of vital organs and tissues, adequate perfusion must be maintained. Measurement of the blood pressure is therefore vital in the monitoring of the critically ill woman. First attempted by Stephen Hales in 1733, the non-invasive measurement of blood pressure became possible with the development of the blood pressure cuff by Scipione Riva-Rocci in 1896. Whilst it is possible to form some idea of a patient's blood pressure by observation (a radial pulse requires a systolic pressure of > 80 mmHg and capillary reflexes greater than 2 seconds suggest inadequate perfusion); no numerical data can be obtained without apparatus.

Technology

The basic equipment used to measure blood pressure is a sphygmomanometer. A cuff is applied to the woman's arm level with the heart; it is then inflated to a pressure higher than the expected reading. This will be shown on a dial. Mercury-filled apparatus should not be used due to the potential health and safety risks of mercury spillage. By means of using a stethoscope over the brachial artery; as the cuff is slowly released, tapping noises (Korotkoff sounds) can be heard (Ur & Gordon 1970). These will manifest in five phases: an initial sound, an increasing intensity, maximum intensity, progressive muffling and an absence of sound. The emergence of the initial tapping sound represents the systolic pressure, whilst the point of disappearance represents the diastolic pressure. A variation of this theme is the oscillotonometer, developed by Von Recklinghausen, which uses two cuffs – the smaller of the two amplifies pulsations caused as the larger cuff is released. By controlling a hand leaver, readings are shown on a dial as the pressure comes down.

More common in the modern health care scenario is the DINAMAP (indirect non-invasive automatic mean arterial pressure) machine. A microprocessor controls the inflation and deflation of the cuff. Pressure changes are detected by a transducer, which results in a digital reading being displayed. This concept is often inbuilt into the multifunction monitors seen for use in both routine and critical care. Monitors range from integrated critical care modules to smaller units that wrap around the wrist.

Use: performing non-invasive blood pressure monitoring

The woman should be in a non-disturbed area and either seated or lying down so that the mid-point of the upper arm is at the level of the heart. Cuffs should be selected in relation to the size of the woman's anatomy. In adults, the internal bladder of the cuff should encircle 80% of the arm's circumference. The width of the cuff should cover approximately two-thirds of the upper arm. The centre of the cuff should overlay the brachial artery. Large adult-size cuffs of 35–44 cm should always be available to prevent inaccurate readings being obtained from ill-fitting equipment. If a cuff is wrapped too loosely, it will produce a falsely high reading. Conversely, if the cuff is too tight, the reading will be seen as falsely low (Manning et al. 1983). Ensure manual equipment is set at zero prior to starting. Automatic monitors will self-test and calibrate. Any inadvertent stress or exercise during measurement is likely to give a higher reading. If using a stethoscope to detect Korotkoff sounds, ensure it is well fitting and in good order and that manual equipment is at eye level to provide accurate sightings.

Complications

Blood pressures differ between individuals and are subject to many facets of the person's condition. It is important to establish what is to be considered as 'normal' for each individual, prior to commencing any measurements. Individual measurements on the same person are also subject to change, so it is best to take more than one reading, so as to confirm the data obtained as being fair and accurate. It is not unusual to find that your referral for hypertension is sometimes based on anxiety or technique, as opposed to any direct clinical condition. Careful assessment and application of correct procedure is important when taking vital signs. To reduce the potential for error, the equipment, patient and clinician should all be considered when faced with readings that on initial examination appear to be outside those bounds that have been established as normal for the current phase of the patient's condition. It is also important for staff to maintain their skills of manual blood pressure measurement, despite the now commonplace usage of automated equipment, as it is an invaluable tool with which to corroborate those readings that are a cause for concern.

Peripheral venous cannulation

Venous cannulation is of vital importance when dealing with any critical care situation and should be maintained at all times. To this end, careful thought should be applied prior to cannula selection and insertion. In the standard setting, intravenous access is required principally for routine drug and fluid administration.

As such, it is not anticipated that the cannula will remain *in situ* for any long period of time, or be expected to allow rapid infusion. In this instance, a smaller gauge cannula may be acceptable, as would the selection of a vein of smaller lumen.

In cases of haemodynamic instability, long-term drug or infusion therapy or a potential for sudden deterioration in the patient's condition, venous cannulation requires more in-depth consideration. Cannulae larger than 18 G are best suited for rapid infusion, with larger cannulae up to 14 G allowing higher infusion rates to be achieved. As peripheral veins become obstructed or shut down, it requires the clinician to locate broader lumens, which are harder to cannulate. If a perfectly good vein is rendered unusable by failed cannulation, the situation is made more difficult, so increasing the risk potential of the patient. All staff with responsibility for cannulation should therefore receive formal training and maintain their practical skills.

Use: performing peripheral venous cannulation

- Determine the level of urgency and use for which the cannula is required. If there is someone better suited to the task, have them either perform the procedure or be available to provide assistance.
- Use an aseptic technique and employ universal precautions, ensuring you have a full range of cannulae and sundries available. Use types of cannulae that you feel comfortable with when possible (e.g. winged styles or those that employ a 'bloodless' insertion technique).
- Apply a tourniquet that prevents venous return, whilst allowing arterial flow to the area. This can be checked by the palpation of a pulse, distal to the applied tourniquet.
- Study the anatomy. Only what you see is available for use in the first instance, so take your time in selection. Whilst choosing a vein, try to optimise the following criteria:
  - Make sure the vein is proportionate in size to the cannula you wish to insert and away from jointed areas that might compromise the patency of flow in flexion. Do not waste a large vein access site (e.g. the median cubital vein or the larger veins of the forearm) by inserting cannulae that are too small to perform the required function. Seek assistance if needed.
  - Ensure the vein has a length that will accommodate the cannula, and which is free from obstructions such as evident valves or narrowing and as straight as possible.
  - The vein should be as healthy in appearance as the patient's condition permits. This reduces the likelihood of vascular rupture ('blowing') or shortened life of the cannula.
  - In palpation, the vein should be stable in its surrounding tissues to reduce movement. Gentle traction on the surrounding skin area can aid stabilisation. Stimulation of the vein through a rubbing or gentle tapping technique can induce spasm of the wall of the vessel, so giving form and structure to the target. Note that excessive force in technique is painful and should be avoided.

- The use of alcohol wipes to disinfect the local area is debatable with regard to the reduction of infection rates (Franklin 1999). In dark skin there is the added benefit that vasculature becomes more readily visible as light is reflected from the shining, curved surfaces. Ensure that any applied cleansing solution has dried prior to venepuncture. With smaller cannulae especially, the predominant pain experienced by patients occurs not directly from the penetration, but from the reaction of alcohol with the skin tissue as it is introduced by the cannula.
- Venepuncture can best be achieved by careful visualisation of the anatomy. A positive, brisk insertion of the cannula at an angle of approximately 15–20° should ensure that the skin is fully penetrated. Insertion continues until a flashback of blood is seen in the central chamber of the cannula, indicating that the tip of the cannula is in the vascular lumen. Gentle withdrawal of the introducer leaves the atraumatic cannula positioned for insertion up the vein. If resistance is met, ensure that attempts to continue insertion do not compromise the vessel. It is better to have a cannula that is only partially inserted but patent, as opposed to a failed attempt. This can be used and maintained until a more optimal access is established. After two failed attempts at cannulation, assistance should be sought prior to proceeding. If no success is achieved in transdermal cannulation, venous cut-down by a medical practitioner may need to be considered.
- Cannulae should be properly maintained and checked, so as to ensure patency of function and reduce the incidence of phlebitis. If a cannula needs to be replaced, it is best to site the new cannula prior to the old one becoming unusable, so ensuring that venous access is present at all times.

Complications

Known complications of intravenous therapy fall into three main categories (Campbell 1997):

- *Phlebitis.* This inflammation of the vessel can be caused by a number of factors. The size and material of the catheter, the manner in which it was inserted and also the type, duration and rate of infusion, will all influence the longevity of the cannula, together with any inflammation resulting from infection. Redness, pain or irritation may be early indicators of phlebitis and may require new access to be established. Changing the cannula every 1–2 days is recommended where practical.
- *Infection.* Contamination of the intravenous site or line can result from inadequate skin preparation, poor on-going cleansing, contaminated infusions and host factors. The introduction of these contaminants often stems from poor technique on the part of the carer.
- *Extravasation.* The stability of intravenous cannulae depends upon various factors. The age of the woman may reflect skin or tissue condition and the conscious care of the woman in regard to ensuring the device remains firmly *in situ* and undisturbed. If the cannula is sited in an awkward position such as the

dominant hand, in a high profile area prone to being caught, or directly over a mobile joint such as the wrist or antecubital fossa, then there is a greater potential for displacement. If on-going infusions are present, these might also provide another area where inadvertent traction or catching can displace the cannula. Care must be taken to ensure that the entire intravenous line is secure, and that the woman is fully aware of the various components that may inadvertently become caught or dislodged.

Arterial cannulation

Arterial cannulation is a clinical procedure that is generally reserved for situations where the potential for rapid variations in blood pressure is anticipated. It is also employed where non-invasive blood pressure monitoring is not possible (e.g. morbid obesity, trauma or burns) (Anderson 1997). Whilst *in situ*, the presence of an arterial cannula facilitates easy sampling of arterial blood for gas analysis and acid base balance, so preventing repeated arterial perforation. Women with arterial cannulae require close supervision as the mere employment of the technique indicates an unstable and potentially life-threatening condition. In addition to this, should the line become disconnected, there is the danger of massive haemorrhage occurring.

Technology

A cannula is inserted into an artery. This is connected to a sterile system, primed with heparinised saline and fitted to a transducer. The tubing of the system must be non-compliant so as to ensure that pressures remain constant from the point of reception to the point of transduction. Pulsations that reflect the arterial pressure pass through the system until they reach a membrane. The reverberation against this membrane is detected by sensors and is transduced into an electronic impulse that is displayed on a monitor in both waveform and digital reading.

Technique and practicalities of the procedure

It is often peripheral arteries that are selected for the placement of arterial lines. Whilst larger arteries such as the femoral artery are usually readily accessible, should significant damage occur to the vessel, the blood supply to the distal limb can be compromised if the chosen artery is the sole or principal supply. Commonly, therefore, the radial and ulnar arteries are often chosen for their convenience, clean location and the fact that they are not end arteries. It is imperative, however, to establish that a collateral supply exists between them in case of inadvertent damage being caused. In testing, 3% of hospitalised patients have an inadequate collateral flow. This is commonly established by performing Allen's test (Husum & Berthelsen 1981):

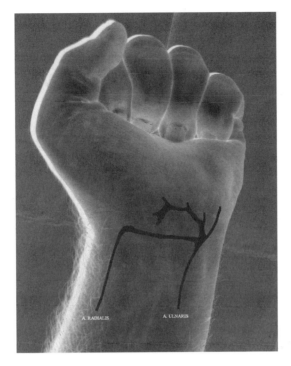

A. RADIALIS   A. ULNARIS

Figure 10.1   Position of the radial and ulnar arteries.

- Palpate both the radial and ulnar arteries (Fig. 10.1).
- Occlude both arteries with the patient's hand both raised and clenched. After 20 seconds, significant blanching should occur.
- Release one side and watch for refill within 5–7 seconds. Repeat for the other side.
- An even refill will indicate a safe colateral supply. If the test is negative, do not proceed.

The following items are required for arterial cannula insertion: sterile gloves, skin preparation, arterial cannula, dressing ± suture and heparinised saline flush.

Once the area has been cleaned and infiltrated with local anaesthetic as required, the cannula may be inserted in one of two ways. By the direct puncture method, the same technique as used in venous cannulation is employed. The cannula is advanced until flashback is obtained and then, as the introducer is withdrawn, passed up the lumen of the vessel. Using the transfixion technique, the cannula is advanced until flashback is seen and then advanced further, so transfixing the artery. The introducer is then removed. The cannula is then slowly withdrawn until clear pulsatile blood flow is obtained, and then advanced up the lumen.

Having ensured there is no air present in the system and that it is boldly marked as arterial, the system can be connected. It is important to ensure that the system is pressurised so that it does not fall below that exerted within the artery. The system must then be set at 'zero'. This will calibrate it to atmospheric pressure (760 mmHg at standard sea level). Close the system to the patient input and open the transducer tap to allow air entry. Zero the transducer at the monitor. Close the transducer tap and ensure it is returned to allow patient line input. With the transducers set at the level of the heart, a pressure wave produced by a left ventricular systole will be seen. It is transmitted faster than the arterial blood flow. The standard waveform will commonly display an initial peak (marking systolic pressure), a descent, interrupted by the dicrotic notch (closure of the aortic valve) and a final trough that marks diastole. Normal values in females (age 19–50 years) range respectively from 100–140 mmHg systolic to 60–90 mmHg diastolic. Levels above this threshold are considered as hypertensive (National Institute of Clinical Excellence 2004). Abnormal waveforms can indicate aortic stenosis, regurgitation or left ventricular failure. If a patient is hypovolaemic, the dicrotic notch will appear lower in its placement on the curve of the downstroke. Collapsing waveforms can show a hyperdynamic circulation sometimes seen during sepsis, anaemia, aortic regurgitation or pregnancy. Arterial blood gas analysis shows the partial pressures of gasses contained in the sample. The range of normal values (as seen in 95% of healthy adults) is as follows:

- Pao_2: 11.3–14.0 kPa/85–105 mmHg
- $PaCO_2$: 4.7–6.0 kPa/35–45 mmHg
- SaO_2: 95–99%
- H^+ concentration: 36–43 nmol/L
- pH: 7.35 7.45
- Bicarbonate: 20–30 mmol/L

Transducer set-up

The following items are required for the set-up of most modern transducers: 500 ml NaCl + heparin at 1 iu/ml, single/double transducer set and a pressure infusion bag (only arterial lines need to be pressurised unless wedge pressure monitors are to be used).

Close all three-way taps and clamps prior to starting. Insert the system inlet into the bag port and fill the chamber. Run through each section in turn ensuring all air is displaced in an upward direction (air rises and will interfere with readings if not removed). Maintain an aseptic technique at all times so as not to contaminate the system.

Complications

Disconnection and subsequent haemorrhage are a very real risk to women with arterial monitoring. Whilst we might normally presume that we will notice any significant haemorrhage, arterial cannulae once disconnected can provide a patent pathway for blood loss. Under arterial pressure this can be very rapid. To put this into perspective, 280 ml is the approximate circulating blood volume of a 3.5 kg baby. This can be lost within 1 minute. It only takes a short period of distraction to miss a potentially fatal occurrence.

Inadvertent arterial drug administration can occur if the set-up is not clearly labelled. Most systems are colour coded; however great care should be taken to ensure that all monitoring and infusion lines are kept in an ordered manner. In an emergency, a three-way tap on the arterial line might look just like any other, so always err on the side of caution.

Arterial occlusion occurs in less than 50% of cases and, as has been outlined in discussing the criteria for insertion site selection, can have grave consequences in single-supply arteries. Other potential complications associated with arterial lines include embolisation and infection or contamination. Aneurysm formation relative to the size and condition of the femoral artery has also been reported. Haematoma upon insertion/withdrawal is common; however, it should be noted that whilst bleeding at a site such as the radial artery can be readily observed and controlled, vessels such as the femoral artery can often be more difficult to view as they often lie deeper in the tissues and thus present a restricted access for the application of direct pressure in the control of haemorrhage.

Inaccurate sample readings can lead to missed diagnoses or inappropriate treatment being undertaken, so it is important that samples are drawn in a controlled manner. To obtain a sample, the three-way tap closest to the woman should be closed. Using a sterile 10 ml syringe, aspirate the system so that the distal section is filled with fresh blood. The volume of the dead space should then be drawn off a minimum of five times, prior to the sample being taken. The technique will depend upon the equipment or method used for processing the sample. Having checked for the presence of air or clotting, the system can then be flushed and zeroed to recommence monitoring.

Central venous cannulation and central venous pressure monitoring

Central venous pressure (CVP) was first recorded in a horse by Stephen Hales in 1733. Experimental progression to human recording was not achieved until 1902, and in 1910 the introduction of CVP measurement in the clinical setting was seen (Kalso 1985). In 1945, the first polythene venous catheters were introduced, so establishing CVP insertion as a common practice although the more common aim at the time was for resuscitation as opposed to routine clinical measurement. There is the ability, however, to use the line for rapid infusion, whilst monitoring the volaemic state.

As previously established, whilst an ECG recording gives an image of the electrical conductivity across the heart, it provides no information with regard to cardiac output. CVP measurement, in reflecting right atrial pressure, provides a means of assessing a patient's haemodynamic status. Cardiac performance may be determined by the combined relationship between preload, afterload and contractility. Preload is the level of ventricular filling and pressure generated by venous return in the left ventricle following diastole. Afterload represents the pressure against which the flow from the left ventricle is subjected at the end of the systolic phase. Both of these are dependent upon the function of the heart and the vascular system. Contractility reflects upon the cardiac tissue alone. The net result from the interaction of these three factors is the stroke volume (volume ejected per minute from the left ventricle). This then circulates in the normal manner. Although catheters are positioned on the right side of the heart, placement of a catheter in the pulmonary artery reflects left ventricular pressures as during diastole the pulmonary venous bed and the left ventricle are in direct communication.

The preload relationship between right atrial pressure and ventricular output are described in Starling's law which states that cardiac output increases as left ventricular end-diastolic volume increases. There is a limit, however, as to how high the filling pressure can be increased. This is due to the tensile limitations of myocyte fibres. Also, and perhaps more commonly, seen is the process that large increases in left ventricular filling pressure (and subsequently increased pulmonary venous pressure) can lead to the occurrence of pulmonary oedema. It has been shown, however, that when patients are undergoing mechanical ventilation in the intensive care setting as a direct result of cardiogenic pulmonary oedema, normal pulmonary artery wedge pressures (PAWPs) have been recorded after ventilation was initiated. In such a case, patients may benefit from additional fluid challenges, despite the presence of pulmonary oedema. The oedema is quickly resolved when cardiac function and performance improves, often within the first 24 hours.

Vasodilatory drugs may be directly monitored for their right-sided effects, so allowing informed titration and optimal control. Parenteral nutrition and concentrated drugs also benefit from the high flow rates and subsequent rapid dilution into the central venous system, so reducing the incidence of local irritation.

Figure 10.2 shows the cardiac cycle in relation to CVP and the ECG.

Technique and practicalities of the procedure

CVP insertion

The internal jugular vein (IJV) is often the favoured point of insertion for CVP lines. A lesser risk of pneumothorax exists in this technique, as the point of insertion is further away from the apex of the lung during the initial stage of the procedure when traumatic introducers and dilators are used. Insertion into the IJV has a less direct path than the subclavian technique. Whilst easy to compress in the event of haemorrhage, a higher incidence of arterial puncture exists as it lies lateral to the common carotid artery and may also prove difficult to cannulate in hypovolaemic patients. The site is also prone to infection, possibly as a result of catheter or neck movement (Hocking 2000).

Whilst the alternative subclavian route tends to increase patient comfort post-placement and allows a more direct route to the heart, it has incurred a high rate of morbidity due to the incidence of damage to the pleural, vascular and neural tissues encountered during insertion. In considering the placement site, poor coagulopathy may render bleeding difficult to control, and the potential for lung damage during insertion may further compromise those with existing lung disease or impaired oxygenation. Catheters in the region of 20 cm in length are used for IJV and subclavian insertion. If femoral or brachial veins are to be

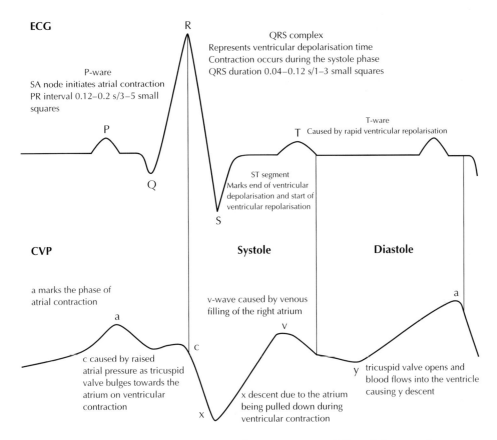

ECG

R

QRS complex
Represents ventricular depolarisation time
Contraction occurs during the systole phase
QRS duration 0.04–0.12 s/1–3 small squares

P-ware
SA node initiates atrial contraction
PR interval 0.12–0.2 s/3–5 small squares

P

T-ware
T   Caused by rapid ventricular repolarisation

Q

ST segment
Marks end of ventricular depolarisation and start of ventricular repolarisation

S

CVP

Systole

Diastole

a marks the phase of atrial contraction

a

v-wave caused by venous filling of the right atrium

v

a

c caused by raised atrial pressure as tricuspid valve bulges towards the atrium on ventricular contraction

c

x descent due to the atrium being pulled down during ventricular contraction

x

y tricuspid valve opens and blood flows into the ventricle causing y descent

Figure 10.2   Cardiac cycle in relation to central venous pressure (CVP) and electrocardiograms (ECGs).

considered, longer catheters of 60 cm are required to ensure that the tip of the catheter reaches the correct placement area.

For neck or subclavian placement, the woman is placed in the Trendelenberg position or supine with a support placed between the shoulders. An aseptic field is established and it is important to monitor that this is maintained throughout the procedure. With long guidewires and multiple lumen catheters, it is easy to contaminate items that will then be passed directly into the central system. Each component of the chosen line is then checked and flushed, and the local area can be infiltrated with local anaesthetic as required. Full monitoring should be in operation and good venous access established prior to starting the insertion procedure.

Insertion technique is commonly limited to two methods. Direct cannulation, as used in peripheral cannulation, allows simple insertion with relatively little ancillary equipment. The catheter is passed over the needle and so reduces the bleeding from the insertion site due to its greater size. The diameter of the needle however, is also relatively large, and carries an increased risk of over-insertion and bleeding from accidental arterial puncture.

The more common method of insertion, especially for multilumen catheters is the Seldinger technique, which employs the use of a guidewire to direct the catheter placement (Hocking 2000). The chosen vein is located with a small-diameter needle. Once in the vein, a guidewire is inserted, and the needle removed. The tip of the wire is commonly J-shaped and flexible, so as not to perforate or traumatise the vessel as it passes through the lumen. Care should be taken not to kink the guidewire as this can cause damage to both the vessel and the catheter as it passes over. It may also prevent the catheter being inserted and require either a new guidewire or abandonment of the procedure. Overinsertion of the guidewire may cause cardiac arrhythmias. In this case, a slight withdrawal should stop stimulation and allow insertion to continue. A dilator can then be passed over the guidewire to open the puncture site to enable the larger catheter to be passed. The dilator (if used) is then removed and the catheter inserted. The guidewire (in multilumen catheters) will appear through the central lumen as the catheter is passed and is removed once correct placement is confirmed. The catheter is then sutured to prevent kinking and movement, and a sterile dressing applied.

A possible third technique of passing the catheter through a large-diameter needle for antecubital insertion is seldom used. The size of the needle leads to bleeding at the point of insertion, and if the catheter needs to be withdrawn through the needle, there is the risk of catheter embolisation should part of the catheter be sheared off by the needle tip.

Once *in situ*, the catheter may be connected to a primed monitoring system. This may be a simple fluid manometer that consists of a line from the woman, a monitoring limb and infusion set, controlled by a three-way tap. Once the entire system is primed, and the monitoring limb filled slightly above the estimated CVP reading, the tap is closed to the infusion set, allowing passage from the CVP line to the monitoring limb. The fluid in the column is then balanced against the CVP and a reading obtained by measurement of the top of the fluid against a scale. If the porous plug at the top of the column is blocked, measurements will be incorrect as the fluid movement will be restricted. It is vital that the base of the system at the level of the three-way tap is level with the woman's heart. This effectively 'zeros' the system against atmospheric pressure to ensure an accurate reading (Woodrow 2002).

More common, however, is the electronic transducer system that converts the action of fluid pressure against a membrane to an electronic signal, so providing both a waveform and numerical data. Opening pressures should then be recorded along with the woman's other observations. Infusion bags should be changed every 24 hours, with system components being changed at least every 72 hours. All waveforms achieved will share the principle of a-, c- and v-waves, with x-y descents.

Interpreting a CVP recording

- A *normal CVP range* is 3–10 mmHg (5–12 cmH$_2$O) (Mooney & Comerford 2003).
- A *low CVP reading* is usually a sign of hypovolaemia or dehydration. This can be as a consequence of haemorrhage or excessive diuresis.

- A *high CVP recording* can indicate the following:
  - Hypervolaemia: defined as an abnormal increase in the volume of blood circulating in the body and often a result of excessive fluid infusion.
  - Cardiac failure, for example right ventricular failure.
  - Pulmonary embolism.
  - Mitral valve failure/regurgitation.
  - Cardiac tamponade.
  - Catheter lumen occlusion/obstruction, for example thrombus, or the catheter lying against the vein wall.

CVP removal

The catheter should be removed with the woman lying flat and having fully exhaled in an attempt to reduce the risk of air entering the catheter upon removal thus causing an air embolus. Withdrawal should be constant and direct pressure applied for at least 5 minutes to the puncture site to prevent bleeding. If any difficulty is experienced during the process, appropriate assistance should be sought (Drewett 2000).

Pulmonary artery pressure monitoring

All too often in the treatment of the critically ill woman, unstable haemodynamics, pulmonary compromise and changing cardiac output require the placement of invasive monitoring to direct the continuing balance of treatment therapies. To obtain optimal data in regard to cardiac output, a pulmonary artery (PA) catheter may be inserted. Often performed in the intensive care setting, the safe use of PA catheters has been documented for many years with good effect. However, recent evidence has suggested that the use of PA catheters has neither increased overall mortality rates nor conferred benefit for critically ill patients (Hall 2005; Shah et al. 2005). A balloon-tipped catheter is inserted through a central vein and 'floated' through the right side of the heart until it comes to rest in the pulmonary artery. Multiple lumens allow for measurement at different levels and the options for infusion or pacing if required. The inflation of the balloon effectively 'wedges' the branch of the pulmonary artery and records the pulmonary capillary wedge pressure (PCWP) or pulmonary artery wedge pressure (PAWP). The use of PA or Swan–Ganz catheters provides the following:

- Indirect measurement of left ventricular end-diastolic pressure
- Central vascular pressures in the presence of decreased cardiac output
- Access to mixed venous blood samples to determine the degree of blood passing unoxygenated from the lungs to the left atrium

Combined, these assist in the determination of shock levels and fluid volume status, the presence of heart disease and any compromise in cardiac output.

CVP can be measured via the proximal port sited 30 cm from the catheter tip. The port is often colour coded blue and can also be used for intravenous infusion. Continual PA pressures are measured via the distal port, which is often coded yellow. Pressures are differentiated as PAS (pulmonary artery systolic) and PAD (pulmonary artery diastolic). This port should never be used for infusions or medication administration. When the balloon is inflated, PAWP is also measured (McHale 1997; Bindels et al. 1999). The balloon port is situated in the distal end of the catheter. Inflated with 0.8–1.5 ml of air (never liquid); the port is usually coded red. Using slow inflation with the specialist syringe supplied with the system (this will not allow itself to be filled with more than 1.5 ml of air), the balloon should inflate using 1.25–1.5 ml of air. Less than this indicates that the catheter has advanced too far into the PA. If the balloon is overinflated, the balloon lumen may rupture. Measurement should not exceed periods of 2–3 respiratory cycles or 10–15 seconds, with the measurements taken being kept to a minimum. If PAWP and PAD are similar (within 4 mmHg difference), then PAD readings can be substituted for PAWP, so reducing the number of required measurements and potential harm being caused. By removing the syringe from the port, the balloon will passively deflate and the PA pressure trace will return. Do not actively withdraw air as this can damage the balloon. Once deflated, the gate port or tap can be closed to avoid inadvertent inflation of the balloon. To prevent loss of the restricted syringe, leave it attached. This will also guard against staff using the port for incorrect purposes.

Table 10.1 lists the expected range of recordings for cardiac monitoring.

Changes in pressure measurements can be caused and influenced by changes in preload, afterload and contractility and can therefore have different indications. It is vital, however, from the onset of treatment to establish what is normal for the woman in question.

A low CVP might indicate a decreased venous return or hypovolaemia due to haemorrhage or polyuria. In shock scenarios, this will be partially offset by peripheral vasoconstriction. Fluid challenges or fluid resuscitation may raise CVP

Table 10.1   Expected range of recordings for cardiac monitoring.

Reading	'Normal' range
CVP (right atrial pressure)	3–10 mmHg
Right ventricular pressure	20–30 mmHg (systolic) and 0–5 mmHg (diastolic)
PA pressure (mean)	10–25 mmHg
PAS pressure	20–30 mmHg
PAD pressure	08–12 mmHg
PAWP	05–15 mmHg

Whilst these figures represent a range within which 'normal' readings can fall, it should be recognised that 'normal' is subject to a combination of many variant factors. As such, pressures should be looked at in regard to trend patterns and the patient's response to therapeutic measures such as fluid challenges, not in a rigid comparison to 'normal' values.

CVP, central venous pressure; PA, pulmonary artery; PAD, pulmonary artery diastolic; PAS, pulmonary artery systolic; PAWP, pulmonary artery wedge pressure.

readings to high levels, and once partial peripheral dilatation occurs, values can appear normal. In conditions of full peripheral dilatation, however, especially with the influences of general anaesthesia, the CVP can then plummet to expose a large volume deficit. Spinal anaesthesia can also have a dramatic effect upon central pressures, as can sepsis, vasodilator overdoses and systemic dysfunction.

A raised CVP can indicate many possible causes. Cardiac factors include left or right heart failure and valve disease. Sympathetic nervous stimulation can give a raised reading, as can increases in venous and cardiac muscle tone. Other cardiac-related causes are tamponade, pulmonary vascular hypertension and embolism. In cases of constrictive pericardial disease, the CVP will rise on inspiration and fall during expiration, in paradox to normal observations. Hypervolaemia resulting from overvigorous fluid therapy is a common source of raised pressures. Intrathoracic causes include intermittent positive pressure ventilation, C-PAP (continuous positive airway pressure) and obstructive airway disease. Whilst no formula exists to calculate the effect of these pressures, if they remain constant in application, then the resulting trends should also remain constant. In the critical care setting, haemo- or pneumothorax should not be ruled out. Other raised pressures can result from abdominal splinting, pregnancy or ascites.

PA catheters can be used to derive a large amount of variable data that cannot otherwise be predicted by clinical examination. Cardiac output (using thermo-dilution techniques) or stroke volume is measured in millilitres or in beats. Increased stroke volume can indicate increased circulating volume or the use of inotropic agents. Decreases can indicate compromised valve function or cardiac contractility. This could progress to heart failure. Systemic vascular resistance figures can be computed; however, figures are dependent on variable factors such as peripheral resistance and heart rate. Much information can be obtained by analysing the waveforms. As previously discussed, invasive pressure waveforms have similar characteristics, but tend to differ in form in relation to the measurement point.

Complications

The potential complications arising from CVP and PA catheters are similar to those covered under arterial pressure monitoring. Haemorrhage, occlusion and false readings are commonly shared with all invasive monitors. In addition, the placement of lines in the heart can lead to dysrhythmias and altered cardiac function and circulation, with possible cardiac arrest. Bleeding and perforation or rupture can cause haemopneumothorax, cardiac tamponade and pulmonary artery haemorrhage, rupture or infarction. Should the woman cough up blood, or blood be noticed in the airway, a pulmonary artery rupture should always be suspected and expert help sought immediately. Whilst a CVP catheter can be flushed regularly, a PA catheter can rupture the pulmonary artery if flushed for longer than 2 seconds whilst under pressure (Connors 1983; Cruz & Franklin 2001).

Due to the complex nature of PA catheters, equipment can fail with examples such as balloon rupture or microshock, which stems from exposure of the thermistor connector tip. Air or thromboembolisms can also occur. It cannot be stressed enough that if invasive monitoring is genuinely required, then women should be placed in a critical care setting, where staff are familiar with the procedures to be undertaken and their on-going management. In all cases of shock, the initial treatment is fluid therapy. This should not be curtailed for fear of the emergence of pulmonary oedema, and is indeed preferable to the use of vasoactive drugs. As the body redistributes fluids, pulmonary oedema often settles very quickly with any excess fluids being dealt with naturally by the kidney or by giving reducing agents such as nitrates or diuretics. The complex relationships that govern cardiac function need direct study and careful analysis to ensure that findings are taken in the context of a woman's condition and the therapeutic measures undertaken in the course of treatment.

Conclusion

Midwifery practitioners may perform intensive monitoring for the critically ill woman on an infrequent basis. However, the skills and knowledge required to use and interpret the results remain a crucial part of accurate and prompt diagnosis and management. It is important to ensure that such attributes are updated on a frequent basis. If practitioners experience difficulties in undertaking monitoring, it may be easier for experienced practitioners to support midwives within the maternity environment (Ball et al. 2003) or for women to be transferred to a unit which provides such care and management on a regular basis.

References

Aehlert, B. (2002) *ECGs Made Easy* (2nd edn). Mosby, St Louis.

Anderson, J. (1997) Arterial cannulation. *British Journal of Hospital Medicine*, **57** (10): 497–9.

Antunes, E., Brugada, J., Steurer, G., Andries, E. and Brugada, P. (1994) The differential diagnosis of a regular tachycardia with a wide QRS complex on the 12 lead ECG: ventricular tachycardia, supraventricular tachycardia with abberant intraventricular conduction, and supraventricular tachycardia with antegrade conduction over an accessory. *Pacing and Clinical Electrophysiology*, **17**: 1515–24.

Ball, C., Kirkby, M. and Williams, S. (2003) Effect of the critical care outreach team on patient survival to discharge from hospital and readmission to critical care: non-randomised population based study. *British Medical Journal*, **327**: 1014.

Bindels, A., Van der Hoeven, J. and Meinders, A. (1999) Pulmonary artery wedge pressure and extravascular lung water in patients with acute cardiogenic pulmonary oedema requiring mechanical ventilation. *American Journal of Cardiology*, **84** (10): 1158–63.

Campbell, J. (1997) Intravenous cannulation: potential complications. *Professional Nurse*, **12** (Suppl. 8): S10–3.

Connors, A. (1983) The role of right heart catheterisation in the care of the critically ill: benefits, limitations and risks. *International Journal of Cardiology*, **4** (4): 474–7.

Cruz, K. and Franklin, C. (2001) The pulmonary artery catheter: uses and controversies. *Critical Care Clinics*, **17** (2): 271–91.

Drewett, S. (2000) Complications of central venous catheters: nursing care. *British Journal of Nursing*, **9** (8): 466–78.

Fearnley, S. (1995) Pulse oximetry. *Update in Anaesthesia*, Issue 5: Article 2.

Franklin, L. (1999) Skin cleansing and infection control in peripheral venepuncture and cannulation. *Nursing Standard*, **14** (4): 49–50.

Hall, J. (2005) Searching for evidence to support pulmonary artery catheter use in critically ill patients. *Journal of the American Medical Association*, **294** (13): 1693–4.

Hocking, G. (2000) Central venous access and monitoring. *Update in Anaesthesia*, Issue 12, Article 13. http://www.nda.ox.ac.uk/wfsa/html/u12/u1213_01.htm

Husum, B. and Berthelsen, P. (1981) Allen's test and systolic arterial pressure in the thumb. *British Journal of Anaesthesia*, **53** (6): 635–7.

Kalso, E. (1985) A short history of central venous catheterisation. *Acta Anaesthesiologica Scandinavica*, **81** (Suppl.): 7–10.

Lee, J. (2000) ECG monitoring in theatre. *Update in Anaesthesia*, Issue 11. http://www.nda.ox.ac.uk/wfsa/html/pages/up_issu.htm

Manning, D., Kuchirka, C. and Kaminski, J. (1983) Miscuffing: inappropriate blood pressure cuff application. *Circulation*, **68** (4):

Marieb, E. (2003) *Human Anatomy and Physiology* (6th edn). Addison Wesley, San Francisco.

McHale, L. (1997) Obtaining a pulmonary artery wedge pressure. *Critical Care Nurse*, **17** (5): 94–5.

Mooney, G. and Comerford, D. (2003) What you need to know about central venous lines. *Nursing Times*, **99** (10): 28–9.

National Institute of Clinical Excellence (2004) *Hypertension: Management of hypertension in adults in primary care.* Clinical Guideline No. 18. National Institute of Clinical Excellence (NICE), London.

Pedersen, T., Dyrlund Pedersen, P. and Moller, A. (2004) Pulse oximetry for peri-operative monitoring. *Cochrane Library*, Issue 4.

Resuscitation Council UK (2005) *Advanced Adult Life Support.* Resuscitation Council UK, London.

Schamroth, L. (1990) *An Introduction to Electrocardiography* (7th edn). Blackwell Scientific, Oxford.

Shah, M., Hasselblad, V., Stevenson, L. et al. (2005) Impact of the pulmonary artery catheter in critically ill patients: meta-analysis of randomized clinical trials. *Journal of the American Medical Association*, **294** (13): 1664–70.

Thelan, L., Urdan, L., Lough, M. and Stacy, K. (1998) *Critical Care Nursing: Diagnosis and management* (3rd edn). Mosby, St Louis.

Tortora, G. and Derrickson, B. (2005) *Principles of Anatomy and Physiology.* Wiley & Sons, Chichester.

Ur, A. and Gordon, M. (1970) Origin of korotkoff sounds. *American Journal of Physiology*, **218**: 524–9.

Woodrow, P. (1998) An introduction to the reading of electrocardiograms. *British Journal of Nursing*, **7** (3): 135–42.

Woodrow, P. (2002) Central venous catheters and central venous pressure. *Nursing Standard*, **16** (26): 45–51.

11 Anaesthesia and Resuscitation of the Critically Ill Woman

Mary Billington and Mandy Stevenson

This chapter considers the two separate but related topics of midwifery involvement with critically ill women who undergo anaesthesia or experience cardiopulmonary arrest. Anaesthesia may be required for management of a woman who is critically ill, or alternatively it may be the cause of critical illness. Similarly, cardiopulmonary arrest may occur in a woman who is critically ill, or it may be an unanticipated event which precipitates critical illness.

Part 1: Anaesthesia

Midwives may appear to have little or no input in the anaesthetic process other than as a support for the woman. However, with any urgent situation such as emergency anaesthesia, there is no room for complacency. Midwives have a valuable role in providing support to anaesthetic and other theatre staff, in addition to being involved in preoperative preparation and immediate post-operative care of the woman who was or who becomes critically ill.

Assumed prior knowledge

- Physiological changes of pregnancy
- Basic preoperative and postoperative care

Introduction

The administration of any form of anaesthesia needs to be undertaken safely and with thorough preparation. Proficient working practices and unit protocols should be in place to ensure that the woman's and practitioner's wellbeing are maintained, such as determining and managing any identified risk factors. For example non-detection of allergies such as to latex, may result in an unexpected allergic or anaphylactic reaction which then necessitates urgent delivery (Health and Safety Executive 2006).

Shibli and Russell (2000) recognise that the optimal anaesthesia for a caesarean section is a regional block, especially for women with pre-eclampsia (National High Blood Pressure Education Program Working Group 2000). However, there will always be situations when a general anaesthetic will be necessary, often in emergency situations where a regional block has 'failed' or for a deteriorating maternal or fetal condition.

General anaesthesia is not performed without risk and statistics from the most recent Confidential Enquiry into Maternal Deaths (CEMD) (Lewis 2004) indicate that six maternal deaths were directly due to the administration of anaesthesia. This figure increases with 20 more deaths recognised as having an 'anaesthetic contribution'. This mortality rate is consistent with the previous report which reported that the 'challenges presented to the obstetric anaesthetist were increasing in number, complexity and severity' (Lewis 2001).

This percentage of maternal deaths needs to be viewed cautiously and lessons need to be learnt. Lack of multidisciplinary cooperation and communication has been acknowledged as a major concern, and, in particular, not involving the anaesthetist at an appropriate time.

Midwives caring for women who may become physiologically challenged and require medical input are required by the *Code of Professional Conduct* (Nursing and Midwifery Council (NMC) 2004a) to 'co-operate with others in the team'. Effective written and prompt verbal communication between all the members of the multidisciplinary team should promote this issue.

Implications of physiological changes of pregnancy

When caring for ill women, who are already physiologically compromised, midwives have a responsibility to ensure that optimal care is provided (NMC 2004a). Physiological changes may occur that worsen the disorder and necessitate delivery more promptly than expected. Hence knowledge of such pregnancy-related physiological adjustments is important as they may not only impact upon the disorder but also upon the anaesthetic process.

Cardiovascular system

The increase in maternal blood volume leads to a decreased haemoglobin level, and an increase in platelets and coagulation factors. Further pathophysiological changes in pre-eclampsia include an increase in cardiac output and an increase in blood pressure. Inaccurate measurement and recording preoperatively of the blood pressure and vital signs may encourage inappropriate fluid management intraoperatively or post-delivery, especially in women with pre-eclampsia who are at risk of fluid overload and the associated problems such as pulmonary oedema (Torr & James 1998).

Nervous system

Pregnant women tend to be more sensitive to anaesthetics, and thus have a decreased requirement for inhalational agents by 25–40% (Palahnuik et al. 1974). This is beneficial for the woman's recovery time but the potential effects upon the fetus must be considered. These vary depending on factors such as length of anaesthesia and surgery, and the drugs utilised. This needs to be taken into account when caring for a neonate with reduced responses in order to instigate appropriate management according to whether the condition is due to the underlying pathology or simply due to the effects of maternal anaesthesia (Datta 2000).

Furthermore, hormonal influences may alter nerve responses to local anaesthetics and therefore decrease the local anaesthetic need by 25% in regional techniques (Levy, cited by Liu 2003).

Respiratory system

These changes include an increase in tidal volume, respiratory rate, oxygen consumption and Pao_2, whereas a reduction in $Paco_2$, compliance and resistance occurs. These alterations may affect the expected values returned during a woman's unconscious state. However, with the effects of pre-eclampsia, and the potential for laryngeal or pulmonary oedema, attention needs to be given to the disease rather than treating it as pregnancy-related changes.

Care and preparation

Preoperative preparation

In any situation, whether planned or emergency, where an anaesthetic is to be administered a formal preanaesthetic assessment needs to be undertaken. This should comprise more than an 'any loose teeth or allergies' question as the woman is rushed into the unfamiliar environment of the operating theatre.

The preoperative appraisal should comprise of:

- *Written consent.* The woman has a right to offer or withhold consent. This decision should be based upon information made available, enabling a choice to be formulated free from interference or persecution from health care practitioners. Information giving to ill women in childbearing may be perceived to be difficult in relation to the depth of information required and the severity of the situation. However, this should not preclude an informed decision being made by the woman after valuable information has been delivered to her by the appropriate personnel. Dimond (2003) proposes that verbal consent is as valid as consent in writing. However one should remain cautious when considering the validity of such decisions as such judgements may be difficult to prove legally. It may be viewed as the word of two opposing people, and unless witnesses were present, who can confirm/refute the accuracy of the conversation? Was the issue discussed adequately and did the woman consent to all eventualities such as a hysterectomy? Verbal consent may be appropriate in certain situations; however, for surgical interventions such as a caesarean section where the risk of requiring a general anaesthetic and the loss of neurological capacity is heightened, perhaps documented evidence is the best form of agreement.

- *Availability of recent blood results.* The last haemoglobin estimation and the difference from previous values must be established as any reduction in oxygen-carrying capacity may affect the anaesthetic used. Saved serum also needs to be available in the laboratory in case urgent cross-matching for transfusion is required.
- *Presence of any systemic disorders.* The presence of conditions such as pre-clampsia, HELLP syndrome (*h*aemolysis, *e*levated *l*iver *e*nzymes, *l*ow *p*latelets), coagulopathy, diabetes, sickle cell disorder, obesity or Scoline apnoea may impact upon the anaesthetic process and thus need to be identified.
- *Presence of anatomical abnormalities.* Certain hazards to the airway may hinder intubation. Obesity, a short neck or arthritis may reduce the patient's ability to flex their neck. Poor dentition such as loose teeth may be dangerous as these foreign bodies can be inadvertently displaced into the trachea.
- *Use of antacids.* Preoperative preparation should include medication to reduce the risk of fluid/particle aspiration (Chan 2006). An H2 antagonist such as ranitidine 50 mg i.v. given within 1 hour pre-operatively can reduce the production of gastric acid secretions. It is often given in conjunction with 30 ml sodium citrate (which can decrease the pH in the stomach).

In 40% of labouring women, solid food has been identified in the stomach 12–24 hours after starvation (Blouw et al. 1976). Gastric motility is reduced due to the elevated progesterone levels, and the cardiac sphincter tone is also reduced. Even if women have been fasting, there remains a risk of a fasting gastric volume of more than 25 ml, and a gastric fluid pH less than 2.5. This increases the risk of Mendelson's syndrome, also recognised as aspiration pneumonitis, which is caused by aspiration of the acidic gastric medium. A resulting disruption of the normal composition of surfactant may then lead to pulmonary oedema and eventually to acute respiratory distress syndrome (ARDS). With the aspiration of solid particles, a similar neutrophilic reaction occurs in the bronchioles and alveolar ducts, and the large particles may produce frank obstruction of the large airways.

All the above areas should be considered by the anaesthetic team in relation to making an informed decision regarding the choice of anaesthesia.

The options remain as either a regional block or general anaesthetic (GA). In deciding between the two techniques, the urgency of the procedure and the health of the mother and fetus should be taken into account. However, the desires of the mother must also be considered. Although there are few contraindications to a GA, regional anaesthesia is preferred to avoid the risks of airway management including difficulties in intubation and maternal aspiration. In cases of acute fetal distress or severe maternal haemorrhage, there may not be sufficient time or maternal compensatory ability to perform a regional anaesthetic. In addition, regional anaesthetics may not provide the adequate uterine relaxation necessary for a difficult breech extraction or retained placenta.

Perioperative care

Positioning

Once transferred to theatre, correct positioning on the operating table is crucial. Accurate client positioning will allow maximum safety to be maintained (e.g. no client contact with metal surfaces to reduce the risk of diathermy burns), with adequate exposure of the operating site. A further aim of correct positioning is to prevent avoidable postoperative problems (e.g. pressure sores, deep vein thrombosis (DVT)). The supine position is used, with the head and neck in the neutral position. However, a major concern regarding this position is that of aortocaval occlusion (supine hypotensive syndrome). A reduction in venous return and a fall in cardiac output are produced by the weight of the pregnant uterus pressing on, and partly occluding, the inferior vena cava. It should be noted that reduced placental perfusion may have occurred before the fall in the woman's blood pressure is apparent.

The effects of supine hypotension can be reduced by undertaking one of two procedures – a left lateral tilt of 15° with a wedge or a full lateral tilt using the table mechanisms. Evidence is variable regarding best practice. Wilkinson and Enkin (1996) found that Apgar scores and neonatal pHs were higher with the use of a lateral tilt. Rees et al. (2002) concur with this (following spinal anaesthesia) but also consider that if a quicker onset from a regional block is required, a tilt position will enable the block to disperse more rapidly.

The correct positioning of arm retainers also needs to be considered, as radial nerve damage can occur by incorrect placement or pressure of the retainer against the middle of the humerus. It is also important to ensure that the woman's elbow does not overlie the edge of the mattress as damage to the ulnar nerve can occur. One area often forgotten is the placement of the blood pressure cuff. The median nerve can be damaged in the antecubital fossa if the elbows are extensively flexed.

Correct heel elevation should reduce venous stasis (and risk of DVT); however practitioners need to ensure that the device is not hard as this can also increase the pressure risk. Many units utilise pneumatic calf compression devices in addition to the use of compression stockings (Thomas 1999a, 1999b).

Lithotomy positioning can also cause concerns. Extremes of rotation and flexion must be avoided to reduce the risk of sciatic and femoral nerve damage. Also, calf veins can be compressed in the lithotomy position.

Monitoring

Once prepared and positioned, urgent consideration needs to be placed upon effective management of the woman's physiological state with the induction of anaesthesia. Deviations from normality may occur as a reaction to any anaesthetic drugs, hence it is crucial that previous adverse reactions are clearly documented in the woman's medical notes. Deviations can be detected through effective use of the measurement and monitoring of vital signs. Both processes are closely linked but are not one and the same. A measuring instrument becomes a monitor when it is capable of delivering a warning when the variable being measured falls outside the preset limits.

The degree of monitoring will depend upon varying factors such as the current and previous health of the woman, the anaesthetic technique to be used, the equipment available and the anaesthetist's ability to use it.

Basic maternal monitoring whilst on the operating table should include cardiac monitoring, oxygen saturation and blood pressure monitoring. One should, however, consider the placement of the equipment, e.g. electrocardiogram (ECG) electrodes do not occlude the area where surgery will take place. If a central venous line is in place, its recording can be returned to the monitor for immediate interpretation to provide valuable results in relation to cardiac capacity and on-going management. However, practitioners should not rely upon the monitor's ability to provide accurate information pertaining to the maternal condition, as monitors can always malfunction. One needs to retain basic sensory skills such as observation and auscultation.

Once effective monitoring is in place, the anaesthetic process can commence with preoxygenation; 100% oxygen is administered via a facial mask. This is essential for pregnant women due to their decreased lung functional capacity and increased oxygen consumption (Gee et al. 1967). The increased intake of oxygen may help minimise the risk of desaturation often seen during prolonged attempts at intubation. Preoxygenation via a clear facemask may reduce any maternal concerns regarding claustrophobia.

Induction of anaesthesia

Induction is usually with drugs such as thiopentone (sodium pentothal) or propofol (Diprivan). Both drugs have systemic effects working on the following systems:

- Central nervous system – causing sedation, loss of consciousness and anaesthesia. Cerebral metabolism, blood flow and intracranial pressure are reduced.
- Cardiovascular system – causing hypotension secondary to myocardial depression.
- Respiratory system – apnoea is common. The woman's response to carbon dioxide and ventilation are depressed.

After intravenous administration of either drug, consciousness is lost in little more time than it takes for these drugs to travel from the site of administration to the brain (arm–cerebral circulation time), where they cross the brain–blood barrier with potential ease as they are lipid soluble. They inhibit the conduction of cellular activity potential and synaptic transmission. As well as inhibiting activity, both agents can rapidly cross the placenta, but do not appear to depress the fetus (Finster et al. 1972).

Airway maintenance

Once sleep has been induced, airway management needs to be undertaken. Intubation is the most advantageous method used to secure and protect the woman's airway (particularly for those at risk of aspiration). The pregnancy-related physiological changes, especially in woman with pre-eclampsia, present greater degrees of oedema, consequently the ease of vocal cord visualisation and accurate intubation may be substantially reduced.

Once anaesthesia has been successfully induced, muscle relaxants will need to be administered to facilitate the ease of intubation. Suxamethonium (Scoline) is administered as a short lasting but quick acting muscle relaxant to enable the endotracheal tube to be passed. Scoline administration causes a depolarisation at the neuromuscular junction, and as this occurs small twitches will be observed as the cell membranes depolarise and the last messages arrive at the peripheral muscles (fasciculation).

Mechanisms need to be employed to ensure swift and accurate intubation takes place and to reduce the risk of desaturation often seen during prolonged attempts at intubation. Although with high risk women, oral intake is often significantly reduced, to prevent the risk of regurgitation, cricoid pressure needs to be applied as anaesthesia is induced and this should not be released until the endotracheal tube is correctly placed and secured. The aim of Sellick's manoeuvre (application of cricoid pressure) is to exert pressure digitally, pushing the cricoid cartilage against the oesophagus and compressing it against the body of the sixth cervical vertebrae, thus preventing passive regurgitation up the oesophagus (Carrie et al. 2002). If, during the procedure, the woman starts to vomit, the pressure should be released to minimise the risk of the oesophagus rupturing, and the woman turned to minimise aspiration. Evidence confirms that cricoid pressure application is widely practiced but is often applied variably. Incorrectly applied pressure can interfere with laryngoscopy (Cook et al. 2000).

If intubation fails, cricoid pressure must be maintained. Failed intubation is an emergency that requires prompt and calm action. Barnardo and Jenkins (2000) propose that failed intubation in the pregnant population is perhaps 8–10 times higher than in the non-pregnant one. The reasons offered in the review included the failure to follow an accepted protocol for failed intubation. If the process fails, the anaesthetist may chose to utilise a regional block (spinal/epidural). The option to maintain the airway with a Guedal airway and facemask for abdominal surgery is exceptionally limited as muscle relaxation and paralysis with assisted ventilation will be required.

Although there is always the expectation that intubation will be successful, complications can occur which need early detection and prompt management. Such complications include:

- Unrecognised oesophageal intubation. Oxygen and anaesthetic gases are delivered directly into the stomach with the woman becoming increasingly oxygen depleted. Carbon dioxide analysis must always be made available at induction, and should detect gas imbalances. Pulse oximetry will only detect late recordable changes, especially if the woman has been preoxygenated, and hence is not a good indicator for incorrectly placed endotracheal (ET) tubes.

- Failed ventilation as a result of the ET tube becoming kinked, disconnected or inserted too far into the main bronchus.
- Aspiration of regurgitated gastric contents, which in turn can cause a direct blockage of the airway.

Once intubation has taken place, usually with an ET tube with an internal diameter of 7.5–8 FG, anaesthetic maintenance will be required. This occurs with the administration of a dose of longer acting muscle relaxant (when muscle power returns), volatile inhalational agents such as isoflurane, carrier agents (oxygen and nitrous oxide) and analgesics (morphine derived). All volatile agents deepen the anaesthetic but will also directly affect the uterus by causing relaxation, and hence should only be used in small concentrations for caesarean sections.

Although rare, severe drug reactions (anaphylaxis) may occur and should be recognised and managed promptly. Practitioners should consider the causes and distinguish the clinical manifestations of such reactions. These include widespread flushing with an erythematous rash due to histamine release, vasodilatation and increased cardiac permeability, through to respiratory distress/obstruction due to bronchospasm, laryngeal oedema or laryngospasm.

Management of such acute situations depends upon prompt action in the form of administering 100% oxygen with the aim of preventing hypoxia from any resulting respiratory or cardiovascular disturbances. Intravenous medication (or, in exceptional cases of no intravenous access, endotracheal doses) of adrenaline, steroids or antihistamines can be utilised to counterbalance the resulting physiological responses such as bronchospasm or hypotension. (Adrenaline produces bronchodilatation and vasoconstriction to revert the problem to normality.)

Careful monitoring with ECG and oxygen saturation (SpO_2) recordings should be considered as the basic minimum. Arterial blood gases and pH may need to be measured to identify the presence of acidosis, hypoxaemia or hypercarbia. Invasive monitoring in the form of arterial and central venous pressure (CVP) lines needs to be established, and renal function assessed through urinary output monitoring.

Fluid management

Perioperative fluid management needs to be cautiously considered. The type and volume of fluid administered may be variable but should take into account:

- Any deficit the woman has accrued (this may be simply due to starvation preoperatively or from vomiting, haemorrhage or pyrexia). The volume required to replace this should equate to 1.5 ml/kg/h taken from the point of starting the fast.
- Any losses due to surgery (e.g. via evaporation of water during open surgery, tissue damage that results in fluid movement such as third space loss, or any acute blood loss) should then be replaced with an appropriate volume of either crystalloid or colloid solution.

For further guidance see Chapter 9.

Vital sign monitoring, peripheral perfusion and urinary output will offer an indication of the adequacy of the fluid replacement.

Anaesthetic reversal

Towards the end of the surgery, GA drug administration will need to be reduced to promote the return of the reflexes and neuromuscular activity. Muscle relaxant drugs can be reversed by the administration of a combination of neostigmine and glycopyrolate (neostigmine alone can cause bradycardia). Inhalational agents will be reduced and oxygenation increased to promote a return to a conscious state. Upon completion of the surgery and once the protective responses are present with good respiratory effort (i.e. gag or cough reflex or attempting to move), the ET tube can be removed. Careful suctioning will need to take place to reduce the risk of triggering an episode of laryngeal spasm and thus further intervention in the form of reintubation.

Once the woman is responsive, transfer on to a tilting patient trolley with suction/oxygen immediately available should occur. Correct client positioning post-surgery is of the utmost importance to prevent the tongue falling back and occluding the airway. The recovery position (left lateral) will ensure that this does not occur.

Postoperative care

Close observation of the recovering woman in an appropriately equipped area is the most efficient way to monitor, identify and treat problems in the recovery period. An unconscious woman should never be left unattended. Holmes and Morton (cited by Morton 1997) provide an *aide-mémoire* in the form of an A to F list to ensure safe recovery following surgery:

- Airway
- Breathing
- Circulation
- Conscious level
- Drains, dressings, drugs
- Elimination
- Fluid balance – fluid input and output including accurate documentation

Post-anaesthesic complications

With any clients after surgery, there will always be the potential for complications to occur. Consideration of 'airway, breathing and circulation' will ensure timely detection of systemic problems to enable early appropriate treatment to take place.

Assessment of respiratory function

Pulse oximetry should reveal any decline in a woman's oxygen saturation levels. Technology should not, however, replace the need for close clinical observation. Problems which may occur following anaesthesia include:

- Airway obstruction. This is recognised as see-saw, inconsistent movements of the chest and abdomen with strident breathing noises. It may be caused by the tongue, foreign bodies or debris and can be remedied by treating the causative factor by either suctioning or head repositioning.
- Acute bronchospasm due to irritation of either the larynx or trachea, or as a severe drug reaction. Medication will be required to reduce the effects. Hence it is important that midwives are clear regarding the whereabouts of emergency drugs such as salbutamol.
- Pulmonary oedema. This is exhibited by dyspnoea, tachypnoea and tachycardia. Care needs to be taken when managing pre-eclamptic women with regard to their fluid management to prevent severe fluid overload occurring and the risk of pulmonary oedema developing. CVP monitoring will enable haemodynamic values to be ascertained and correct management implemented. Management of pulmonary oedema will depend upon the severity or the causative factors of the situation.

Assessment of cardiovascular function

Hypotension is the most common problem post-surgery, usually due to hypovolaemia. Lost volume will need to be restored. Again, CVP and urinary output recordings will indicate the level of success in achieving adequate replacement and conversely indicate that fluid overload is not occurring.

Other causative factors of hypotension need to be considered in the absence of fluid depletion, such as reduced myocardial contractility due to the fact that most anaesthetic agents have the potential to reduce contractility. The management is to reverse the drugs used or simply, under close observation, allow the drugs to wear off. Cardiac dysrhythmias may be seen after anaesthesia, often in the presence of hypoxia or an electrolyte imbalance. The specific problem will need to be addressed to allow spontaneous resolution to occur.

Other concerns post-anaesthesia

Women who have experienced an emergency delivery for maternal/fetal compromise may have the additional concern of their neonate's health and wellbeing. However, with the systemic effects of a general anaesthetic, this reaction may be delayed. Upon return to the recovery room, information should be made available as required, but most importantly opportunities should be made in the days after surgery to debrief and explain any concerns.

Nausea and vomiting are common complications post-surgery, occurring in up to 80% of clients. A variety of factors can increase the incidence, such as the type of operation (surgery to the abdomen), administration of opioid analgesics and also clients with a tendency to motion sickness (Hatfield & Tronson 2001). Treatment should include the prescription of antiemetic medication.

Other complications which may occur include the following (Carrie et al. 2002):

- The risk of haematoma following cannula removal – thrombophlebitis may occur
- Trauma from intubation, such as trauma to the lips, teeth, pharynx or larynx resulting in a sore throat
- Muscular skeletal pain may occur which may be attributed to the administration of suxamethonium

Part 2: Resuscitation

Cardiopulmonary arrest may occur in a woman who is critically ill as a complication of her underlying condition, or it may be an unanticipated event that precipitates critical illness. Thus all midwives, including those who work mainly in community settings, need to be skilled in basic or immediate life support (BLS or ILS) and also to be able to assist the advanced life support (ALS) team with measures to treat or reverse the cause of arrest (Resuscitation Council UK 2001).

"The key to resuscitation of the child is resuscitation of the mother" (International Resuscitation Guidelines 2000, p. 294). This applies both before the age of fetal viability, when fetal survival depends on maternal survival, and after 24 weeks' gestation when the potentially viable fetus must also be considered.

Assumed prior knowledge

- Resuscitation Council UK adult basic life support algorithm (Handley 2005)
- Physiological changes in the cardiovascular and respiratory systems in pregnancy

Introduction

The incidence of cardiopulmonary arrest in pregnancy is rare (approximately 1:30 000) and is most commonly related to events at the time of birth, but it may also be related to physiopathological changes of pregnancy (International Resuscitation Guidelines 2000).

Outcomes from cardiac arrest in pregnancy are poor due to the physiological and pathological changes of pregnancy which make it difficult to secure an adequate airway, breathing and circulation (Morris & Stacey 2003). These are considered in more detail later in the chapter.

However, approximately 50% of maternal deaths are potentially preventable (Advanced Life Support in Obstetrics (ALSO) 2000) and the ALS algorithm for management of cardiac arrest in adults identifies eight potentially reversible causes of cardiac arrest – the four 'Hs' and the four 'Ts' (Deakin et al. 2005):

- Hypoxia
- Hypovolaemia
- Hyperkalaemia/hypokalaemia and metabolic disorders

Table 11.1   Potentially reversible causes of cardiopulmonary arrest (adapted from Deakin et al. 2005).

Potential cause	Pregnancy/childbirth-related condition
Hypoxia	Pulmonary oedema (HELLP syndrome, tocholysis) Eclampsia Status epilepticus Mendelson's syndrome Intubation difficulties High spinal block Cardiac or respiratory disease
Hypovolaemia	Antepartum or postpartum haemorrhage, disseminated intravascular coagulopathy Severe hyperemesis gravidarum
Hyperkalaemia/hypokalaemia and metabolic disorders	Renal failure
Hypothermia	
Tension pneumothorax	Trauma (e.g. road traffic accident) Complication of insertion of central venous pressure or pulmonary artery catheter Asthma
Tamponade	Chest trauma Complication of insertion of pulmonary artery catheter
Toxic/therapeutic disturbances	Magnesium sulphate toxicity Anaphyaxis (e.g. Jectofer, latex) Septic shock
Thromboemblic/mechanical obstruction	Pulmonary embolism Amniotic fluid embolism Air embolism

- Hypothermia
- Tension pneumothorax
- Tamponade
- Toxic/therapeutic disturbances
- Thromboembolic/mechanical obstruction

Examples of conditions related to pregnancy and childbirth are shown in Table 11.1. Midwives will recognise many of them as the major causes of maternal death in recent reports of the CEMD (Lewis 2001, 2004).

Effective cardiopulmonary resuscitation

The principles of management of maternal cardiopulmonary arrest are as for any adult, but modifications must be made to compensate for the physiological changes of pregnancy. Senior obstetric and paediatric staff should be involved at an early stage to provide expertise in the management of any pregnancy-related cause of cardiopulmonary arrest and of neonatal resuscitation, respectively.

The interventions that lead to the most successful outcome following cardio-pulmonary arrest are summarised in the 'chain of survival' (Resuscitation Council UK 2000a). This comprises:

- Early access to the emergency services (out-of-hospital arrest) or cardiac arrest team (in-hospital arrest)
- Early basic life support
- Early defibrillation (if applicable)
- Early advanced life support

The purpose of BLS is to maintain adequate ventilation and circulation until the arrival of the personnel and equipment needed to initiate defibrillation and ALS, which aims to reverse the underlying cause of the arrest. In the absence of BLS, oxygen stores are depleted within 4–6 minutes of collapse (Handley 2005). However, the physiological changes of pregnancy lead to an even more rapid onset of hypoxia, as outlined below. BLS is basically a 'holding operation' and even when performed optimally in a non-pregnant adult, does not achieve more than 30% of normal cardiac output and cerebral perfusion (Handley 2000). These facts reinforce the importance of the 'chain of survival'.

Midwives have an important role to play to ensure that all links of the 'chain of survival' are strong. The close contact that they have in caring for critically ill women means that they are in a prime position to recognise deterioration of the woman's condition and to initiate early intervention to prevent arrest, or to recognise the onset of arrest and rapidly mobilise the cardiac arrest team and prepare equipment, such as the cardiac arrest trolley and defibrillator. Their role also involves early imple-mentation of effective BLS, and effective team-working once ALS is available.

Specific management of underlying causes of, or conditions associated with, cardiopulmonary arrest should take place concurrently with resuscitation. This includes securing two routes of intravenous access with wide-bore cannulae (if not already present). Central veins provide the optimal route as they allow drugs to be delivered rapidly into the central circulation, but the technique has a variety of complications (see Chapter 10). Peripheral venous cannulation is quicker and safer, but drugs administered by the peripheral route can take 1–2 minutes to reach the central circulation (Kuhn et al., cited by Jevon & Raby 2001). However, their delivery to the central circulation can be speeded up by flushing with at least 20 ml 0.9% saline (Deakin et al. 2005) and by raising the limb (Resuscitation Council UK 2002). Ultimately the route chosen will depend on the skills and equipment available.

Suction and oxygen should be readily available and, most importantly, all procedures should be carried out with the woman in an appropriate position to reduce aortocaval compression (see the section on circulation below).

BLS should be undertaken according to the Resuscitation Council UK algorithms for BLS (Handley 2005) or in-hospital resuscitation (Soar & Spearpoint 2005), but in the second half of pregnancy consideration must be given to factors affecting airway, breathing and circulation, as outlined below.

Airway

Specific considerations include:

- An increased risk of regurgitation of stomach contents due to reduced gastric emptying, the relaxing effect of progesterone on the cardiac sphinctor and the pressure of the gravid uterus on the stomach.
- The risk of inhalation of regurgitated stomach contents, which may result in Mendelson's syndrome.
- Difficulty with trachael intubation due to:
    - Obesity of the neck.
    - Breast enlargement.
    - Laryngeal oedema (particularly in the presence of hypertensive disorders of pregnancy).

Early endotracheal intubation by an experienced anaesthetist is therefore required, with the application of cricoid pressure until the airway has been secured with a cuffed ET tube. In order to assist the anaesthetist, the midwife should ensure the availability of the following (Morris & Stacey 2003):

- At least one pillow, to flex the neck and extend the head in preparation for intubation
- A short-handled laryngoscope or one with the blade mounted at an angle of more than 90°, which may help overcome difficulties of intubation caused by the anatomical changes of pregnancy
- A laryngeal mask airway, which may be effective if tracheal intubation is unsuccessful

Breathing

Specific considerations include:

- Breathing movements are more difficult to assess due to enlarged breasts and abdomen.
- A more rapid onset of hypoxia. Oxygen requirements increase by 20% in pregnancy due to a 10–15% increase in maternal basal metabolic rate (Llewellyn-Jones 1999) and the added effects of fetal metabolism. Thus irreversible brain damage from anoxia may occur in a shorter time period than the 3–4 minutes for a non-pregnant adult (Morris & Stacey 2003).
- Mechanical effects of the gravid uterus on the:
    - *Diaphragm*, leading to splinting and reduced chest compliance – higher inflation pressures may be required.
    - *Lung bases*, leading to a 200 ml reduction in expiratory reserve volume (de Swiet 1998) and thus a reduced ability to withstand hypoxia.

Early and effective ventilation using 100% oxygen is therefore required.

Circulation

Specific considerations include:

- Cardiac output increases by 30–50% by the end of the second trimester of pregnancy due to increased blood volume and an increase in heart rate of up to 15 beats/min (Llewellyn-Jones 1999). This needs to be maintained during cardiopulmonary resuscitation (CPR).
- A supine position during the second half of pregnancy causes compression of the inferior vena cava, which reduces venous return leading to a reduction in cardiac output by up to 25% (Kerr, cited by Jevon & Raby 2001).
- In the supine position, venous return depends upon collateral blood flow via the azygous and paraspinal veins, which is insufficient for CPR to be effective (Thomson & Greer 2000).
- Effective chest compressions are difficult to implement because:
  - The ribs are flared – the subcostal angle widens from 68 to 103° (de Swiet 1998)
  - The diaphragm is raised by 4–7 cm (ALSO 2000)
  - The abdomen and breasts are enlarged.

In order maximise the effectiveness of chest compressions, compression of the inferior vena cava must be reduced, and indeed it has been suggested that attempts at resuscitation are futile if this compression is not relieved (Morris & Stacey 2003). This can be achieved by using sandbags, pillows, the back of an upturned chair or a laminated wooden wedge, such as the Cardiff resuscitation wedge, to effect a left lateral tilt, or in the absence of suitable equipment, a rescuer can kneel behind the woman and act as a 'human wedge' (Morris & Stacey 2003). Other alternatives are to elevate the woman's right hip by 15° (Campbell & Klocke 2001) or to manually displace the uterus by lifting it to the left and towards the woman's head (Morris & Stacey 2003).

Rees and Willis (1988) examined the efficacy of chest compressions with varying degrees of lateral tilt and found that at an angle of 27°, 80% of the maximal force of chest compressions could be delivered, along with significant relief of compression of the vena cava. A tilt of more than 30° makes it difficult to carry out chest compressions as a pregnant woman has a tendency to roll forwards (Thomson & Greer 2000; Morris & Stacey 2003). However, Kiss and Arvieux (2004) believe that, because chest compressions are more effective in the supine position, use of the supine position with manual displacement of the uterus is likely to be more effective.

Chest compressions should be performed higher on the sternum to allow for the upward movement of abdominal contents, but there are no guidelines on the exact hand position (International Resuscitation Guidelines 2000).

Once the trachea is intubated, chest compressions (at a rate of 100/min) should continue uninterrupted during ventilations (at a rate of 10/min), as a pause in chest compressions allows coronary perfusion to fall substantially (Deakin et al. 2005). Chest compressions that are uninterrupted for ventilation result in a substantially higher mean coronary perfusion pressure.

Emergency caesarean section

The overview of physiological changes of pregnancy presented above indicates the difficulties of providing effective oxygenation and circulation in women who experience cardiopulmonary arrest in the second half of pregnancy. Thus the Resuscitation Council UK (2000a) recommends emergency caesarean section if resuscitation is unsuccessful after 5 minutes. This is not only an attempt to save the unborn baby, but is also important for maternal survival (Morris & Stacey 2003). Emptying the uterus removes many of the obstacles to effective resuscitation. In particular, it relieves compression on the inferior vena cava (which is only partially reduced by a left lateral tilt or manual displacement of the uterus) and allows for more effective ventilation of the lungs.

Once the decision for caesarean section has been made, speed is of the essence and, in view of the time taken to prepare theatre packs, a scalpel is all that is initially required (Morris & Stacey 2003). Cox and Grady (1999) suggest that a vertical abdominal and uterine incision provides the quickest route, although Bobrowski (1999) believes that this is a matter of personal preference, and that a low transverse incision is associated with less blood loss and quicker closure.

Most babies who survive maternal cardiopulmonary arrest are born within 5 minutes of its occurrence (Morris & Stacey 2003) but there are reported cases of babies being born neurologically intact after 20 minutes of maternal CPR (Katz et al., cited by Jevon & Raby 2001). Mitchell (1995) suggests that this may be due to the 'all or nothing' phenomenon of fetal hypoxic injury – i.e. fetal death follows hypoxic cerebral damage, whereas survival with no detectable damage indicates that the maternal hypoxic episode was not associated with hypoxic damage to the fetal brain.

Physiological adaptations of the fetus that facilitate adequate fetal cerebral oxygenation in the presence of maternal hypoxia are peripheral vasoconstriction, which diverts circulation to the vital fetal organs such as the heart and brain, and the higher oxygen saturation of fetal haemoglobin (Jevon & Raby 2001). Thus Bobrowski (1999) suggests it is reasonable to undertake a caesarean section up to 25 minutes after maternal cardiopulmonary arrest if signs of fetal life are present.

Maternal and neonatal prognosis is improved if CPR is continued during the caesarean section (Morris & Stacey 2003), and transabdominal open cardiac massage may be considered to help compensate for aortocaval compression (Cox & Grady 1999). However, perinatal outcome is extremely poor following postmortem caesarean section (Cox & Grady 1999; Lewis 2004), although the current CEMD report showed a significant increase in babies surviving perimortem caesarean section due to improved resuscitation techniques, particularly when the woman collapsed in a well-equipped and staffed delivery room or theatre (Lewis 2004).

The midwife's role includes anticipation of a decision to deliver by caesarean section wherever the woman is situated, and the preparation of appropriate personnel and equipment (including neonatal resuscitation).

Advanced life support

ALS involves the use of more specialised equipment (including drugs) and techniques to support breathing and circulation, as well as measures to attempt to restore cardiac output (Jevon & Raby 2001).

Heart rhythms associated with cardiopulmonary arrest can be divided into those for which early defibrillation is indicated (ventricular fibrillation (VF) and pulseless ventricular tachycardia (VT)) and those for which it is not (asystole and pulseless electrical activity (PEA)) (Deakin et al. 2005). (See Chapter 10 for further information on ECGs.)

VF/pulseless VT

VF and pulseless VT are the commonest arrhythmias of cardiac arrest in adults, and they have a better prognosis than other rhythms. However, their incidence is lower in pregnancy than in the non-pregnant population as they are mainly associated with ischaemic heart disease (Jevon & Raby 2001; Smith 2005). A single precordial thump may be effective in instances where the cardiopulmonary arrest is witnessed or an ECG at the time of arrest shows VF, but *rapid* defibrillation is the definitive treatment. Its chances of success decline by 7–10% for each minute after arrest as myocardial energy reserves are quickly depleted, although this process can be slowed by effective BLS (Davies 2005). However, BLS must not delay shock delivery. The priority should be to quickly establish an ECG trace, using either an ECG machine or defibrillator paddles, and early defibrillation if indicated.

Defibrillation

Defibrillation is defined as the 'termination of fibrillation or, more precisely, the absence of VF/pulseless VT five seconds after shock delivery' (Resuscitation Council UK 2002). During defibrillation an electrical current is passed across the myocardium with the aim of causing depolarisation of a critical mass of the cardiac muscle, which then allows spontaneous sinoatrial node activity to resume. Two paddles are placed on the chest, one to the right of the sternum below the right clavicle and the other over the apex, which allows the maximum current to flow through the myocardium. Gel pads are used to improve conduction and minimise the risk of skin burns.

Defibrillation is not contraindicated in pregnancy as there is no significant transfer of current to the fetus (International Resuscitation Guidelines 2000) and there are reported cases of it being used without adverse fetal effects (Jevon & Raby 2001). However, it can be difficult to apply the apical defibrillator paddle when the woman is tilted laterally, and care must be taken that the breast does not come into contact with the hand holding the paddle. This can be avoided by using adhesive electrodes (Morris & Stacey 2003).

As soon as a shockable rhythm is identified, one shock is given (150–200 J biphasic or 360 J monophasic) followed by immediate resumption of chest compressions and ventilations at a ratio of 30:2 without reassessing rhythm or pulse.

CPR is continued for 2 minutes, followed by reassessment of rhythm and a second shock (at the same energy as the first) if required. This sequence is repeated as long as VF/pulseless VT persists (Deakin et al. 2005).

A study by Nanson et al. (2001) demonstrated that the standard energy requirements for adults are appropriate for use in pregnancy as, although it has been suggested that the physiological changes of pregnancy might alter transthoracic impedance (TTI) (and therefore affect current pathways during defibrillation), there was no significant difference between TTI at term compared with 6–8 weeks' postnatally.

Safety issues that the midwife should be aware of during defibrillation are that direct or indirect contact with the mother (for example, via the bed or a drip stand) should be avoided, and that open sources of oxygen should be temporarily removed as arcing in the presence of oxygen can cause fire (Resuscitation Council UK 2002).

Automated external defibrillators

As stated above, rapid defibrillation is the definitive treatment for VF/pulseless VT. However, the use of manual defibrillators requires the presence of personnel who have been trained in their use and who are skilled in the interpretation of ECGs. This may lead to delay in defibrillation beyond 8 minutes, which is associated with poorer prognosis (Liddle et al. 2003).

The use of automated external defibrillators (AEDs), which analyse the cardiac rhythm, provide instructions to the operator via a screen or voice prompts, and deliver shocks at a preset level, can help reduce this delay. Training to use AEDs is much simpler than training to use a manual defibrillator. The Resuscitation Council UK recommends that any personnel who may have responsibility for management of cardiac arrest in hospital or community settings should be trained in the use of AEDs, with the aim of providing a shock within 3 minutes of collapse in a hospital setting (Davies 2005).

Non-VF/VT

Defibrillation is not indicated for arrhythmias such as asystole and PEA, when management is continued CPR and appropriate drug therapy. Outcomes are relatively poor unless a reversible cause can be found and treated effectively (Deakin et al. 2005). PEA is a common presenting arrhythmia in pulmonary embolism, hypovolaemia and amniotic fluid embolism (Nanson et al. 2001).

Drugs used during cardiopulmonary resuscitation

The role of drugs is secondary to defibrillation and cardiopulmonary resuscitation as there is limited evidence for the use of a small number of drugs during early management of cardiopulmonary arrest (Resuscitation Council UK 2002). Their use is summarised in Table 11.2.

Table 11.2 Drugs used during cardiopulmonary resuscitation (from Resuscitation Council UK (2002), unless otherwise indicated).

Drug	Dose	Action	Comments
Adrenaline (epinephrine)	1 mg (10 ml of 1:10 000) i.v., every 3–5 minutes 2–3 mg diluted to a volume of 10 ml (sterile water) via an ET tube (followed by five ventilations to disperse the drug and aid absorption by the bronchial tree)	Vasoconstriction – increases coronary and cerebral perfusion Uteroplacental vasoconstriction may have adverse fetal effects (Lee et al., cited in Levon & Raby 2001) but when cardiac output is low vasoconstriction is more likely to improve uteroplacental blood flow (Maternal and Child Health Research Consortium 2000)	First drug used in cardiac arrest from any cause Caution when cardiac arrest is associated with cocaine or other sympathomimetic drugs
Amiodarone	300 mg diluted in 5% dextrose to a volume of 20 ml Prefilled syringe	Antiarrhythmic Used when defibrillation fails to correct VF or pulseless VT Side effects: hypotension and bradycardia	Administration via central line is preferable to peripheral vein Cannot be given via an ET tube
Lidocaine (lignocaine)	Initial dose of 100 mg Additional bolus of 50 mg if necessary	Antiarrhythmic	Used when amiodarone is not available
Atropine	Symptomatic bradycardia: 0.5–1 mg i.v. Asystole or PEA: 3 mg i.v. or 6 mg in a volume of 10–20 ml via an ET tube	Blocks action of vagus nerve on sinoatrial node and AV node; increases sinus automaticity and facilitates AV node conduction	No conclusive evidence of its value, but anecdotal accounts of its success Dose does not cause fixed, dilated pupils
Other drugs	Magnesium sulphate: 1–2 g (2–4 ml of 50%) i.v., given over 1–2 minutes	VT or VF associated with hypomagnesaemia	Only used if electrolyte imbalance is a factor in arrhythmia or arrest
	Calcium chloride: 10 ml of 10% i.v.	For PEA caused by hyperkalaemia, hypocalcaemia or overdose of calcium channel-blocking drugs (e.g. magnesium sulphate)	Calcium and sodium bicarbonate cannot be given together as it causes precipitation of calcium carbonate
	Sodium bicarbonate: 50 mmol i.v. (50 ml of 8.4%)	For severe acidosis (pH < 7.1; base excess <−10 (Cox & Grady 1999)), hyperkalaemia or overdose of tricyclic antidepressants	

ET, endotracheal tube; PEA, pulseless electrical activity; VF, ventricular fibrillation; VT, ventricular tachycardia.

Training needs

Cardiac arrests are rare in pregnancy, but a key factor for successful resuscitation is that all staff are skilled in CPR (Department of Health 2004). The *Midwives Rules and Standards* (NMC 2004b) places the onus on midwives to ensure that they are appropriately prepared to be able to carry out emergency procedures such as resuscitation. However, Davies and Gould (2000) cite several studies indicating that a health care professional's competence in resuscitation, in terms of both knowledge and skills, is often poor.

Retention of skills has been shown to be particularly poor amongst staff who very rarely use them in practice (Morris & Stacey 2003), which includes most midwives. However, Wynne et al. (1999) assert that there is no evidence that experience acquired through involvement with cardiopulmonary arrests improves theoretical knowledge or skill in performing resuscitation. Thus the Resuscitation Council UK (2000b) recommends that hospital staff should have updates yearly as a minimum, and that specific training for cardiac arrests in special circumstances, such as pregnancy, should be provided for staff working in these areas. This is echoed by the CEMD (Lewis 2004), which suggests that emergency drills for maternal resuscitation should be regularly practised in clinical areas in all maternity units. Attending an annual update should realistically be achievable by midwives (Jevon & Raby 2001), although Davies and Gould's (2000) review of studies on retention of knowledge and skills suggests the optimum period is no longer than 6 months.

In addition to attending annual resuscitation updates, midwives' training needs can also be met through programmes such as the Advanced Life Support in Obstetrics (ALSO) course, and trust-specific training courses on obstetric emergencies that include CPR. These may be designed specifically for midwives (Jevon & Stewart 2001) or for the multiprofessional team (Cro et al. 2001), the latter emphasising simulation of 'real' situations to improve clinical effectiveness, confidence and team-working skills.

Presence of relatives

The presence of relatives and significant others during resuscitation is the subject of much discussion. This is related mainly to accident and emergency and intensive treatment unit settings, with nothing being found specific to childbearing women who require resuscitation. However, it is valuable for midwives to have an appreciation of the main lines of argument to better inform decisions about whether or not to suggest that birth companions remain or leave the room in the event of maternal collapse.

The suggested possible benefits of relatives' presence are as follow (Barrett & Wallis 1998; Offord 1998; Hadfield-Law 1999; Boyd 2000; Resuscitation Council UK 2000a; Ardley 2003; Kidby 2003):

- Witnessing the extent of attempts at resuscitation has more impact than being told that everything possible is being/was done.

- Relatives may find it more distressing to be separated from their family member than to witness the attempts at resuscitation, as imagining possible procedures may be worse than the reality.
- Patients who survive may find comfort from relatives' presence during transient periods of consciousness.
- It may help the medical team to decide when to discontinue resuscitation.
- It may help relatives to come to terms with death or disability.

The suggested possible disadvantages of relatives' presence are as follow (Fulbrook 1998; Resuscitation Council UK 2000a; Ardley 2003; Kidby 2003):

- Relatives may become distressed and could physically or emotionally hinder the resuscitation attempt.
- A legal claim for compensation may be presented in the event of relatives suffering protracted nervous shock or psychological injury.
- Confidentiality may be breached as relatives may see and hear things of a personal nature.
- Relatives may be physically hurt due to the pace of procedures, restricted space available and number of health care professionals attending the woman.

Counter to these suggestions, it is argued that rather than leading to litigation, the presence of relatives may be a sound risk management strategy as many claims are associated with a lack of information and poor communication which, in this situation, could result from relatives feeling that they were excluded from the resuscitation attempt (Hadfield-Law 1999; Boyd 2000).

A further suggested disadvantage of relatives being present during resuscitation is that it may increase stress for staff (Offord 1998; Kidby 2003), but Boyd and White (1998) found that there was no difference in perceived stress levels for staff whether or not relatives were present. Hadfield-Law (1999) draws an interesting parallel between many of the objections made by staff to the presence of relatives during resuscitation and the objections that were raised in the past about fathers being present at the birth – distressing sights, unnecessary pressure on staff, getting in the way or fainting!

As each situation is unique, there is no right or wrong answer about whether or not relatives should be present during resuscitation. Appreciation of the suggested advantages and disadvantages of relatives' presence can help the midwife take appropriate action for the situation. When relatives are present during resuscitation, the Resuscitation Council UK (2000a) recommends that they are accompanied at all times, are given the option of leaving the room at any stage, and are provided with clear explanations and the opportunity to have questions answered. Midwives have a valuable role in both providing, and facilitating provision of, these supportive measures to the woman's relatives.

References

Advanced Life Support in Obstetrics (ALSO) (2000) *Advance Life Support in Obstetrics Provider Manual* (4th edn). American Academy of Family Physicians, Kansas City.

Ardley, C. (2003) Should relatives be denied access to the resuscitation room? *Intensive and Critical Care Nursing*, **19**: 1–10.

Barnardo, P. and Jenkins, J. (2000) Failed tracheal intubation in obstetrics: a 6 year review in the UK region. *Anaesthesia*, **55** (7): 690–4.

Barratt, F. and Wallis, N. (1998) Relatives in the resuscitation room: their point of view. *Journal of Accident and Emergency Medicine*, **15**: 109–11.

Blouw, R., Scatliff, J. and Craig, D. (1976) Gastric volume and pH in postpartum patients. *Anaesthesiology*, **45**: 456–7.

Bobrowski, R. (1999) Trauma in pregnancy. In: D. James, P. Steer, C. Weiner and B. Gonik (Eds) *High Risk Pregnancy: Management options*. W.B. Saunders, London.

Boyd, R. (2000) Witnessed resuscitation by relatives. *Resuscitation*, **43** (3): 171–6.

Boyd, R. and White, S. (1998) Does witnessed cardiopulmonary resuscitation alter perceived stress levels in Accident and Emergency staff? *Journal of Accident and Emergency Medicine*, **15**: 394–5.

Campbell, L. and Klocke, R. (2001) Update in nonpulmonary critical care: implications for the pregnant patient. *Americal Journal of Respiratory Critical Care Medicine*, **163**: 1051–4.

Carrie, L., Simpson, P. and Popat, M. (2002) *Carrie's Understanding Anaesthesia*. Butterworth Heinemann, Oxford.

Chan, Y.K. (2006) *Aspiration prophylaxis*. http://www.frca.co.uk/SectionContents.aspx?sectionid=72#

Cook, T., Godfrey, I., Rockett, M. and Vanner, R. (2000) Cricoid pressure: which hand? *Anaesthesia*, **55** (7): 648.

Cox, C. and Grady, K. (1999) *Managing Obstetric Emergencies*. BIOS Scientific Publishers, Oxford.

Cro, S., King, B. and Paine, P. (2001) Practice makes perfect: maternal emergency training. *British Journal of Midwifery*, **9** (8): 492–6.

Datta, S. (2000) *The Obstetric Anaesthesia Handbook* (2nd edn). Mosby, St Louis.

Davies, N. and Gould, D. (2000) Updating cardiopulmonary resuscitation skills: a study to examine the efficacy of self-instruction on nurse's competence. *Journal of Clinical Nursing*, **9** (3): 400–10.

Davies, S. (2005) The use of automated external defibrillators. In: Resuscitation Council UK (Ed.) *Resuscitation Guidelines 2005*. Resuscitation Council UK, London.

Deakin, C., Nolan, J. and Perkins, G. (2005) Adult advanced life support. In: Resuscitation Council UK (Ed.) *Resuscitation Guidelines 2005*. Resuscitation Council UK, London.

Department of Health (2004) *Maternity Standard, National Service Framework for Children, Young People and the Maternity Services*. Department of Health, London.

Dimond, B. (2003) *Legal Aspects of Midwifery* (2nd edn). Books for Midwives, London.

Finster, M., Morishima, H. and Boyes, R. (1972) Tissue thiopental concentrations in the fetus and newborn. *Anesthesiology*, **36**: 155.

Fulbrook, S. (1998) Legal implications of relatives witnessing resuscitation. *British Journal of Theatre Nursing*, **7** (10): 33–5.

Gee, J., Packer, B., Millen, J. and Robin, E. (1967) Pulmonary mechanics during pregnancy. *Journal of Clinical Investigation*, **46**: 945–52.

Hadfield-Law, L. (1999) Do relatives have a place in the resuscitation room? *Care of the Critically Ill*, **15** (1): 19–22.

Handley, A. (2000) Adult basic life support. In: Resuscitation Council UK (Ed.) *Resuscitation Guidelines 2000*. Resuscitation Council UK, London.

Handley, A. (2005) Adult basic life support. In: Resuscitation Council UK (Ed.) *Resuscitation Guidelines 2005*. Resuscitation Council UK, London.

Hatfield, A. and Tronson, M. (2001) *The Complete Recovery Room Book*. Oxford University Press, Oxford.

Health and Safety Executive (2006) About latex allergies. http://www.hse.gov.uk/latex/index.htm

International Resuscitation Guidelines (2000) Part 8: Advanced challenges in resuscitation. Section 3: Special challenges in ECC. 3F: Cardiac arrest associated with pregnancy. *Resuscitation*, **46**: 293–5.

Jevon, P. and Raby, M. (2001) *Resuscitation in Pregnancy: A practical approach.* Books for Midwives, Oxford.

Jevon, P. and Stewart, S. (2001) Delivery suite emergencies: a new training opportunity for midwives. *Practising Midwife*, **4** (8):14–16.

Kidby, J. (2003) Family-witnessed cardiopulmonary resuscitation. *Nursing Standard*, **17** (51): 33–6.

Kiss, G. and Arvieux, C. (2004) Remarks on guidelines ERC 2000: cardiac arrest associated with pregnancy (Letters to the editor). *Resuscitation*, **61**: 367.

Lewis, G. (2001) *Why Mothers Die 1997–1999: The Confidential Enquiries into Maternal Deaths in the United Kingdom.* Royal College of Obstetricians and Gynaecologists (RCOG) Press, London.

Lewis, G. (2004) *Why Mothers Die 2000–2002: Report on Confidential Enquiries into Maternal Deaths in the United Kingdom.* RCOG Press, London.

Liddle, R., Davies, S., Colquhoun, M. and Handley, A. (2003) ABC of resuscitation: the automated external defibrillator. *British Medical Journal*, **327**: 1216–18.

Liu, D. (2003) *Labour Ward Manual* (3rd edn). Churchill Livingstone, London.

Llewellyn-Jones, D. (1999) *Fundamentals of Obstetrics and Gynaecology.* Mosby, London.

Maternal and Child Health Research Consortium (2000) *Confidential Enquiry into Stillbirths and Deaths in Infancy: 7th annual report.* Maternal and Child Health Research Consortium (MCHRC), London.

Mitchell, L. (1995) Cardiac arrest during pregnancy: maternal–fetal physiology and advanced cardiac life support for the obstetric patient. *Critical Care Nurse*, **Feb**: 56–60.

Morris, S. and Stacey, M. (2003) ABC of resuscitation: resuscitation in pregnancy. *British Medical Journal*, **327**: 1277–9.

Morton, N. (1997) *Assisting the Anaesthetist.* Oxford University Press, Oxford.

Nanson, J., Elcock, D., Williams, M. and Deakin, C. (2001) Do physiological changes in pregnancy change defibrillation energy requirements? *British Journal of Anaesthesia*, **87** (2): 237–9.

National High Blood Pressure Education Program Working Group (2000) Report of the National High Blood Pressure Education Program Working Group (NHBPEPWG) on high blood pressure in pregnancy. *American Journal of Obstetrics and Gynecology*, **183**: S1–S22.

Nursing and Midwifery Council (2004a) *Code of Professional Conduct: Standards for conduct, performance and ethics.* Nursing and Midwifery Council (NMC), London.

Nursing and Midwifery Council (2004b) *Midwives Rules and Standards.* NMC, London.

Offord, R. (1998) Should relatives of patients with cardiac arrest be invited to be present during cardiopulmonary resuscitation? *Intensive and Critical Care Nursing*, **14**: 288–93.

Palahnuik, R.J., Shnider, S.M. and Eger, E.I. (1974) Pregnancy decreases the requirement for inhaled anaesthetic agents. *Anaesthesiology*, **41**: 82–3.

Rees, G.O., Thurlow, J.A., Gardner, I.C., Scrutton, M.J.L. and Kinsella, S.M. (2002) Maternal cardiovascular consequences of positioning after spinal anaesthesia for Caesarean section: left 15° table tilt vs. left lateral. *Anaesthesia*, **57** (1): 15–20.

Rees, G. and Willis, B. (1988) Resuscitation in late pregnancy. *Anaesthesia*, **43**: 437–9.

Resuscitation Council UK (2000a) *Advanced Life Support Manual.* Resuscitation Council UK, London.

Resuscitation Council UK (2000b) *CPR Guidance for Clinical Practice and Training in Hospitals.* Resuscitation Council UK, London.

Resuscitation Council UK (2001) *Cardiopulmonary Resuscitation: Guidance for clinical practice and training in primary care.* Resuscitation Council UK, London.

Resuscitation Council UK (2002) *Immediate Life Support Course Manual.* Resuscitation Council UK, London.

Shibli, K. and Russell, I. (2000) A survey of anesthetic techniques used for caesarean section in the UK in 1997. *International Journal of Obstetric Anaesthesia,* **9**: 160–7.

Smith, G. (2005) Prevention of in-hospital cardiac arrest and decisions about cardiopulmonary resuscitation. In: Resuscitation Council UK (Ed.) *Resuscitation Guidelines 2005.* Resuscitation Council UK, London.

Soar, J. and Spearpoint, K. (2005) In-hospital resuscitation. In: Resuscitation Council UK (Ed.) *Resuscitation Guidelines 2005.* Resuscitation Council UK, London.

de Swiet, M. (1998) The respiratory system. In: G. Chamberlain and F. Broughton Pipkin (Eds) *Clinical Physiology in Obstetrics.* Blackwell Science, Oxford.

Thomas, S. (1999a) Graduated compression and the prevention of deep vein thrombosis – part 1. *Journal of Wound Care,* **8** (1): 41–3.

Thomas, S. (1999b) Graduated compression and the prevention of deep vein thrombosis – part 2. *Journal of Wound Care,* **8** (2): 93–5.

Thomson, A. and Greer, I. (2000) Non-haemorrhagic obstetric shock. *Bailliere's Clinical Obstetrics and Gynaecology,* **14** (1): 19–41.

Torr, G. and James, M. (1998) The role of the anaesthetist in the management of pre-eclampsia. *Update in Anaesthesia,* Issue 9, Article 4. http://www.nda.ox.ac.uk/wfsa/html/u09/u09_012.htm

Wilkinson, C. and Enkin, M. (1996) Lateral tilt for caesarean section. *Cochrane Database of Systematic Reviews,* Issue 1.

Wynne, G., Gwinnutt, C., Bingham, B., Van Someren, V., Colquhoun, M. and Handley, M. (1999) Teaching resuscitation. In: M. Colquhoun, A. Handley and T. Evans (Eds) *ABC of Resuscitation.* BMJ Books, London.

12 Pain Management of the Critically Ill Woman

Pat Jackson

Pain is a common experience for critically ill women (Puntillo et al. 2001; Pasero 2003; Puntillo 2003) and it is suggested that most critically ill women experience moderate to severe pain (Carroll et al. 1997). It is often continuous pain from the disease or condition causing the critical illness, or from surgery undertaken in response to the critical episode. Frequently this is interspersed with many painful procedures such as endotrachael suctioning, tube replacement and injections (Puntillo et al. 2001; Stanik-Hutt et al. 2001; Pasero & McCaffery 2002). This chapter provides an overview of concept and physiology of pain, and aspects of management relevant to the care of critically ill childbearing women.

Assumed prior knowledge

- Anatomy and physiology of the neurological system
- Understanding of conditions that may be associated with pain during childbearing

Introduction

Pain is a complex subject that has been defined by the International Society for the Study of Pain (1979) as "an unpleasant sensory and emotional experience associated with actual or potential tissue damage or described in terms of such damage." One individual's pain cannot be compared to another's experience, as McCaffery's (1968) definition states "Pain is whatever the experiencing person says it is, existing whenever he or she says it does."

It is a subjective experience that has biological, psychosocial, physical and emotional dimensions, making it a unique experience for each individual. This is dependent on several elements including culture, anxiety and stress levels, previous experience, age and genetic factors. Culture is important as sets of behaviours and attitudes within a group will affect behaviour and beliefs around illness (Walker et al. 1995; Park 2001). Stereotyping, however, should be avoided (Martinelli 1987; East 1992) as it can lead to delay in diagnosis and treatment especially in women from ethnic minorities (Lewis 2004). Anxiety has a strong cultural overlay and falls into two groups. The first is a temporary response to a specific situation and in the second group it is a characteristic of an individual's personality. Personality affects how a person will express their pain, with introverts being more stoical and less likely to complain. Extroverts complain more freely with the result that staff caring for these patients often respond more promptly. Therefore, relief tends to come more quickly, but at the risk of them being labelled as a difficult patient (McIntosh 1990).

An individual's ability, or lack of it, to withstand stress can adversely affect the functioning of the body and how they perceive and cope with pain. Previous experience can lead to an expectation of pain and can be influenced by their own experience or that of friends and family. Observation of others and information provided about the pain experience may lead to an expectation that may be significantly different from the reality (Hiscock 1993), especially with the critically ill woman. Pain memory can impact on someone's reaction to pain so it is necessary to modify expectations and current experiences of pain by appropriate and accurate information (Carr & Thomas 1997). Age has been found to have little influence except when caring for children or the elderly, so it is less of a factor in women of childbearing age although it may be significant in that they may have developed some coping strategies for dealing with pain (Walker et al. 1995). Genetic factors affect the nocireceptor pain reception in nerve cells (Stamer et al. 2005) and therefore pain thresholds and tolerance varies from one person to another. A genetically determined variation in drug metabolism and the individual's response to analgesics also influences pain management.

Normal physiology

Pain is felt when specialised nerve endings (nocireceptors) are stimulated and transmit information along nerve pathways. The purpose is mainly protective, to act as a warning that tissues are being damaged, but the pain may persist even after the stimulus is removed as the chemicals produced take time to dissipate. There are two types of pain – somatic and visceral – and the recognition of the type and intensity occurs mainly in the cerebral cortex. Somatic pain arises from the skin, muscles and joints and can be superficial or deep. Superficial somatic pain tends to be localised and sharp or pricking in nature and is transmitted via large myelinated fibres. Deep somatic pain is more diffuse and is expressed as burning or aching with the impulses being transmitted along small unmyelinated C-fibres (Ndala 2005).

Visceral pain originates in the internal organs, which are supplied with nerve fibres that transmit pain only and pass along the visceral sympathetic nerves into the spinal cord. The pain is felt away from the stimulated organ in an area of the body innervated by the same segment of the spinal cord using the same pathways as pain signals from the skin. The position in the cord to which the visceral afferent fibres pass from each organ depends on the part of the body from which the organ developed embryologically (Guyton & Hall 2000). As a result, the location of the pain is not over the visceral organ involved but presents as 'referred pain' felt in the skin or a surface area away from the stimulated area. The person feels the pain and reports it as originating from an area of the body away from the visceral organ affected and potentially this causes confusion for the process of reaching a diagnosis (Pocock & Richards 2006).

Secondary physiological changes

Pain leads to fear and anxiety, which increases stress and provokes a reduced tolerance to pain and produces secondary physiological changes. Severe, acute pain accompanied by physical exhaustion exacerbated by sleep deprivation, hunger, nausea and physical and mental exertion will affect homeostasis. In the case of the critically ill woman an awareness of danger to self, and in pregnancy the additional risk to the fetus/baby, creates anxiety and fear about the outcome.

Stress in these situations causes stimulation of the sympathetic nervous system to release the hormonal neurotransmitters noradrenaline and adrenaline. These catecholamines mediate the response that allows the 'fright, fight or flight' response leading to an increase in the heart rate and raised cardiac output followed by hyperventilation and a decrease in cerebral and uterine blood flow due to vasoconstriction. Blood is diverted from the splanchnic bed, which includes the uterus, to the skeletal muscles, causing a rise in the blood pressure. There is an increase in the metabolic rate leading to a rise in blood glucose and an alteration in the acid base balance of the blood, causing maternal alkalosis, which in pregnancy will give rise to fetal hypoxia. The fetus may already be compromised and this situation may exacerbate any fetal distress. Vasoconstriction causes the woman's pupils and bronchioles to become dilated and she will perspire. Reduced gastrointestinal motility and slower gastric emptying impairs the function of the gastrointestinal tract and leads to ileus, which has implications for pain management. The muscoskeletal system responds by contractions, spasm and rigidity of the muscles. This leads to the patient being reluctant to move, causing other problems from immobility with implications for pain assessment and management.

Cardiovascular responses in the woman are also already compromised during labour as the cardiac output increases as labour progresses which can make the recognition of the severity of the illness more difficult in the critically ill woman.

Critically ill women and pain

Pain and anxiety act in a synergistic and cylindrical fashion to exacerbate each other (Cullen et al. 2001). Bryant and Yearby (2004) described how the anticipation of normal labour can often create anxiety which is hard to adequately dispel, and although for most women they would not anticipate a situation where they become critically ill, when the occasion arises their anxiety levels increase dramatically. The hospital environment may also create anxiety, heightened if treatment is required in critical care settings with equipment and personnel adding to the intensive surroundings. This will distract the woman from identifying and adopting her usual coping mechanisms which play a vital role in reducing the need for pharmacological pain relief. Complications may occur if pain is not adequately treated as the woman will be unwilling to move even if able to. Lack of movement can lead to respiratory infection, and venous stasis and platelet aggregation that can predispose to deep venous thrombosis.

The perception of pain due to an acute clinical illness undergoes substantial processing at supraspinal levels and these mechanisms play a major role in the representation and modulation of the pain experience.

Pharmacology

Drugs given concurrently may exert their effects independently or they may interact (Siney 2004). Interactions may be due to potentiation or antagonism of one drug by another or occasionally some other effect. Pharmacokinetic interactions occur when one drug alters the absorption, distribution, metabolism and excretion of another; this reduces or increases the amount of drug available to produce its pharmacological effects. Competition at receptor sites or drugs acting on the same physiological system may change the effects a drug has on the body. Pregnancy alters the therapeutic situation, both because it alters how a drug is absorbed, metabolised and excreted as well as the actions of a drug. Many drugs are reversibly bound to plasma proteins and in pregnancy the blood volume increases, affecting the blood concentration of some drugs as they are diluted in a larger volume of fluid and may be less effective than in a non-pregnant woman (Siney 2004).

Absorption

Most oral drugs are absorbed in the small intestine, so the process is accelerated by gastric emptying which in pregnancy is reduced slightly and in labour markedly, especially if pethidine has been given, thereby reducing the effectiveness of oral drugs. Delayed absorption of drugs given orally shortly before labour may lead to greatly increased plasma levels postpartum and can contribute to a fall in drug clearance that may be observed in the puerperium (Hytten & Chamberlain 1991).

Following an intramuscular injection there will be a period of uptake from the muscle when the blood concentration will not have reached a sufficient level to provide pain relief to the woman. This period will vary from client to client. On reaching a level of analgesia the concentration will continue to rise so that there may be oversedation in the mother leading to maternal and, before the birth, fetal side effects. This pattern of provision of analgesia leads to peaks and troughs of analgesic blood concentration, or 'roller coaster' analgesia (Austin et al. 1980). The systemic use of opioid analgesics to alleviate labour pain necessitates a specific compromise between using sufficient drugs to provide effective analgesia, without increasing harmful side effects in the mother and fetus/neonate (Heelbeck 1999).

Metabolism/excretion

Specific variations in drug metabolism and excretion and the response of the individual may alter in pregnancy, and is further complicated by critical illness. Liver metabolism is increased and so drugs that depend on the activity of liver enzymes are eliminated more quickly than usual (Siney 2004) but there is no change in the rate of elimination of drugs that rely on blood flow in the liver. However, increased blood flow in the kidneys in normal pregnancy leads to a quicker elimination of some drugs. In women with renal insufficiency, which may occur within critical illness, dosage adjustment is necessary and the treatment of pain must be modified and adapted to allow for the impaired renal function (Launay-Vacher et al. 2005). During pregnancy there is a risk of harming the embryo or fetus by exposing it to a teratogenic substance which may cross the placenta. The development, growth or function of the fetus may be affected depending on the period of gestation.

Management of pain

The consequences of poorly controlled pain are well known but still the condition is undertreated. Although there have been advances in the management of pain there is still a lack of scientific evidence on which to base treatment (Smith et al. 1999). Pain needs to be managed effectively in order to minimise the potentially adverse effects to the critically ill woman and, in pregnancy and labour, to her fetus/baby. Unrelieved or inadequately controlled pain is common and can lead to major physiological and psychological stress (Pasero et al. 1999; Pasero 2003; Puntillo 2003). The nervous system responses may exacerbate the signs and symptoms of the existing disease processes and lead to some deterioration in the woman's physical condition. Uncontrolled pain will also trigger emotional stress responses that will increase the risk of complications and inhibit the healing processes. Effective treatment is therefore required to ensure that the woman is kept pain-free in order to reduce any consequential adverse effects. This need is balanced with the requirement to ensure that any analgesia given does not mask any vital signs and symptoms which may lead to changes in the woman's condition going undiagnosed. Critically ill women under the care of a consultant obstetrician may benefit from care and treatment from the specialised pain management team.

During the antenatal period and labour, up to the birth of the baby, the management of any condition has to take into consideration the effect on the fetus. Benefits to the woman must outweigh the risks to the fetus/neonate when analgesic drugs are being prescribed. The nature of any medication that a woman may be on long-term for a pre-existing condition must be considered when assessing and evaluating pain management in the individual client, along with other short-term medication prescribed for the critical episode. These drugs can include immunosuppressants, antidepressants, antibiotics or anticonvulsants (Siney 2004). Pain relief has to include an evaluation of the potentially adverse effect on the fetus of the analgesic drug against the effect of the maternal condition and the possible secondary physiological effects on the fetus.

In a situation where the fetus is still alive, the need to facilitate delivery as soon as possible to alleviate the maternal condition or allow life-saving treatment to the mother or baby may also need to be considered. In this event the need to ensure that the neonate has appropriate care at birth to minimise the adverse effects from the maternal condition must also take into account the analgesic drugs used. For women with pregnancy-related complications, analgesia and anaesthesia may be essential to ensure maternal safety. Analgesia and anaesthesia can also benefit the fetus by relieving maternal distress and reducing the disordered physiology which would follow. This can increase the probability of delivering the neonate in a good condition. Where the fetus has already died *in utero* the wellbeing of the mother is the only concern when managing pain relief during the delivery of the stillbirth.

Little or no research has been undertaken about pain relief for the critically ill pregnant woman. A Cochrane systematic review (Neilson 2003) to assess the effectiveness and safety of any intervention for the care of women and/or their babies following a diagnosis of placental abruption found no trials to show which forms of pain relief were best. Other recommendations for pain relief in relation to maternal medical conditions or obstetric emergencies lack research evidence to support them. For some complications, such as cardiac disease, an epidural may be the method of choice (Yerby 2005).

Pain assessment

Pain assessment is the important first step in order to ensure effective management. There are unique challenges in the process of assessing the pain of the critically ill woman as she may be intubated, have received medication such as neuromuscular blocking agents or sedation that will interfere with her ability to communicate effectively, or else be too ill to report her pain (Pasero & McCaffery 2002). Regular pain assessment and documentation using appropriate tools is essential.

The use of a hierarchy of pain intensity measures may be suitable in this situation as it provides a guide to health care providers in the assessment and management of pain (McCaffery & Pasero 1999). Self-report is the most reliable indicator and is the first in the hierarchy of pain intensity measures. A visual analogue scale is most frequently used to quantify the pain, with the 0–10 numerical scale being the commonest. It is important that the critically ill patient is given plenty of time to reply to questions (Kwekkeboom & Herr 2001) as she may have difficulty processing information and responding (Pasero 2003). Clinicians should assume that certain procedures are painful and use other basic measures to assess the pain intensity if the patient is unable to self-report.

Behavioural indicators such as restlessness and grimacing form part of the hierarchy, as well as physiological indicators including increased heart rate and blood pressure. They can be used by carers as cues to determine the presence and intensity of pain. However, carers tend to underestimate the pain and provide inadequate pain relief. The woman's response should be monitored during the procedure to assess the effectiveness of the pain relief. Medication to relieve anxiety will sedate a patient but will not relieve the pain.

From their study into post lower segment caesarean section pain, Lorimer et al. (2002) reported that visual analogue scores reliably predicted the requirement for further analgesia and showed less variability for pain on movement than for pain at rest. They concluded that assessment of pain on movement is a more reliable indicator of analgesic need than pain at rest and therefore may be the better guide to analgesia requirements.

Strategies for managing pain in the critically ill should include the administration of the drugs promptly at the intervals allowed by the prescription, even if the woman is pain-free. Pain level should be assessed 30–45 minutes after drug administration to evaluate the effectiveness. If not pain-free, then the prescription should be reassessed to increase the dose or changed to a more effective drug or combination of drugs.

Complementary and alternative therapies

For pain management in pregnancy and childbirth, non-pharmacological treatment options should be considered where possible before analgesic medications are used. Their place in the care of the critically ill woman may be limited depending on the nature of the critical episode. Midwives should ensure that they are familiar with the *Midwives Rules and Standards* (Nursing and Midwifery Council (NMC) 2004b) which state that "Homeopathic and herbal medicines are subject to the licensing provisions of the Medicines Act 1968. A number of these, however, have product licences but have not been evaluated for their efficacy, safety or quality and you should look to the best available evidence to inform women."

Continuous or one-to-one support by a midwife or trained layperson during labour has been found to reduce analgesic use, operative delivery and dissatisfaction, especially if the support person is not a member of the hospital staff and is present from early labour, particularly if an epidural analgesia service is not available (Hodnett et al. 2003). Transcutaneous electrical nerve stimulation (TENS) does not reduce pain in labour, but there is evidence for a weak analgesia sparing effect (Carroll et al. 1997). Hypnosis increases satisfaction with pain relief and acupuncture decreases the need for analgesics (Smith et al. 2003). Hypnosis in labour also leads to a decrease in the requirement for pharmacological analgesia, an increase in the incidence of spontaneous vaginal delivery and a decrease in the use of labour augmentation (Cyna et al. 2004). Entonox is a versatile analgesic that can be used for immediate short-term analgesia or as supplementation to systemic analgesia. It is rapid acting and also rapidly eliminated from the blood stream and there is no risk of overdose (Street 2000).

Pharmacological analgesia

Opioids are still the main analgesics used for acute pain; however they do not always provide sufficient pain relief and can have adverse effects, and tolerance and addiction can compromise the outcome (Kalso 2005). Recent research indicates that individual variation in opioid responses is substantial. This is explained by different mechanisms of pain and genetic factors, which are responsible for the availability of functional opioid receptors, pharmacogenetic factors that regulate the transport of opioids to the target receptors and the metabolism of opioids. The Human Genome Project has provided data on the genomic variation that may influence the pharmacological responses (Stamer et al. 2005). Screening for variations in the drug-metabolising enzymes has been suggested as a way of improving patient medication. Genetic factors may also be a major reason for adverse drug reactions and the involvement of genes in pain perception, pain processing and pain management are under investigation.

Opioid effectiveness can be improved by individualising doses, route of administration and the drug. Oral is usually not the route of choice for a critically ill childbearing woman even if she is conscious and able to take oral medication (Hytten & Chambelain 1991). Pethidine is the most commonly used intramuscular opioid for the relief of labour pain but concerns have been raised about its effectiveness and also the effect of the drug on the respiratory system of the newborn baby (Elbourne & Wiseman 2003). Intravascular administration has greater efficacy than equivalent intramuscular dosing (Isenor & Penny-MacGillivray 1993). A Cochrane systematic review to assess the effects of different opioids and different doses of the same opioid administered intramuscularly in labour concluded that there was not enough evidence to evaluate the comparative efficacy and safety of the various opioids used as analgesia in labour (Elbourne & Wiseman 2003).

Epidural analgesia is more effective in reducing pain than non-regional methods of analgesia (Liu & Sia 2004; Anim-Somuah et al. 2005). The combined spinal–epidural technique has been introduced in an attempt to reduce the adverse effects reported from the traditional epidural techniques. A Cochrane systematic review (Hughes et al. 2003) to assess the relative effects of combined spinal-epidural versus epidural analgesia in labour specifically concluded that the only proven benefit was a faster onset of effective pain relief from the time of injection. Both techniques are associated with similar obstetric and neonatal outcomes (Hughes et al. 2003) and a similar incidence of hypotension and transient fetal heart rate changes (Patel et al. 2003). The addition of opioids to an epidural local anaesthetic improves the quality and duration of pain relief and reduces local anaesthetic requirement (Lyons et al. 1997); it also improves maternal satisfaction (Murphy et al. 1991).

A more recent Cochrane systematic review (Ng et al. 2004) to assess the relative efficacy and side effects of spinal versus epidural anaesthesia in women having caesarean sections found that both spinal and epidural methods can achieve effective regional anaesthesia for the operation. However, spinal anaesthesia allows surgery to begin earlier, which may be advantageous in the critically ill woman where time may be important in order to improve the outcome for her and/or the fetus. A study in New Zealand looked at the optimal dosing interval for epidural pethidine after lower segment caesarean section. The study challenged the authors' own 3-hourly minimum dosing interval (Lorimer et al. 2002).

Rectal analgesia can be used but the slow absorption means delayed onset of pain relief and there is reduced patient acceptability. A Cochrane review of rectal analgesia for pain from perineal trauma following childbirth concluded that it provides short-term pain relief but more research is required to assess the long-term effect (Hedayati et al. 2003).

Efficacy of pain relief can be increased or adverse effects reduced by combining other drugs that modulate opioid receptor-mediated effects. Tissue damage, such as that associated with infection, inflammation or ischaemia, produces an array of chemical mediators that act either directly to activate and/or sensitise nociceptors. Therefore non-steroidal anti-inflammatory drugs (NSAIDs) can be used to lower peripheral pain by reducing prostaglandin production. They are relatively safe in early and mid pregnancy but they are associated with an increased risk of miscar-riage (Nielsen et al. 2001; Li et al. 2003) and can precipitate fetal cardiac and renal complications in late pregnancy (Ostensen & Skomsvoll 2004). Fetal exposure to NSAIDs has been associated with persistent pulmonary hypertension in the neonate (Alano et al. 2001). Caution is required in critically ill women with renal, cardiac or hepatic impairment or those undergoing anticoagulent therapy.

Lactation

A number of general principles apply when providing analgesic drugs for pain management during lactation. If the neonate is compromised then the ideal nutrition is breast milk, and if the mother's condition will allow then she should be encouraged to breastfeed her baby. The choice of drugs should be based on knowledge of their potential impact on breast feeding and on the breast-fed infant secondary to transfer in human milk. However, there is little research into the effects of many drugs during lactation, which means that clinical decisions have to be made on evidence derived from pharmacokinetic or observational studies, case reports and anecdotes (Australian and New Zealand College of Anaesthetists and Faculty of Pain Medicine 2005).

The lowest effective dose of analgesic is recommended and breast feeding should be avoided when the drug concentration in milk would be at peak levels. Neonates should be observed for any effects of any medication transferred in breast milk. The principles of the passage of drugs via human milk (Ilett et al. 1997), including drugs relevant to pain management, have been reviewed (Rathmell et al. 1997; Spigset & Hagg 2000; Bar-Oz et al. 2003). High lipid solubility, low molecular weight and low protein binding encourage secretion through breast milk although the neonatal exposure is usually low, 0.5–4% of the maternal dose. However, if the drug metabolism in the neonate is impaired, the excretion of the drug may be slow. During the early postpartum period when small amounts of colostrum are secreted, breast feeding is unlikely to pose a risk, even from ana-lgesics administered in the intrapartum period. The amount of paracetamol trans-ferred to the neonate was found by Notarianni et al. (1987) to be approximately

2%. Although neonatal glucuronide conjugation may be reduced, the drug is considered safe and there have been no reports of adverse effects. This dose is much less than the recommended single infant dose of 10 mg/kg.

NSAIDs must be considered individually, but usually the levels in milk are low. Ibuprofen has a low transfer – less than 1% of the maternal dose – is short acting and has the best documented safety. Diclofenac and ketorolac are also secreted in small amounts in breast milk and short-term or occasional use is compatible with breast feeding (Rathmell et al. 1997). They are licensed for postoperative use (British Medical Association & the Royal Pharmaceutical Society of Great Britain 2003).

Role of the carer

Caring for a woman in pain can be a challenging task requiring up-to-date knowledge and skills (Carr & Thomas 1997). There is research evidence to suggest that the approach used by the midwife providing care for women in labour can enhance a women's personal control. Continuity of care is vital with communication being the key as both verbal and non-verbal communication can help to relieve anxieties. Critically ill women will be extremely anxious and may not know what has happened to them or why they require intensive care. They will be anxious about themselves and also the welfare of their family (Park 2001), and should be encouraged to be involved in their care whenever possible and to express their feelings with all members of the multidisciplinary team. Ideally the midwife will be suitably trained and experienced in providing care in the high risk situation. Her role and responsibility is clearly laid down in the *Midwives Rules and Standards* (NMC 2004b) in Rule 6.

The guidance notes include the reminder that 'practice should be based on the best available current evidence' and that 'Each practitioner is accountable for her own practice. Good team working is in the interests of the woman and baby and can only be achieved by mutual recognition of the respective roles of midwives and others who participate in their care. Practice must be based upon locally agreed evidence based standards to ensure that effective communication and co-operation will benefit the care of the woman and baby' (NMC 2004b).

In New Zealand, Barton et al. (2004) found in a survey of midwives' pain knowledge and attitudes that those working regularly with an acute pain service were more knowledgeable about analgesics, non-drug pain management and addiction issues. An acute pain service was shown to have a positive influence on pain management practice.

Rule 7 (NMC 2004a) of the *Guidelines for the Administration of Medicines* states that "A practising midwife shall only supply and administer those medicines, including analgesics, in respect of which she has received the appropriate training as to use, dosage and methods of administration."

Further guidance is given in these guidelines (NMC 2004a) to midwives about their accountability and the need for appropriate records. Record-keeping is also covered in Rule 9 (NMC 2004b) and affirms that "A practising midwife shall keep, as contemporaneously as is reasonable, continuous and detailed records of observations made, care given and medicine and *any form of pain relief administered by her to a woman."*

Each woman needs appropriate counselling, education and support from her carers related to her individual situation in order to minimise or prevent post-traumatic stress disorder (see Chapter 14).

Conclusion

All critically ill women should have the right to adequate analgesia and management of their pain as indicated by Jacobi et al. (2002). Many patients continue to suffer unrelieved pain and inappropriate attitudes and beliefs of staff may contribute to this phenomenon (Clarke et al. 1996), but there continues to be an improvement in the understanding of pain mechanisms. Aspects of genetic differences influencing efficacy, side effects and adverse outcomes of pharmacotherapy will be of importance for pain management in the future (Stamer et al. 2005). Pain and its relief must be assessed and documented on a regular basis. Pain intensity should be regarded as a vital sign and the response to treatment and side effects should be recorded as regularly as other observations such as pulse or blood pressure. The prescription of analgesic drugs and pain-relieving techniques should be reviewed regularly to ensure that analgesia is effective and appropriate to the level of pain experienced by the woman (UK Royal College of Anaesthesists 2003). On-going analgesic use requires close liaison between the obstetric team and the medical practitioner managing the pain so that appropriate levels of pain relief are provided for the critically ill woman.

References

Alano, M., Ngougmna, E. and Ostrea, E. et al. (2001) Analysis of nonsteroidal anti-inflammatory drugs in meconium and its relation to persistant pulmonary hypertension of the newborn. *Pediatrics*, **107**: 517–23.

Anim-Somuah, M., Smyth, R. and Howell, C. (2005) Epidural versus non-epidural analgesia for pain relief in labour. *Cochrane Database of Systematic Reviews*, Issue 3. http://www.mrw.interscience.wiley.com/cochrane/clsysrev/articles/CD000331/frame.html (last accessed Feb 2006)

Austin, K., Stapleton, J. and Mather, L. (1980) Multiple intramuscular injections: a major source of variability in analgesic response to meperidine. *Pain*, **8**: 47–62.

Australian and New Zealand College of Anaesthetists and Faculty of Pain Medicine (2005) *Acute Pain Management: Scientific evidence* (2nd edn). Australian and New Zealand College of Anaesthetists, Melbourne.

Bar-oz, B., Bulkowstein, M. and Benyamini, L. (2003) Use of antibiotic and analgesic drugs during lactation. *Drug Safety*, **26**: 925–35.

Barton, J., Don, M. & Foureur, M. (2004) Nurses and midwives pain knowledge improves under the influence of an acute pain service. *Acute Pain*, **6** (2): 47–51.

British Medical Association and the Royal Pharmaceutical Society of Great Britain (2003) *British National Formulary*, No. 46. British Medical Association and the Royal Pharmaceutical Society of Great Britain, London.

Bryant, H. and Yearby, M. (2004) Relief of pain during labour. In: C. Henderson and M. Macdonald (Eds) *Mayes' Midwifery: A textbook for midwives* (13th edn). Bailliere Tindall, London.

Carr, E. and Thomas, V. (1997) Anticipating and experiencing post-operative pain: the patients' perspective. *Journal of Clinical Nursing*, **6**: 191–201.

Carroll, D., Tramer, M., McQuay, H. et al. (1997) Transcutaneous electrical nerve stimulation in labour pain: a systematic review. *British Journal of Obstetrics and Gynaecology*, **104**: 169–75.

Clarke, E., French, B., Bilodeau, M., Capasso, V., Edwards, A. and Empoliti, J. (1996) Pain management knowledge, attitudes and clinical practice: the impact of nurses' characteristics and education. *Journal of Pain and Symptom Management*, **11**: 18–28.

Cullen, L., Greiner, J. and Titler, M. (2001) Pain management in the culture of critical care. *Critical Care Nursing Clinics of North America*, **13** (2):151–66.

Cyna, A,, McAuliffe, G. and Andrew, M. (2004) Hypnosis for pain relief in labour and childbirth: a systematic review. *British Journal of Anaesthesia*, **93**: 505–11.

East, E. (1992) How much does it hurt? *Nursing Times*, **88** (40): 48–9.

Elbourne, D. and Wiseman, R. (2003) Types of intra-muscular opioids for maternal pain relief in labour. *Cochrane Database of Systematic Reviews*, Issue 4. John Wiley & Sons, Chichester. http://www.mrw.interscience.wiley.com/cochrane/clsysrev/articles/CD001237/frame.html (last accessed Feb 2006)

Guyton, A. and Hall, J. (2000) *Textbook of Medical Physiology* (10th edn). W.B. Saunders, Philadelphia.

Hedayati, H., Parsons, J. and Crowther, C. (2003) Rectal analgesia for pain from perineal trauma following childbirth. *Cochrane Database of Systematic Reviews*, Issue 3. John Wiley & Sons, Chichester. http://www.mrw.interscience.wiley.com/cochrane/clsysrev/articles/CD003931/frame.html (last accessed Feb 2006)

Heelbeck, L. (1999) Administration of pethidine in labour. *British Journal of Midwifery*, **7** (6): 372–7.

Hiscock, M. (1993) Setting up a patient-controlled analgesia service. *British Journal of Intensive Care*, **April**: 149–52.

Hodnett, E., Gates, S., Hofmeyer, G. and Sakala, C. (2003) Continuous support for women during childbirth. *Cochrane Database of Systematic Reviews*, Issue 3. John Wiley & Sons, Chichester. http://www.mrw.interscience.wiley.com/cochrane/clsysrev/articles/CD003766/frame.html (last accessed Feb 2006)

Hughes, D., Simmons, S., Brown, J. and Cyna, A. (2003) Combined spinal-epidural versus epidural analgesia in labour. *Cochrane Database of Systematic Reviews*, Issue 4. John Wiley & Sons, Chichester. http://www.mrw.interscience.wiley.com/cochrane/clsysrev/articles/CD003401/frame.html (last accessed Feb 2006)

Hytten, F. & Chambelain, G. (Eds) (1991) *Clinical Physiology in Obstetrics* (2nd edn). Blackwell Scientific, Oxford.

Ilett, K., Kristensen, J. and Wojnar-Horton, R. (1997) Drug distribution in human milk. *Australian Prescriber*, **20**: 35–40.

International Association for the Study of Pain (1979) Pain terms: a list with definitions and notes on usage. *Pain*, **6**: 249.

Isenor, I. and Penny-MacGillivray, T. (1993) Intravenous meperidine infusion for obstetric analgesia. *Journal of Obstetrics, Gynaecology and Neonatal Nursing*, **22**: 329–56.

Jacobi, J., Fraser, G., Coursin, D. et al. (2002) Clinical practice guidelines for sustained use of sedative and analgesics in the critically ill adult. *Critical Care Medicine*, **30** (1): 119–41.

Kalso, E. (2005) Improving opioid effectiveness from ideas to evidence. *European Journal of Pain*, **9** (2): 131–5.

Kwekkeboom, K. and Herr, K. (2001) Assessment of pain in the critical ill. *Critical Care Nursing Clinics of North America*, **13** (2): 181–94.

Launay-Vacher, V., Karie, S., Fau, J., Izzedine, H. and Deray, G. (2005) Treatment of pain in patients with renal insufficiency: the World Health Organization three-step ladder adapted. *Journal of Pain*, **6** (3): 137–8.

Lewis, G. (2004) *Why Mothers Die 2000–2002: Report on Confidential Enquiries into Maternal and Child Health*, 6th Report. Royal College of Obstetrics and Gynaecologists (RCOG) Press, London.

Li, D-K., Liu, L. and Odouli, R. (2003) Exposure to non-steroidal anti-inflammarory drugs during pregnancy and risk of miscarriage: population based cohort study. *British Medical Journal*, **327**: 368.

Liu, E. and Sia, A. (2004) Rates of caesarean section and instrumental vaginal delivery in nulliparous women after low concentration epidural infusions or opioid analgesia: systematic review. *British Medical Journal*, **328**: 1410.

Lorimer, M., Pedersen, K. and Lombard, W. (2002) Optimal dosing interval for epidural pethidine after Caesarean section. *Acute Pain*, **4** (1): 27–31.

Lyons, G., Columb, M. and Hawthorne, L. (1997) Extradural pain relief in labour; bupivacaine by extradural fentenyl is dose dependent. *British Journal of Anaesthesia*, **78**: 493–7.

Martinelli, A. (1987) Pain and ethnicity: how people of different cultures experience pain. *Association of Operating Room Nurses' Journal*, **46** (2): 273–81.

McCaffery, M. (1968) *Nursing Practice Theories Related to Cognition Bodily Pain: Man–environment interactions.* University of California at Los Angeles Students Store, Los Angeles.

McCaffery, M. and Pasero, C. (1999) Assessment: underlying complexities, misconceptions and practical tools. In: M. MCaffery and C. Pasero (Eds) *Pain: Clinical manual* (2nd edn). Mosby, St Louis.

McIntosh, J. (1990) Models of childbirth and social class: a study of 80 working class primigravidae. In: S. Robinson and A. Thomson (Eds) *Midwives, Research and Childbirth*, Vol 1. Chapman & Hall, London.

Murphy, J., Henderson, K., Bowden, M. et al. (1991) Bupivacaine versus bupivacaine plus fentanyl for epidural analgesia: effect on maternal satisfaction. *British Medical Journal*, **302**: 564–7.

Ndala, R. (2005) Pain relief in labour. In: D. Stables and J. Rankin (Eds) *Physiology in Childbearing with Anatomy and Related Biosciences* (2nd edn). Elsevier, Edinburgh.

Neilson, J. (2003) Interventions for treating placental abruption. *Cochrane Database of Systematic Reviews*, Issue 1. John Wiley & Sons, Chichester. http://www.mrw.interscience.wiley.com/cochrane/clsysrev/articles/CD003247/frame.html (last accessed Feb 2006)

Nielsen, G.L., Sorensen, H.T., Larsen, H. and Pedersen, L. (2001) Risk of adverse birth outcome and miscarriage in pregnant users of non-steroidal anti-inflammatory drugs: population based observational study and case-control study. *British Medical Journal*, **322**: 266–70.

Ng, K., Parsons, J., Cyna, A. and Middleton, P. (2004) Spinal versus epidural anaesthesia for caesarean section. *Cochrane Database of Systematic Reviews*, Issue 2. Wiley & Sons, Chichester. http://www.mrw.interscience.wiley.com/cochrane/clsysrev/articles/CD003765/frame.html

Notarianni, L., Oldham, H. and Bennett, P. (1987) Passage of paracetamol into breast milk and its subsequent metabolism by the neonate. *British Journal of Clinical Pharmacology*, **24**: 63–7.

Nursing and Midwifery Council (2004a) *Guidelines for the Administration of Medicines.* Nursing and Midwifery Council (NMC), London.

Nursing and Midwifery Council (2004b) *Midwives Rules and Standards.* NMC, London.

Ostensen, M. and Skomsvoll, J. (2004) Anti-inflammatory pharmacotherapy during pregnancy. *Expert Opinion on Pharmacotherapy*, **5**: 571–80.

Park, G. (2001) Sedation and analgesia – which way is best? *British Journal of Anaesthesia*, **87** (2): 183–5.

Pasero, C. (2003) Pain in the critically ill patient. *Journal of Perianaesthesia Nursing*, **18** (6): 422–5.

Pasero, C. and McCaffery, M. (2002) Pain in the critically ill patient. *American Journal of Nursing*, **102**: 59–60.

Pasero, C., Paice, J. and McCaffery, M. (1999) Basic mechanisms underlying the causes and effects of pain. *Pain: Clinical manual* (2nd edn). Mosby, St Louis.

Patel, N., Fernando, R., Robson, S. et al. (2003) Fetal effects of combined spinal-epidural (CSE) vs. epidural labour analgesia: a prospective, randomised study. *International Journal of Obstetric Anaesthesia*, **12** (Suppl. 1): 1.

Pocock, G. and Richards, C. (2006) *Human Physiology: the Basis of medicine* (3rd edn). Oxford University Press, Oxford.

Puntilllo, K. (2003) Pain assessment and management in the critically ill: wizardry or science? *American Journal of Critical Care*, **12**: 310–16.

Puntillo, K., White, C., Morris, A. et al. (2001) Patients' perceptions and responses to procedural pain: results from Thunder Project 11. *American Journal of Critical Care*, **10**: 238–51.

Rathmell, J., Viscomi, C. and Ashburn, M. (1997) Management of nonobstetric pain during pregnancy and lactation. *Anaesthetic Analgesia*, **85**: 1074–87.

Siney, C. (2004) Drugs and the midwife. In: C. Henderson and S. Macdonald (Eds) *Mayes Midwifery: a Textbook for midwives* (13th edn). Bailliere Tindall, London.

Smith, C., Collins, C., Cyna, A. and Crowther, C. (2003) Complementary and alternative therapies for pain management in labour. *Cochrane Database of Systematic Reviews*, Issue 2. John Wiley & Sons, Chichester. http://www.mrw.interscience.wiley.com/cochrane/clsysrev/articles/CD003521/frame.html (last accessed Feb 2006)

Smith, G., Power, I. and Cousins, M. (1999) Editorial 1. Acute pain – is there scientific evidence on which to base treatment? *British Journal of Anaethesia*, **82** (6): 817–19.

Spigset, O. and Hagg, S. (2000) Analgesics and breast-feeding: safety considerations. *Paediatric Drugs*, **2**: 223–38.

Stamer, U., Bayerer, B. and Stuber, F. (2005) Genetics and variability in opioid response. *European Journal of Pain*, **9** (2): 101–104.

Stanik-Hutt, J., Soeken, K., Belcher, S. et al. (2001) Pain experiences of traumatically injured patients in a critical care setting. *American Journal of Critical Care*, **10**: 252–9.

Street, D. (2000) A practical guide to giving Entonox. *Nursing Times*, **96** (34): 47–8.

UK Royal College of Anaesthetists (2003) *Pain Management Services: Good practice.* Royal College of Anaesthetists and the Pain Society, London.

Walker, J., Hall, S. and Thomas, M. (1995) The experience of labour: a perspective from those receiving care in a midwife-led unit. *Midwifery*, **11**: 120–9.

Yerby, M. (2005) Cardiac and hypertensive disorders. In: D. Stables and J. Rankin (Eds) *Physiology in Childbearing with Anatomy and Related Biosciences* (2nd edn). Elsevier, Edinburgh.

13

Transfer and Admission to the Intensive Treatment Unit of the Critically Ill Woman

*Terry Ferns**

This chapter will examine how to identify the deteriorating childbearing woman and the safe transfer to level 3 facilities. Level 3 facilities are defined by the Department of Health (2000) as being needed by patients requiring advanced respiratory support alone or basic respiratory support together with the support of at least two organ systems. This level includes all complex patients requiring support for multiorgan failure.

The chapter will also consider acute respiratory distress syndrome (ARDS) as the client requiring transfer will have differing specific needs depending on gestation, whether she is/is not in labour or whether she is pre- or postnatal. An overview of factors to consider for all transfers related to clinical deterioration will be provided.

Assumed prior knowledge

- Physiopathology which may impact upon a woman's condition and cause systemic deterioration
- Knowledge of one's own unit's protocol for transferring critically ill childbearing women to the intensive treatment unit (ITU)
- Knowledge of equipment available in one's own unit to facilitate prompt and safe transfer

* With thanks to Allison Letford, Queen Elizabeth Hosptial Woolwich, for midwifery input.

Identifying the deteriorating client and obstetric emergencies

The first question to pose is who requires transfer? This question can be answered through a comprehensive, systemic, systematic assessment with an emphasis on attention to detail. Recently the Intensive Care Society (2002a) suggested that those at risk of deterioration might be identified by:

- The exhibition of abnormal physical signs and symptoms
- The woman's condition or premorbid history
- Intuition (based on pattern recognition from past experience)

If we add to these assessment criteria the need for further maternal investigations (computed tomography scan, for example) or management (surgery, ventilation or specific organ support, for example), we can offer a reasonable criteria for identifying those requiring transfer. In essence one should always approach the pregnant woman with a high index of suspicion and assume both mother and baby are in distress until an appropriate assessment proves otherwise.

When reviewing current tools such as the early warning score system (Morgan et al. 1997) or the patient at risk team protocol (Goldhill et al. 1999), one can conclude that the following are considered to be the most important factors to consider when identifying those requiring transfer:

- Airway: can the woman maintain her airway?
- Breathing: what is the rate, depth and pattern of breathing?
- Circulation: what is the woman's blood pressure and pulse? What is the woman's perfusion: How warm are they? What is their temperature? What is their colour? What is their urine output?
- Neurology: is the woman conscious, orientated and pain-free?

Plus, is there any evidence of fetal compromise (cardiotocograph, ultrasound scan)?

If one is satisfied that the woman meets 'normal' criteria for the above, one can reasonably assume the woman is stable unless the woman has an underlying condition that has already raised cause for concern. The further away from normal the woman's vital signs, the more concern one should have, as a fundamental goal of the midwife should be to identify deterioration as early as possible in order to implement the appropriate care.

With childbearing women, deterioration can be sudden and catastrophic, therefore team members will need to consider whether they have time to initiate the controlled transfer as detailed below. There may be circumstances where time is extremely short. However, such incidents can be minimised by appropriate screening and continuous monitoring of high risk pregnancies by a high quality coordinated multidisciplinary team.

Guidelines for transfer to ITU

Take a few moments to consider this question before reading on:

If I was coordinating a transfer to manage clinical deterioration what would I need to do to ensure that transfer is safe?

A significant proportion of women experiencing clinical deterioration will require surgical intervention prior to intensive care admission. Therefore, an enforced detour from the obstetric department to theatre may be required before the woman presents in the intensive care department. This section will deal primarily with intrahospital transfers although the same principles will apply to hospital to hospital transfers. The early stages of this chapter rely heavily on recommendations by the Intensive Care Society (2002a, 2002b) and Wallace and Ridley (1999). Above all, the important principle of transportation is 'do no further harm' (Advanced Trauma Life Support 1997).

Theoretical frameworks must guide clinical practice, and client assessment requires a systematic strategy. Professional transfer is no exception to this rule. Any critically ill woman requires extensive assessment, intervention and monitoring equipment originally guided by the acronym below (adapted from Resuscitation Council UK 2000):

- **M**: *m*onitor, *m*ode of transfer and equipment
- **O**: *o*xygen and airway management
- **V**: *v*enous access
- **E**: *e*xpertise

Monitor

The minimal monitoring equipment that is required for a safe transfer includes the following.

- *Electrocardiograph monitor*. A portable electrocardiograph monitor is a fundamental requirement, which allows the observation of cardiovascular indices such as heart rate and rhythm (Docherty 2002). However, such equipment is no substitute for regular pulse checks as, for example, pulseless electrical activity can give a false indication of cardiovascular stability in the absence of a cardiac output. Ability to record non-invasive blood pressures is further recommended.
- *Arterial line*. Women should ideally be connected to an invasive arterial line allowing for continuous, accurate blood pressure monitoring. Subsequently, team members will be able to continuously monitor systolic, diastolic, mean and pulse pressures. Arterial line access will also allow for the opportunity to withdraw regular blood samples. Prior to transfer arterial lines should be zeroed, calibrated and transduced and checked to ensure a quality pressure wave reading. Poor trace reading can be the result of inadequate pressure in the circuit, blocked cannulae, air bubbles or leaks in the system (Webster 2003). Staff should also resist the temptation to compare non-invasive blood pressure readings with invasive as the general consensus of opinion is that providing the invasive mode is utilised correctly its values are superior in terms of accuracy to non-invasive measurements, particularly in the suboptimal, low cardiac output state. A good non-invasive reading in the presence of a poor invasive measurement should be treated with caution; do not be tempted to gravitate towards whichever mode of measurement produces the higher reading.

- *Pulse oximetry.* Women should also be connected to pulse oximetry via a saturation probe to enable the early recognition of hypoxaemia. Team members are given an immediate warning of deterioration, which is not the case when observing for unreliable symptoms such as cyanosis (Spyr 1990). Szaflarski (1996) notes that cyanosis is an unreliable indicator of hypoxaemia, occurring only when the SpO_2 is lower than 67%. Pulse oximetry is a highly valuable technique but its accuracy is very dependent on correct use (Tittle & Flynn 1997). Accuracy can depend on perfusion, haemoglobin, temperature or skin pigmentation (Goodfellow 1997) and pulse oximetry should be viewed as an adjunct to careful, detailed, systematic assessment not as a replacement.
- *Temperature monitoring.* Peripheral or core temperature monitoring should also be considered as a reflection of tissue perfusion as there is an increased gradient between core and peripheral temperature in shocked states (Webster 2003). However, once again, monitoring equipment is no substitute for feeling the woman's skin for indicators of impaired perfusion such as excessive vasoconstriction or dilatation.
- *Catheterisation and nasogastric tubes.* Women may also be considered for urethral catheterisation and nasogastric tube insertion prior to transfer. Urinary output can be a good indicator of cardiac and renal function as a drop in cardiac output of 10–20% can have a direct effect on the glommerular filtration rate by up to 20% (Darovic 1995). Nasogastric tube insertion will allow for stomach emptying to avoid aspiration, a potentially catastrophic complication that must be strenuously avoided if possible, which is a particular concern during pregnancy due to anatomical and physiological changes. Further, nasogastric drainage offers information that may help to guide fluid and electrolyte replacement. However, we must consider the altered anatomy and physiology of pregnancy, which predisposes the woman to epistaxis, for example, and the potential for invasive lines such as nasogastric tubes to become focal sites for infection. As we shall see, expertise in the decision-making process for the safe transfer of childbearing women cannot be overemphasised. Frequently, interventions and actions must be weighed up between the potential advantages and disadvantages of withholding or implementing therapy.
- *Fetal heart rate monitoring.* Also, for the purpose of transfer, if the woman is pregnant, fetal heart rate monitoring needs to be considered. Such monitoring requires personnel who can interpret fetal heart rate tracings, emphasising the importance of the practical involvement of midwives in the transfer process. Often transfers involve multiple personnel and midwives must make sure that, if necessary, they elbow their way to the woman's side!

Mode of transfer and equipment

The transfer of any critically ill woman can be simplified and made less traumatic for patients and staff alike if the team considers the practical logistics of the transfer. Simple steps like being familiar with hospital design and layout can prevent apprehension. Departments may be on different floors at different ends of the hospital and staff should not rely on colleagues to guide them to their destination, but should have conducted practice runs to make the transfer run smoothly. Often, routine trolleys are too narrow to accommodate equipment and specialist trolleys designed specifically for transfers should be available.

Frequently, complicated invasive monitoring, infusions and therapies are attached to patients prior to and during transfers and such equipment should be safely secured and clearly visible to the team members. Staff experienced in caring for childbearing women may not be familiar with portable equipment utilised during transfer and therefore it is imperative that colleagues comfortable with the process of transferring critically ill women are utilised. In the United Kingdom, the implementation of outreach services has led to individual members of the multidisciplinary team being frequently involved in transfers and such staff should be involved in transfers. Practically, outreach service staff frequently take responsibility for the storage, electrical charging and availability of transfer equipment as they tend to utilise such equipment the most frequently; therefore it seems reasonable to involve such personnel at the earliest available point. Further, the remit of outreach services includes staff education and training, and a clear link between the maternity department, theatre or critical care can be bridged by such a service.

Oxygen

Women requiring transfer to critical care areas would be expected to be receiving high doses of empirical oxygen as respiratory distress is a frequent indicator for transfer. The ability of the woman to maintain her airway needs to be considered and prophylactic intubation may be considered. Hypoxia develops more rapidly in the pregnant woman, and anatomical and physiological changes may make ventilation and intubation more difficult. The aim is to stabilise the woman for transfer and avoid any possibility of sudden deterioration during the transfer. If intubation is required, a portable ventilator with disconnection alarms is a prerequisite (Wallace & Ridley 1999). Mechanically ventilated patients require monitoring of oxygen supply, inspired oxygen concentration, ventilator settings, airway pressures and end tidal carbon dioxide (Intensive Care Society 2002b). Sufficient oxygen to complete the journey is a necessity and the airway must be safe and secure prior to departure.

Intubated women will require suitable analgesia, sedation and perhaps paralysis so any prescriptions should ensure that chosen drugs have a minimal cardiovascular effect.

Venous access

Intravenous access is an absolute priority. Women in high dependency areas should not routinely be cared for without patent intravenous access. There may be a dilemma regarding a woman deteriorating who does not have intravenous access. Two large-bore catheters for fluid resuscitation should suffice (Intensive Care Society 2002b). Central venous access may be appropriate for large-volume resuscitation or a necessity for inotrope administration, but there are dangers in the emergency situation of siting central venous lines – such as causing a pneumothorax, cardiac arrhythmia or cardiac tamponade (Woodrow 2002). Also, central venous pressure (CVP) line readings have lost credibility except in exceptional circumstances of profound hypovolaemia or fluid overload. Clinical judgement is required to weigh up the options of taking the time to insert the line, against delaying the treatment of the cause of the deterioration. Ensuring women viewed as high risk have patent access will negate the dilemma of insertion of access in an emergency situation.

Expertise

It cannot be emphasised enough that the quality of an obstetric department team is dictated by the quality of the personnel in it. Midwives are educated to perform as autonomous practitioners and as such, through their careers, become comfortable with taking responsibility and making decisions. However, the obstetric emergency is a situation that occurs unpredictably, so experience must be quantified by level of education and number of clinical experiences as opposed to length of time practising in a department or length of time qualified. Critical care admissions are conducted consultant to consultant. Subsequently, Wallace and Ridley (1999) recommend that individual hospitals should have a designated consultant responsible for transfers. Such a model should apply to intrahospital transfers.

The medical team has a responsibility to ensure that channels of communication are clear and appropriate personnel are informed of imminent decisions to transfer. A close relationship between anaesthetic staff, intensivists, midwives, neonatologists, operating department personnel and theatre/critical care nurses is vital. Midwifery and nursing staff should liaise through operational meetings, for example, to ensure that all team members are clear about their roles in the run up, imminent move, transfer and post-transfer. Support services such as portering should also be briefed regarding the importance of a swift, coordinated transfer. In particular, staff conducting transfers should be suitably qualified and be aware of other team members' skills and limitations.

The transfer of critically ill childbearing women requires anticipation, vision, coordination, resource allocation and leadership. Wallace and Ridley (1999) emphasise that the 'scoop and run' principle is not appropriate for moving critically ill women. In the recent past authors such as Mackenzie et al. (1997) or Vyvyan et al. (1991) have noted that in relation to interhospital transfers, junior staff are frequently utilised, which might subsequently result in higher incidences of life-threatening complications; such comments should be considered when embarking on all hospital transfers.

As noted above, clear clinical and organisational leadership cannot be over-emphasised. In an ideal situation the woman who deteriorates should quickly be reviewed by outreach services and anaesthetic doctors trained in intensive care/obstetric medicine. It is much more appropriate for such staff to stabilise women prior to transfer, and then transfer, as opposed to a situation where critically ill women arrive at the doors of the intensive care department lacking stable vital signs, intravenous access, monitoring and so on. Although the process of transferring critically ill women may be primarily managed by experienced anaesthetic and nursing staff, midwifery personnel should also accompany women to offer practical assessment and to monitor a potentially distressed fetus and to ensure thorough handover to receiving personnel. Depending on the woman's conscious levels a familiar, competent professional midwife can offer valuable reassurance to women experiencing extremely frightening and life-threatening situations. Further, midwifery staff will be familiar and comfortable in the transferring obstetric department, knowing its layout and equipment availability, and will be a vital constituent of the team if significant stabilisation and monitoring needs to take place prior to departure. Also, accurate record keeping frequently requires a nominated scribe and the collection of contemporaneous records.

Immediate preparation prior to transfer

Subsequently, the team should gather prior to transfer and ensure that an adequate assessment has been conducted, appropriate monitoring and supportive therapy initiated, and relevant clinical investigations completed. Particular attention should be given to ensuring a safe airway and that appropriate fluid resuscitation or inotrope therapy has been implemented as the hypovolaemic woman tolerates transport poorly and volume loading is usually a prerequisite (Wallace & Ridley 1999). In essence investigations required will, to a large extent, be determined by the woman's clinical presentation. The main principles of critical care management revolve around diagnosis and treatment of the cause of the deterioration, and optimisation of cardiac output, arterial blood pH and arterial Pao_2. Some of these variables can be considered through a thorough physical assessment; however cardiac output, for example, cannot be reliably predicted by physical examination (Eisenberg et al. 1984) and subsequent clinical investigations should be ordered during the assessment and management of the woman considered for transfer.

Obviously the clinical presentation of the woman may guide further investigations and an experienced team member can consider which tests are required by simply considering what questions they would ask if they were receiving the woman.

Wallace and Ridley (1999) suggest a checklist for considering if women are ready for transfer. A condensed amended format is shown below. However, one must consider the baseline observations of the woman and the physiological changes associated with pregnancy.

Respiration

- Is the airway safe?
- Are intubation and ventilation required?
- Are sedation, analgesia and paralysis adequate?
- Arterial oxygen pressure > 13 kPa, saturation > 95%
- Arterial carbon dioxide pressure 4–5 kPa (fit young adult)

Circulation

- Systolic blood pressure > 120 mmHg
- Heart rate < 120 beats/min
- Satisfactory perfusion (colour, warmth, urine output)
- Intravenous access confirmed
- Circulating volume replaced
- Confirmation of blood availability
- Identification/management of bleeding

Neurology

- Glasgow coma scale completed
- Pupillary response assessed
- Consideration of analgesia, sedation or paralysis

Monitoring

- Electrocardiography
- Pulse oximetry
- End tidal carbon dioxide measurements
- Invasive/non-invasive blood pressure monitoring
- Temperature monitoring
- Consideration of central line insertion
- Consideration of nasogastric tube insertion
- Consideration of urethral catheterisation

Investigations

- Twelve-lead electrocardiography
- Radiographs
- Arterial blood gases
- Biochemistry
- Haematology
- Microbiology picture

In conjunction with clinical assessment and stabilisation there are essential clerical and practical issues to be considered. Medical and midwifery documentation should be completed, relatives/next of kin notified of transfer, property/valuables documented and packed, and confirmation that the receiving department is notified, ready and consenting to transfer.

A final check that all of the above are accounted for is required. Occasionally women can be ready for transfer but there may be delays, for example, in portering services. A woman's conditions can change rapidly, so never assume that because the woman was stable 10 minutes ago, that 10 minutes later they are ready to leave. Women should always be rechecked immediately prior to transfer.

Practicalities

- Patient secured and safely placed on trolley
- Sufficient oxygen supply
- Monitoring securely attached, alarms set and working appropriately
- Infusions charged, secured and suitable backup medications available
- Drainage devices secured
- Portering services available
- Trolley available
- Transfer charts and all available notes/investigations collected, with times documented
- Contact numbers available
- Receiving department notified of imminent departure and estimated arrival time
- Identification and allergy bracelets visible
- Appropriate availability of portable defibrillator, intubation equipment, suction, spare ventilator tubing, self-inflating re-breath bag and supplementary equipment dressings, syringes, etc.
- Dignity maintained (warm blankets applied, woman suitably covered)

Intradepartmental transfers

The aim of the transfer process is to ensure stabilisation and a standard of monitoring that mimics regular intensive care monitoring (Wallace & Ridley 1999). Movement should be controlled and not rushed. The clinical experts should control the speed of movement not the support staff. Discussions between staff regarding deterioration and the need to return to the original department, detour to another or continue should be conducted though pre-incident training. When travelling, for example, in lifts, consideration should be given to actions in the event of sudden deterioration or lift failure. The woman's next of kin should not directly accompany the transfer team but provision should be given for them to wait in a suitable relatives area, be that within the original department or adjacent to the receiving department (Wallace & Ridley 1999).

Handover

Expert-to-expert handover must be a priority. Subsequently, midwifery staff must accompany transfers although staff will frequently also form part of a team consisting of an anaesthetist, a nurse, operating department personnel and portering staff. The midwife must ensure handover is conducted to a suitably qualified professional, for example a theatre nurse in theatres or a critical care nurse in intensive care. Particular attention should be given to ensuring staff receive all information regarding current levels of information given to relatives and their location. It is a matter of client safety and professional courtesy to hand over patients to colleagues; emergency transfers should not ignore published policies regarding, for example, checking identification. All documentation should be verbally handed over and the transfer team should be completely satisfied that they have handed all information over appropriately. Any changes identified during transfer should be documented. In these situations it is best practice for the transfer team to remain in the receiving department for a short while to allow colleagues to absorb the information given and query any perceived discrepancies. In particular, the delivering and receiving departments must consider the potential stressors involved in accommodating transfers and work to a common goal of client safety and interprofessional collaboration that emphasises continuity of care.

Post-transfer

Well planned and executed transfers allow the multidisciplinary team to project a professional service. Staff should be encouraged to debrief and share experiences to maximise the opportunity for implementing best practice. Staff will benefit from observing transfers prior to being practically involved.

Organisational issues

The Intensive Care Society (2002b) offer comprehensive recommendations regarding the transfer of critically ill adults, and midwifery departments should be familiar with and involved in the implementation of such recommendations at both local and network levels. Midwifery departments need to press for inclusion within critical care networks and ensure that the philosophy of critical care without walls extends into the obstetric facility.

Acute respiratory distress syndrome

Acute respiratory distress syndrome (ARDS) has held its ground against a strong and concerted medical challenge. The original ARDS was described by Ashbaugh et al. (1967), who reported how soldiers injured during fighting in the Vietnam war received non-respiratory trauma but following fluid resuscitation frequently manifested terminal respiratory distress. Mortality rates for patients presenting with ARDS vary in the literature according to the severity of the syndrome and aetiological/coexisting factors (Florence 1997). Thomas (1997) has indicated that mortality rates for ARDS have remained unchanged for the previous 15 years, while McLuckie (2004) considers that the mortality rate has declined worldwide, resulting in survival rates of between 60 and 75% being reported.

The frequent dual diagnosis of ARDS and sepsis means that clients may present with a wide range of symptoms, ranging from respiratory distress to profound shock, making the condition – when further complicated by the life-threatening challenge of obstetric emergency – one of the most difficult critical care experiences.

ARDS is defined by arterial hypoxaemia, bilateral pulmonary infiltrates due to high permeability pulmonary oedema, lung inflammation and decreased lung compliance (Beale et al. 1993; Gattiononi & Pelosi 1996; Repine & Abmaham 1996). Acute onset pulmonary oedema is non-cardiogenic in origin. Annual incidence of ARDS is approximately six cases per 100 000 population (Evans & Smithies 1999).

ARDS and *acute lung injury* are frequently used interchangeably in the literature but there is a clear distinction. ARDS is seen as a severe form of acute lung injury, but is characterised as being non-cardiogenic in origin. In essence, clients can develop pulmonary oedema due to congestive cardiac failure and subsequent back pressure into the pulmonary circulation. This would be viewed as the classic form of pulmonary oedema. ARDS may be classified as a form of pulmonary oedema but the pulmonary oedema manifests due to increased tissue permeability and develops due to an internal pulmonary insult or a systemic event such as severe shock. Childbearing women may present with pneumonia (an acute lung injury) and subsequently deteriorate to a diagnosis of ARDS. Therefore, all women with ARDS have an acute lung injury but not all women with an acute lung injury have ARDS (Bernard et al. 1994).

ARDS is associated with diffuse damage to the alveoli and lung capillary endothelium (Harman 2003). The early stages of the disease are described as exudative, proliferative and fibrotic in nature. The *exudative stage* usually begins within 24 hours of the initial insult and is characterised by fluid leakage and accumulation in the lung tissue. During the *proliferative phase* there is a reduction in surfactant production and fibrin leaks from capillaries causing an inflammatory response, increased respiratory rate and pulmonary hypertension. During the *fibrotic stage*, the lung becomes filled with dense fibrous tissue producing worsening hypoxia and stiff uncompliant lungs. Two distinct sequences of events are currently accepted:

- *Damage to the alveocapillary membrane.* Damage to the alveocapillary membrane develops with increased permeability at the level of the alveocapillary membrane, leading to leakage of fluid through the capillary endothelium and into the interstitial space, and through the alveolar epithelium into the alveoli. The net result of this process is the collection of fluid in the lung interstistum and alveoli spaces, disrupting the efficiency of gas exchange across the capillary–alveoli interface and leading to hypoxia.
- *Increase in alveocapillary membrane permeability.* Increasing alveocapillary membrane permeability leads to interstitial and alveolar oedema, encouraging alveoli collapse. The subsequent development of atelectasis reduces functional residual capacity and, increasingly, circulating blood confronts alveoli containing fluid and exudates. This leads to shunting and decreasing lung compliance that leads to an increase in the amount of energy required to breath.

The combination of oedematous lung tissue, heavy and rigid, increasing alveolar exudates, surfactant loss and fibrosis leads to atelectasis, poor compliance, hypoxia, ventilation/perfusion mismatching, shunting, reduced functional residual capacity, an increased work of breathing, increased energy expenditure and eventual respiratory exhaustion and collapse.

The childbearing woman is at risk of developing ARDS from two perspectives. First, the condition can develop from an intrinsic respiratory insult such as pneumonia or aspiration and, second, can develop due to a secondary systemic event such as shock (e.g. hypovolaemic, septic, anaphylactic), disseminated intravascular coagulopathy (DIC), or as a consequence of medical therapy such as massive blood transfusion. Common causes of acute lung injury in the childbearing woman are pre-eclampsia, eclampsia, obstetric haemorrhage, amnionitis, endometritis and amniotic fluid embolism (Dhond & Dob 2000; Jiva 2000). Multiple organ failure frequently links the two key factors of ARDS and severe sepsis. Sepsis, aspiration and DIC have been reported to be present in 38, 30 and 22% of cases of ARDS in pregnancy, respectively (Theunissen & Parer 1994; Clapp & Capeless 1997). From a systemic perspective the overriding, unifying event that appears to contribute to the development of ARDS is a period of profound hypotension.

Care and management

A successful outcome will only be the case if there is early identification of deterioration, the cause of the syndrome is identified and treated and appropriate monitoring and supportive therapy is initiated. Intubation and mechanical ventilation is a consequence of the development of ARDS, although debate continues to rage over ventilation policy in relation to underventilating to prevent ventilator-induced lung injury or hyperinflation to discourage atelectasis. Positive pressure ventilation is applied within the concepts of a closed, consolidated lung field, a closed but recruitable lung field and an area of open diseased lung. Ventilation should attempt to achieve adequate oxygenation with the lowest possible mean and peak airway pressures; permissive hypercapnia should be considered.

The dilemma one faces is that the increased tissue permeability means that fluid resuscitation to maintain cardiac output frequently compromises and worsens the respiratory picture. The priority of care revolves around prompt resuscitation and achievement of a normal haemodynamic status. Women who are mechanically ventilated should be given adequate pain relief and sedation to minimise oxygen demands, and steps should be taken to control pyrexia. In essence, ARDS should be viewed as a systemic insult and optimalisation of perfusion and ventilation should be the goal. Care should be thoughtful and individualised, and stress-related factors should be limited in specific organs. Management should strive to avoid compounding the problem with excessive oxygenation, overhydration or inappropriate over/underventilation.

Early indications that the syndrome may develop include the identification of causative risk factors and early manifestations of the condition, ranging from dyspnoea with exertion, severe dyspnoea at rest, tachypnea, anxiety, agitation and the need for increasing levels of high concentrations of inspired oxygen (Harman 2003). Jiva (2000) suggests one should be suspicious and consider acute lung injury or pulmonary infection if dyspnea occurs without exertion or is inordinately severe and is accompanied by significant tachypnoea and respiratory distress.

Childbearing women, as noted earlier, have lower threshholds for deterioration and are more difficult to identify due to normal physiological processes during pregnancy. The woman presenting with respiratory failure and requiring positive pressure ventilation and sedation offers particular challenges to medical/midwifery/nursing staff particularly in relation to, for example, supine positioning. Supportive options that may be considered in the management of women presenting with ARDS include diuresis, positive end expiratory pressure ventilation, fluid resuscitation and inotropic agents, which may diminish maternal cardiac output and uteroplacental perfusion (Dhond & Dob 2000). Above all, maternal hypotension should be avoided as this leads to shunting of blood from the placental bed and fetal hypoxaemia (Erickson & Parisi 1990).

Treatment of the underlying cause of ARDS is essential together with supportive respiratory therapy such as oxygen or invasive and non-invasive ventilation. Cardiovascular stability should be maintained and supportive therapy initiated to prevent secondary complications such as renal failure. Early adequate nutrition is now regarded as important to the management of patients presenting with ARDS (Artigas et al. 1998).

Conclusion

This chapter has considered the safe transfer of women to critical care areas and the altered physiology, presentation, assessment and management of women diagnosed with ARDS. The key components to consider are:

- Early identification of the deteriorating woman is a fundamental midwifery goal.
- Midwives require extensive assessment skills to identify the deteriorating client.
- Holistic assessment frameworks are required to conduct a professional assessment.
- Familiarity with published guidelines for safe patient transfer must be adhered to.
- Swift goal-related therapy, treating the cause of the deterioration and comprehensive monitoring must form part of the professional midwife's repertoire.
- Relatives require explanations and support and close liaison between the nursing and midwifery teams is essential.

References

Advanced Trauma Life Support (1997) *Advanced Trauma Life Support Manual* (6th edn). American College of Surgeons, Chicago.

Artigas, A., Bernard, G., Carlet, J., Dreyfuss, D., Gattionini, L., Hudson, L., Lamy, M., Marini, J., Matthay, M., Pinsky, M., Spragg, R. and Suter, P. (1998) The American European Consensus Conference on ARDS. Part 2: Ventilatory pharmacologic supportive therapy, study design strategies and issues related to recovery and remodelling. *American Journal of Respiratory Critical Care Medicine*, **157**: 1332–47.

Ashbaugh, D., Bidgelow, D. and Petty, T. (1967) Acute respiratory distress in adults. *Lancet*, **122** (7511): 319–23.

Beale, R., Grover, E., Smithies, M. and Bihari, D. (1993) Acute respiratory distress syndrome: no more than an acute lung injury? *British Medical Journal*, **307**: 1335–9.

Bernard, G.R., Artigas, A. and Brigham, K.L. (1994) The American–European Consensus Conference on ARDS. *American Journal of Respiratory Critical Care Medicine*, **149**: 818–24.

Clapp, J. and Capeless, E. (1997) Cardiovascular function before, during and after the first and subsequent pregnancies. *American Journal of Cardiology*, **80**: 1469–73.

Darovic, G. (1995) *Haemodynamic Monitoring: Invasive and non-invasive clinical application* (2nd edn). W.B. Saunders, London.

Department of Health (2000) *Comprehensive Critical Care: A review of adult critical care services*. Department of Health, London.

Dhond, G. and Dobb, D. (2000) Focus on obstetrics: critical care of the obstetric patient. *Current Anaesthesia and Critical Care*, **11**: 86–91.

Docherty, B. (2002) Cardio-respiratory physical assessment for the acutely ill: part one. *British Journal of Nursing*, **11** (11): 750–8.

Eisenberg, P., Jaffe, A. and Schuster, D. (1984) Clinical evaluation compared to pulmonary artery catheterisation in the haemodynamic assessment of critically ill patients. *Critical Care Medicine*, **12**: 549–53.

Erickson, N. and Parisi, V. (1990) Adult respiratory distress syndrome and pregnancy. *Semiars in Perinatology*, **14**: 68–78.

Evans, T. and Smithies, M. (1999) ABC of intensive care organ dysfunction. *British Medical Journal*, **318**: 1606–9.

Florence, E. (1997) ARDS mortality is related to initial pathology. *Journal of Respiratory Critical Care Medicine*, **155**: 398.

Gattiononi, L. and Pelosi, P. (1996) Pathophysical insights into acute respiratory failure. *Current Opinion in Critical Care*, **2**: 8–12.

Goldhill, D., Worthington, L., Mulcahy, A., Tarling, M. and Sumner, A. (1999) The patient at risk team: identifying and managing seriously ill ward patients. *Anaesthesia*, **54**: 853–60.

Goodfellow, L. (1997) Application of pulse oximetry and the oxyhaemoglobin dissociation curve in respiratory management. *Critical Care Nurse Quarterly*, **20** (2): 22–7.

Harman, E. (2003) Acute respiratory distress syndrome. http://www.emedicine.com/med/topic70.htm

Intensive Care Society (2002a) *Guidelines for the Implementation of Outreach Services*. Intensive Care Society. London.

Intensive Care Society (2002b) *Guidelines for the Transport of the Critically Ill Adult*. Intensive Care Society, London.

Jiva, T. (2000) Critical care of pregnant women, part 1; pulmonary oedema, ARDS, thromboembolism. *Journal of Critical Illness*, **15** (6): 316–24.

Mackenzie, P., Smith, E. and Wallace, P. (1997) Transfer of adults between intensive care units in the UK. *British Medical Journal*, **314**: 1455–6.

McLuckie, A. (2004) Editorial II: high-frequency oscillation in acute respiratory distress syndrome (ARDS). *British Journal of Anaesthesia*, **93** (3): 322–4.

Morgan, R., Williams, F. and Wright, M. (1997) An early warning scoring system for detecting and developing critical illness. *Clinics in Intensive Care*, **8** (2): 100.

Repine, J. and Abmaham, E. (1996) Challenges in treating the acute respiratory distress syndrome. *Current Opinions in Critical Care*, **2**: 73–8.

Resuscitation Council UK (2000) *Advanced Life Support Handbook*. Resuscitation Council UK, London.

Spyr, J. (1990) Pulse oximetry; understanding the concept, knowing the limits. *Registered Nurse*, **53** (5): 38–45.

Szaflarski, N. (1996) Pre analytical error associated with blood gas/pH measurement. *Critical Care Nurse*, **16** (3): 89–100.

Theunissen, I. and Parer, J. (1994) Fluid and electrolytes in pregnancy. *Clinical Obstetrics and Gynecology*, **37**: 3–15.

Thomas, C. (1997) Use of the prone position, the ventilation perfusion relationship in ARDS. *Care of the Critically Ill*, **13** (3): 96–100.

Tittle, M. and Flynn, M. (1997) Correlation of pulse oximetry and co-oximetry. *Dimensions of Critical Care Nursing*, **16** (2): 88–95.

Vyvyan, H., Kee, S. and Bristow, A. (1991) A survey of secondary transfers of head injury patients in the south of England. *Anaesthesia*, **4**: 728–31.

Wallace, P. and Ridley, S. (1999) A B C of intensive care transport of critically ill patients. *British Medical Journal*, **319**: 368–71.

Webster, N. (2003) Educational review: monitoring the critically ill patient. http://www.rcsed.ac.uk/Journal/Vol44-6/4460010.htm

Woodrow, P. (2002) Central venous catheters and central venous pressure. *Nursing Standard*, **16** (26): 45–51.

14 Psychological Needs and Care of the Critically Ill Woman

Lynne Spencer

This chapter will focus on the psychological needs and care that a woman who is, or who has been, critically ill during childbirth requires to be able to be comfortable with her experience. The purpose of providing psychological care for women in their childbearing year is so that they understand the process that they are living and working through. The childbearing year is a transition with many ups and downs and has been described by Page (1993) as a journey that requires sensitive support from the staff caring for the woman. With sensitive support the woman and her family are able to remain emotionally intact, strong and confident that they will be able to provide good enough parenting for their baby.

The basis of all care provided to women needs to demonstrate that wherever possible the woman is respected. This really means listening to her and her partner to understand her fears and wishes. It is important for a woman to have an element of choice in the care she accepts. This means that care providers need to communicate clearly and accurately what options are available and what may be the outcomes of the options, both the positive and negative, and the likelihood of the outcomes. This needs to be in as calm an environment as possible, with as much time as is possible to give the woman and her partner space to make a decision. Clear communication from a care provider who is compassionate and genuine, will enable a woman and her partner make an informed decision about the care that is offered to them. Having made that decision, the woman and her partner will feel they have some control in the situation even though the option they have chosen is not what they would have preferred in the first instance, but is the choice that is most appropriate in their situation.

Assumed prior knowledge

- The *Changing childbirth* report (Department of Health 1993)
- The effects of loss and the grieving process

Introduction

There are areas that may be new to midwifery practice, such as the triggers for post-traumatic stress disorder (PTSD) as identified by the American Psychological Association (1994). Triggers that are relevant to midwifery practice are:

- An event posing a serious threat to one's life or physical integrity
- An event that presents the possibility of serious threat or harm to one's loved ones

Two other factors not immediately identifiable as relevant to midwifery practice, but which may be linked to the woman and her family, are:

- The sudden destruction of one's environment
- Seeing another person injured or killed as the result of an accident or physical violence

All of the above may be equated to or identified as a result of a difficult childbirth experience. The signs and symptoms of PTSD include:

- Efforts to avoid thoughts or feelings associated with the trauma (in this case the birth or period of critical illness) and thus not speaking about the experience
- Efforts to avoid activities or situations which arouse recollections of the event, such as avoiding hospitals, wanting a home birth or avoiding newborn infants
- Inability to recall an important aspect of the trauma (psychogenic amnesia) such as not being able to recall seeing the baby following the birth
- Markedly diminished interest in significant activities, such as caring for the baby, other children, self or partner
- Feeling of detachment or estrangement from others; for example, not loving or caring for the baby
- Restricted range of emotion, such as being unable to feel happy about the baby
- Sense of a foreshortened future; for example, not expecting the baby to survive or expecting herself or other family members to die
- Recurrent nightmares
- Recurrent and intrusive recollections of the labour, birth or period of critical illness
- Psychological distress at exposure to internal or external cues that symbolise or resemble aspects of the trauma, such as a smear test or vaginal examination at the postnatal examination

Care in pregnancy

For many years social scientists have been challenging the way in which care in pregnancy is provided to women. This has relevance for women who become critically ill during childbearing. Oakley (1984) pointed out that care was ritualised and demanded that women be passive recipients. Care of this nature ignores the individuality of a woman and reduces the accountability of midwives and obstetricians, because they are able to follow routines and procedures, which in turn lull care providers into a false sense of security and important changes in the woman's behaviour and physiology can be missed. This is particularly the case when the care provider repeatedly uses language that will quieten a woman – and thinks wrongly that she has reassured the woman – such as: 'You mustn't be frightened, everything is ok' or 'Don't worry.'

Robinson has, in her observations and reflections in the *British Journal of Midwifery* (BJM), repeatedly provided midwives with examples of what is said to women, but still these comments continue. This author wonders whether the midwives who say such comments ever read the BJM, or whether they skip Robinson's page because it makes uneasy reading. I find that it is often the most sobering and touching page, and makes me stop and think about my behaviour. However, even if there are midwives who do not read Robinson's page, what about the rest of us? If we hear the comments and say nothing we are colluding with them, and are just as accountable as the midwives who make the comments.

Each individual woman has her own subjective experience during pregnancy, and what may seem to be a difficult pregnancy to one woman will seem a breeze to another (Lyons 1998). Each woman needs to be heard and have her anxieties reduced by clear information that is provided calmly, and repeated until she understands what is happening. This will then normalise the experience for her, and reduce the risk of complications for her emotionally following childbirth. A woman who is anxious in pregnancy will have higher levels of stress hormones in her body. These will interfere with the onset and establishment of labour, which will lead to more interventions, and further trauma. It may even lead to emergency procedures where there is little time for clear concise information, further increasing the woman's anxiety because she has not had time to prepare herself for what is to happen; sometimes there is not a midwife who is devoted to explaining exactly what is happening to the mother and partner.

Crisis care

When a woman is critically ill, the first concern must always be for her physical safety. However, her emotional and psychological needs must always be remembered too. During the crisis it is important that the atmosphere be as calm as possible – anxiety is catching. If the care givers are anxious and become irritable this will be picked up by the woman and her family. This will increase their feelings of anxiety, fear, loss of control, vulnerability and panic. A midwife who explains what is happening in language that is appropriate for the woman and her partner or family is invaluable. This will foster a sense of trust in the woman and her family towards the care givers. A woman who is provided with information clearly is more likely to be able to accept the treatment offered or provided much more easily than a woman who is afraid and without an understanding of what is happening to her. She is able to let go and be completely sedated; she has to let go of her mind and enter a state of altered consciousness to a much further extent than a woman in normal labour. To do this she needs to be able to trust the midwife and the doctor. Parratt and Fahy (2003) suggest that women who trust their midwife have an improved sense of self following childbirth. Although this study focuses on normal childbirth, I suggest that if trust is important when the woman is experiencing normal labour it is even more important when she is critically ill.

Yet to get a woman to trust her, the midwife needs to be honest and open about the care the woman is receiving. In 1983, Kirkham identified that midwives spent much of their time filling in forms, and provided very little information to women. If a woman asked a question, the midwife deflected the question and uttered platitudes of 'don't worry' and 'relax'. These responses were not likely to decrease anxiety but to increase it, especially as no information was provided to enable the woman not to worry or relax. The result was that the woman did not speak again, because there was no point. She gave up, and no relationship became established with the midwife.

In addition, if the maternity service is short staffed, will there be enough midwives on duty to always ensure that a midwife is available to be supportive in this manner or will the midwife be caring for more than one woman? Women who are critically ill need to have a midwife in constant attendance; this is reassuring for the woman and her family. Continuity of carer/staff is important at this time. It will minimise conflicting information, and will enhance the woman's ability to remain feeling in control and as if she has some choices – and thus is a positive enhancer to communication between the woman and staff.

Immediate post-crisis care

The environment in which care is provided is important. It must be in a room that is quiet so that the woman can relax and sleep. If her partner is with her, they also need a place to sleep and rest. Minimal noise will reduce the stimulation experienced by the couple so that their stress hormones begin to return to normal. The light needs to be appropriate and controllable.

The woman requires appropriate analgesia offered to her regularly. If a woman is left to ask for analgesia, staff may be perceived as being very unkind by the woman and her partner.

Food needs to be appropriate for an invalid, light but nutritious, and of an adequate portion for a young woman recovering from trauma. Relatives need to be advised as to what food to bring in for the woman as it may be difficult for her to digest the food that she would ordinarily prefer.

Infant feeding and care

When a woman has been critically ill it is likely that her baby has had to be taken to the neonatal unit. The very fact that the two have been separated may be enough to trigger a psychological trauma (Robinson 2002), particularly if the mother has wanted to breast feed her baby. It is important to treat and respond to the mother and infant as a couple. It is likely that the birth has been early and often involves an emergency lower segment caesarean section; this means that the woman's milk production is likely to be delayed. If she is unconscious during the first 48 hours following the birth of the baby, there will not have been any physical stimulation (vision) to encourage her body to respond to the presence of a baby. With the baby in the neonatal unit there will be no auditory stimulation, and with the baby absent there is no physical stimulation (touch) to produce milk. A midwife is unable to gain consent from the woman to stimulate her nipples by touch or her breasts by massage, so the midwife needs to wait until the woman is conscious and able to discuss this rationally with her. Some women will be embarrassed by having another adult massage her breasts and may wish to do this themselves.

It is important that whatever the feed that has been given to the baby, the mother perceives it to be appropriate for the time that it was given. Therefore an explanation needs to be given to the mother and her partner as to the type and amount of feed that the baby tolerated. It is useful if the woman has been unconscious for any period of time for her to be able to have evidence of her baby's survival. A photograph is satisfactory but it is inanimate and is often of poor quality due to the amount of light and reflection from equipment in the neonatal unit (NNU).

As long ago as the 1980s, some neonatal units had video cameras that recorded the baby in the NNU and transmitted this live to the mother on the postnatal ward. This is really positive for the woman. However, if she has been unconscious for 48 hours she has missed many of the very precious hours that a mother spends with her newborn child. Therefore the partner could be encouraged to video the baby intermittently in this time so that when the woman awakes she can see the first few hours of her baby's life, and remove the void that may seem to exist for her.

As soon as possible, mother and baby need to be reunited, either by the baby visiting his or her mother or the mother visiting her baby. It is important to remember that each mother–infant dyad is unique and the way in which their relationship develops will be unique to them. The environment of the NNU with the accompanying bright lights, heat, dry atmosphere and noise from buzzers and beepers mean that neither mother nor baby is likely to enjoy the time in the unit. Babies need to be held emotionally, and the environment in the NNU is not conducive to the emotional or physical stability of babies. They need their mothers. However, the very care that the baby requires necessitates separation and gets in the way of a developing relationship. It can also mean that for many women the experience of having had a baby in the NNU leaves them feeling that they have been excluded from the care and this can leave the mother feeling that something is missing from her relationship with her baby. She may resent the nurses in the NNU because they have been caring for her baby instead of her, and that they respond to her baby in a way that she is not able to.

Many women grow up in northwestern Europe without having experienced caring for a newborn baby, let alone a very small baby. The nuclear family with only two children who are less than 4 years apart does not provide young women with much experience of caring for young babies, and many of the advertisements for baby care products only show beautiful, term babies and perfectly groomed mothers. Women have little preparation for the months of providing care to a baby who gives little or no feedback, and it takes time to learn how to handle even a term baby with confidence.

Babies who spend time in the NNU are, by the nature that they have been in the NNU, more fragile than term babies, so the mother needs support to learn how to handle the baby without causing too much stress. The mother may be sensitive to the baby trying to withdraw from the care being provided by her and feel that she is being rejected, or that she will cause harm. The first is inaccurate and the parents need to discuss these fears with staff so that they feel confident to continue to provide care, but the second may be accurate and again needs to be discussed with the staff. The result may be that parents stop providing care, whereas the staff in the NNU will continue because they have the confidence to do so. This may lead the mother to withdraw from providing care and leave her feeling a failure. McFadyen (1998) suggests that it is important for the staff in the NNU to teach parents how to recognise and understand the baby's signals.

The mother may resent the staff in the NNU for being able to provide care for her baby and may perceive them as being uncaring or too professional, not providing enough love for her baby. In this instance the relationship between care providers and mother will not develop favourably, and the mother may feel unsupported, criticised and her sense of failure may increase. The nurse may not recognise that the mother is experiencing difficulty and may feel unvalued because the mother is not relating well to her. This in turn will affect the mother–infant relationship, causing the mother to withdraw from providing care; this will feedback to the nursing staff who will find it difficult to relate to a mother who seems not to care for her baby. In a situation such as this, the woman may cease to visit her baby.

Parents may be in a state of shock because the birth was unplanned and was associated with critical illness of the mother. They may be too numb to speak about what has happened. They may feel guilty and have a sense of failure because their baby is not the baby they had envisaged, fantasised about and wanted. Instead of feeling warm and loving towards their baby they might be overwhelmed with feelings of helplessness, anxiety and bewilderment, which they project onto their baby and describe him or her as helpless. These feelings block our ability to learn, and to perceive accurately what is being said, so parents require clear information that is conveyed calmly and repeated when necessary and written down so that they can refer to it later.

A good nurse/midwife–mother relationship facilitates development of the parents' confidence and their sense of a relationship with their baby, which will facilitate the mother's recovery and decrease the time that the baby will need to spend in hospital, because the parents will feel confident enough to take their baby home, as soon as he or she is ready to be discharged.

Care of the critically ill woman's family

Care of the partner

When a woman becomes critically ill, her partner is jolted out of mundane life into a tense period when they may be preoccupied as to whether she will survive and how they will cope without her. Partners who are present at traumatic births are affected by the experience – by what they see, hear, smell and feel – both emotionally and physically. The partner being affected in this way is unable to support the woman, and may react by withdrawing and not communicating with the woman, staff or family (Sullivan 1998). It is therefore important to remember that partners will also require support, the same type of support that the woman is receiving, although tailored to their own specific needs. If the woman is unconscious, she is not able to provide support to her partner, so partners can feel extremely vulnerable yet may respond as many people do when feeling vulnerable – with anger to hide their vulnerability. It is important that staff providing care can see past the anger and support the vulnerable individual in front of them, who may be feeling very young, helpless and out of control.

Care of other children

It is important to remember that not all women who become critically ill during childbirth will be expecting their first child. Some will have older children, and some will have stepchildren with their partner. It is therefore important to include these children and enable them to participate in the care of their younger sibling wherever possible and to be able to visit their mother.

Hospitals have never been very exciting or pleasant places to visit, therefore it is important that there is a child-friendly area in the maternity unit where the children can be taken when they get bored with being in the clinical environment.

It is also important for staff to relate well with these children, as they may have many anxieties about their mother and the baby, not least that in some way the illness was their fault and that they are in some way to blame.

Care of grandparents and wider family and friends

At the time of critical illness the focus needs to be on the woman, her partner if she has one and baby. However, there are many people who assume or demand ownership or special status during the birthing period. The staff caring for the woman need to be assertive and calm when they deflect questions and enquiries from people who assume these special statuses; for example, being able to deflect enquiries with:

'I will ask X to contact you as soon as possible; does X have your telephone number? May I take it?'

'No it is not possible for you to visit at this moment in time; X will contact you and inform you when it is appropriate for you to visit, but by all means send flowers and a card.'

It is important to pass on these details as the woman and her family will feel supported and cherished from these well wishers.

It may be appropriate to bring a pay phone into the room so that the woman is able to make her own calls, otherwise calls will have to wait until she leaves the department and is able to use a mobile or land line telephone.

People assume a right to know although they do not have such a right unless the woman and her partner agree to the information being released. Staff have a duty to care for the woman and her partner and confidentiality is part of that care (Nursing and Midwifery Council 2004).

If the woman and her partner agree, then grandparents may be included fully in the care of the baby. Some women will be happy that their mother or mother-in-law provides care for the baby whilst she is incapacitated – others will not. This needs to be identified. Do not assume that because you would be happy with your mother caring for your baby, that the woman wants her mother to care for her baby.

It is also important for the woman and her partner to be able to spend time together alone. There will be many visitors who will want to see her to make sure she is alright, but these need to be limited so that she is able to regain her health.

Neonatal loss

It is important to remember that not all women who have been critically ill will have a living baby when they leave hospital, or that the baby may die later once the mother has left hospital. A woman in this situation not only has to come to terms with her severe and unexpected illness and perhaps lifelong complications, she has also to come to terms with the death of her baby. As with all neonatal losses, the family needs appropriate support at the time and support that is on-going.

The midwife caring for the woman will need to take into consideration how ill the woman has been and whether she knew at the time of the birth if the baby had been stillborn or had died later. When a woman has been sedated for perhaps 48 hours and does not know of her baby's death, one of the first questions she will ask is 'Is my baby alright?' or 'Where is my baby?' The midwife and the woman's family will have had 48 hours to absorb this news, and will be behaving in what may seem to be an odd manner to the woman. The woman needs to be told in a sensitive manner what has happened to her baby, and where her baby is. Her partner may not be the most appropriate person to do this and staff caring for the woman should not leave it for the partner to do, unless this is his/her wish.

With the woman's permission the baby should be collected from the mortuary, and placed in a cot or Moses basket so that she and her partner have time with the baby. The midwife needs to describe clearly what the baby looks like so that the woman and partner are not shocked by what they see. Remember you may have seen a dead baby, but they may have never seen a dead person before. It may be appropriate to remove the clothing from the baby, so that the mother is able to have skin to skin contact and touch and stroke her baby as much as she wants. The baby should be able to remain with the mother for as long as is practical, and the parents will need support from the midwife to undertake what care they want to give their baby. This may mean being able to bath the baby or dress, cuddle and kiss him. The midwife will need to liaise with the mortician to identify how long it is practical to have the baby out of the mortuary, taking into account the time of year, and the temperature in the hospital.

The obstetricians may request for the baby to have a postmortem. It is import-ant to delay this procedure until after the parents have seen and held their baby, and remind the parents that following the procedure their baby will have incisions and sutures. Parents may ask whether any organs will be removed from their baby. The midwife must again liaise with the mortuary to find the answer to this question so that the parents are told the truth at the time, and identify clearly what organs have been retained and why. Failure to do so leaves parents feeling bewildered later when they find out, because they feel deceived by people who were supposed to be caring for them. More importantly trust in the whole organ-isation, the NHS, is lost and may never be regained, leaving parents resentful and antagonistic with any other health care personnel they meet.

The funeral can be delayed until the woman is well enough to attend. This will not delay her grieving process because she will have been grieving appropriately if sensitive support has been offered.

For women whose religion requires that the funeral take place within 24 hours of death, the above may not be possible. However, it is important that sensi-tive photographs are taken for the woman so that she has some knowledge and awareness of her baby. A woman who has been denied the opportunity to see and hold her baby, but whose partner and parents have had this opportunity, may feel resentful towards the family members because they have had an opportunity that she has not, and she may feel excluded from the care (personal communica-tion from clients). If a woman has not been able to see her baby then the midwife or partner can help her visualise her baby by describing in detail what the baby looked like, and its vital statistics, weight, length, head circumference, hair and facial features.

One woman told me several times during our counselling together, 'He was a ginger nut, with big round cheeks.' This was what the obstetrician informed her 72 hours after her son had been born by emergency caesarean section for placental abruption. Her son had been stillborn 25 years prior to the counselling. She had held on to what the obstetrician had said to keep a picture in her head, and keep her son's existence real.

Psychological debriefing

Many midwifery services are now providing women with the opportunity to 'debrief' following their childbirth experience, and many midwives themselves are keen to develop this service. What needs to be kept paramount is that no harm comes to the woman from accessing this service; therefore it is important that midwifery service managers identify clearly that it is to benefit the woman rather than to reduce the number of litigation suits that are pressed on the service.

There is a need for human beings to understand their experiences. The depth of this understanding will vary from woman to woman, and therefore each debriefing will be individual to each woman. Indeed the word 'trauma' is derived from the word 'chaos' and many women will express their confusion as to what happened to them, or why it happened to them. This is part of the normal reflection that occurs after any experience.

In psychological debriefing, the woman needs to tell her story as she herself perceives it. This may mean repeating her story over and over again, so that she pieces it together and can get it in the right order. For a woman who has been heavily sedated over a period of days this will be even more important because she really will have no memory as to what happened while she was asleep. And if her health was deteriorating over a few days she may have difficulty in remembering those days as well. From the repetition, she will begin to make sense of her experience, and 'de-confusion' will occur. This can be assisted by the person facilitating the debriefing having ready access to the woman's notes, so that information can be provided, or the timing of events explained or clarified.

Smith and Mitchell (1996) suggest that debriefing enables a woman to re-evaluate her birthing experience in the presence of someone who is knowledgeable. This is useful, particularly if the person is an empathic listener. One of the difficulties of providing this service is that not all midwives may want to undertake this role, feeling that it is beyond their experience, and yet another skill to develop; some women may be so confused and perhaps angry seeing the midwife who was present during the birth that they may find that the debriefing is not supportive at all. Indeed, Phillips (2003) identified data from a randomised controlled trial suggesting that psychological debriefing either makes no difference or even results in further morbidity. Therefore it is important that the woman undertakes the exploration voluntarily and deliberately to understand her birth experience and re-evaluate it. This may mean that she will need further on-going support and it may not necessarily be appropriate for midwifery services to provide this support, because the midwives may not have the appropriate skills to continue further with the woman.

Lastly, sometimes it is just one or two midwives who provide this service. These midwives develop their skills so much that it is only they who are used, and when they are sick or on annual leave or eventually move on, no-one is left who can provide the service. Therefore, the service provision needs to be reviewed annually to ensure that there are enough midwives available to provide the service.

On-going emotional support

Any woman who has experienced being critically ill during childbirth will have some reservations about future pregnancies or childbirth. It is important that the woman at some point is able to visit an obstetrician and discuss the likelihood of the same complication occurring, and at the same time be able to discuss ways of reducing such a risk. This may or may not be possible depending on the complication, but this information is important to women. Knowledge is power, and this provides a sense of control and safety.

It may well be that the woman was so traumatised following the birth that she is unable to speak about it for months. Inglis (2002) identified that it was often a year following the birth before the woman contacted the midwifery service to discuss her birthing experience, and that some women were already pregnant before contacting the service. Some women contain the experience until after the midwife and health visitor stop visiting on a regular basis and then begin to speak about their experience to friends and family. Friends and family are able to listen for a period of time but often end up withdrawing exhausted, frustrated because nothing they say seems to alleviate the distress, and feeling helpless, which is a reflection of how the woman is experiencing life.

This is the time for the woman to have access to a debriefing or counselling service where she can repeat her story and the person listening to her will be able to reflect back accurately and paraphrase what is being said, to demonstrate understanding and to clarify where necessary. This in turn validates the woman's story because she feels she is being heard, and accepted as telling the truth; the listener absorbs the experience, it is not refuted, denied or received with shock and a look of 'please don't tell me any more' (i.e. shut up). The effect for the woman is she feels contained, she can absorb the experience and she can accept her experience (Kitzinger 2004).

This suggests that debriefing cannot become ritualised, or offered to women on a certain day or time. It can only be undertaken when the woman is ready and when she asks. The time allotted needs to be at least 1 hour, so that the woman is able to ask the questions she needs to ask that will validate her experience, and understand what happened in her care.

In future pregnancies the midwives caring for the woman need to recognise that the woman will bring her previous experience with her, which will impact and influence her feelings in the current pregnancy. This may include feelings of anxiety, fear, dread, hope, hostility and ability to experience pleasure. The woman may be experienced by the midwife as being particularly needy (Spencer 1999) and the midwife may feel drained by encounters with her. The midwife may wish she could shake this woman off her, or refer her to another midwife to escape from her neediness, or just experience a feeling of being stressed and irritable whilst with the woman. Taylor (1991) suggested that midwives require support groups so that they can share feelings in a safe environment. She suggested that this would lead to an increased awareness because midwives would be able to explore their own anxieties and break down their own defences. The group would need to be facilitated by a person who was not only a skilled facilitator but who also had a good knowledge and understanding of midwifery, defence mechanisms, how groups function, and other psychological processes.

Emotional support may need to resume in the next pregnancy when the woman may be reminded by certain changes in her body of what happened previously. Because of her previous experience, she may need more time with the midwife than other multigravid women.

The support required will be different for each woman but the focus needs to be on the woman's perception of her pregnancy and childbirth experience. If this perception is that it is better than the last experience, then any previous trauma may be healed because of the most recent experience. This support is offered in some NHS Trusts by midwife psychotherapists.

Care of midwives

As mentioned previously, midwives need the appropriate skills to support a woman through her exploration of her birthing story. It is unlikely that she will develop her skills adequately in her initial training and will need further skill development. This takes time and money. Many further education colleges offer counselling courses at several levels – introduction, certificate, diploma and postgraduate; and many universities offer postgraduate diplomas or master level courses. A midwife needs to discuss with her supervisor what level of training she requires; will she still be employed as a midwife who is enhancing her functional role of midwife or will she become a counsellor to women? If it is the former then a certificate level course may well be appropriate, but if she is to become a counsellor, then the training needs to be at masters level. The reality of this is that it will take a minimum of 3 years to complete, and the midwife will need supervision or 'consultative support' from a counselling supervisor, once per fortnight for a session that lasts 50 minutes. The cost of this is likely to be a minimum of £35.00 per session. Therefore, the midwife and her supervisor of midwives/midwifery manager need to discuss who is to pay for this requirement of the British Association of Counsellors and Psychotherapists (BACP) and who will be the supervisor. Will the midwife have a choice? Will she be able to choose and go outside of the Trust, or will the midwife be supervised by someone her midwifery manager chooses?

The former is more appropriate because the midwife counsellor will be able to leave the unit for consultative support and have time that is uninterrupted and solely used for support in her functional counselling role. Consultative support from within the Trust may feel to the midwife as if she is being observed, or may feel as though subjective to the Trust's needs not the to the midwife and her clients' needs.

Midwives who undertake debriefing sessions as part of their functional role as a midwife and yet are not seen as counsellors by their clients still need access to consultative support so that they can process the information that they hear from women in a way that is not harmful or overwhelming to themselves. It would not be appropriate for midwives who undertake debriefing to debrief themselves to a peer. The support would be superficial, often snatched during coffee breaks, and would therefore perhaps be less than useful. Consultative support, to be useful to care provider, needs to be undertaken regularly, with intent, in a secure environment where confidentiality of client material can be ensured, and where no interruptions are guaranteed. There is nothing worse than beginning to explore a session with a client, than to have to finish because an emergency has occurred, and staff are being called away.

Clarke (1996) suggested that midwives need to be genuine and warm in their interactions with women. This enables the woman to feel good about herself and increases her self-esteem. The midwife also needs the same from the woman. If not, the midwife loses confidence, withholds her approval from the woman and communicates less and less. This results in the relationship failing, leaving both feeling dissatisfied. The midwife needs to be understanding, compassionate and willing to give and receive love. This generates the woman's trust in the midwife. However, for anyone to behave and relate in this way they need to feel cherished themselves and have the opportunity to discuss their likes and dislikes of clients (transference and countertransference) in a safe environment (Spencer 1999).

Although the focus of this chapter is on the psychological needs and care of the woman and family who have been touched by critical illness during the childbearing year, it is important to remember the impact that caring for a woman who becomes critically ill, or dies, may have on the midwives involved in that care. The recent Confidential Enquiry into Maternal Deaths (CEMD) (Lewis 2004) highlights the devastating effect that an unexpected maternal death may have, to the extent that some staff appeared to blame themselves, even when care was exemplary. Furthermore, some were not offered counselling or support and were left to cope alone with the guilt they felt. It is perhaps unsurprising that a few left their profession as a result. The CEMD recommends that provision must be made for the prompt offer of support and/or counselling (Lewis 2004), and the same points could be made in relation to staff who are involved in the care of any woman who becomes critically ill.

Practice check

- Are women encouraged to write their stories so that midwives and obstetricians are able to read them and reflect upon them?
- Are partners encouraged to video their baby in the neonatal unit on a daily basis?
- Are children of the couple able to visit both mother and baby?
- Are women nursed in a suitable environment for an appropriate period of time?
- Does a dietician liaise with the maternity services to identify an appropriate menu for women recovering from a critically ill period?
- Can the woman's partner stay with her throughout the 24-hour clock?
- Is refreshment provided for partners of critically ill women?
- Are the midwives who provide debriefing clear about their role?
- Would the maternity service benefit from employing a counsellor to provide on-going support to women?
- Are services reviewed on an annual basis?

References

American Psychological Association (1994) *Diagnostic and Statistical Manual of Mental Disorders*. American Psychological Association, Washington.

Clarke, R. (1996) All you need is love. *Modern Midwife*, **6** (7): 30.

Department of Health (1993) *Changing Childbirth: Report of the Expert Maternity Group*. Her Majesty's Stationery Office (HMSO), London.

Inglis, S. (2002) Accessing a debriefing service following birth. *British Journal of Midwifery*, **10** (6): 368–71.

Kirkham, M. (1983) Admission in labour: teaching the patient to be patient. *Midwives Chronicle*, **96** (2): 44–5.

Kitzinger, S. (2004) Flashbacks, nightmares and panic attacks after birth. *British Journal of Midwifery*, **12** (1): 12.

Lewis, G. (2004) *Why Mothers Die 2000–2002: Report on Confidential Enquiries into Maternal Deaths in the United Kingdom*. Royal College of Obstetricians and Gynaecologists (RCOG) Press, London.

Lyons, S. (1998) Post traumatic stress disorder following childbirth: causes, prevention, and treatment. In: S. Clement and L. Page (Eds) *Psychological Perspectives on Pregnancy and Childbirth.* Churchill Livingstone, London.

McFadyen, A. (1998) Special care babies and their carers. In: S. Clement and L. Page (Eds) *Psychological Perspectives on Pregnancy and Childbirth.* Churchill Livingstone, London.

Nursing and Midwifery Council (2004) *The NMC Code of Professional Conduct: Standards for conduct, performance and ethics.* Nursing and Midwifery Council, London.

Oakley, A. (1984) *The Captured Womb.* Blackwell, Oxford.

Page, L. (1993) Redefining the midwife's role: changes needed in practice. *British Journal of Midwifery,* **1** (1): 21–4.

Parratt, J. and Fahy, K. (2003) Trusting enough to be out of control: a pilot study of women's sense of self during childbirth. *Australian Journal of Midwifery,* **16** (1): 15–22.

Phillips, S. (2003) Debriefing following traumatic childbirth. *British Journal of Midwifery,* **11** (12): 725–30.

Robinson, J. (2002) Separation from the baby – a cause of PTSD? *British Journal of Midwifery,* **10** (9): 548.

Smith, J. and Mitchell, S. (1996) Debriefing after childbirth: a tool for objective risk management. *British Journal of Midwifery,* **4** (11): 581–6.

Spencer, L. (1999) *Midwives experiences of their relationships with women.* Unpublished MSC thesis, South Bank University, London.

Sullivan, J. (1998) Men becoming fathers: "Sometimes I wonder how I will cope". In: S. Clement and L. Page (Eds) *Psychological Perspectives on Pregnancy and Childbirth.* Churchill Livingstone, London.

Taylor, M. (1991) Providing emotional support. *Nursing Times,* **87** (2): 66.

Index